Study Guide

Lippincott Williams & Wilkins'

COMPREHENSIVE
Medical Assisting

Study Guide

Lippincott Williams & Wilkins'

COMPREHENSIVE
Medical Assisting

Second Edition

Connie West-Stack, M.ED., MLT, CMA
Medical Assisting Program Director
South Piedmont Community College
Polkton, North Carolina

Brenda Bonham Howe, R.N.
Clinician III, Internal Medicine Triage Nurse
Bend Memorial Clinic, LLP
Bend, Oregon

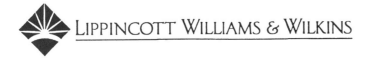
LIPPINCOTT WILLIAMS & WILKINS

Acquisitions Editor: John Goucher
Managing Editor: Rebecca Keifer
Marketing Manager: Hilary Henderson
Production Editor: Christina Remsberg
Compositor: Maryland Composition
Printer: Victor Graphics

To purchase additional copies of this book, call our customer service department at **(800) 638-3030** or fax orders to **(301) 824-7390.** International customers should call **(301) 714-2324.**

Visit Lippincott Williams & Wilkins on the Internet: http://www.LWW.com. Lippincott Williams & Wilkins customer service representatives are available from 8:30 am to 6:00 pm, EST.

05 06 07 08 09
1 2 3 4 5 6 7 8 9 10

PREFACE

This is the *Study Guide* to accompany *Lippincott Williams & Wilkins' Comprehensive Medical Assisting 2e*. It is a learning resource that will help you to retain important information, master skills, and become a success as a medical assistant. To help you get the most out of your studies, we've included a variety of exercises that will help reinforce the material you learned and build your critical thinking skills. This guide is unique in a number of ways and offers features that most study guides do not. Please take a few moments to look through the *Study Guide* and become familiar with the features we've included to enhance your learning experience.

The *Study Guide* is divided into three sections. The first section contains exercises for each chapter. Each chapter includes the following:

- **Chapter competencies,** which will serve as a guide as you review your text. You will be expected to master each learning and performance objective.
- **Chapter outline,** presented in a tabular format to provide a space for you to take notes.
- **Learning self-assessment exercises** including matching, skill drills, multiple choice, and critical thinking practice components. Your instructor has the answer key to these exercises.

- **Key terms** (also included among the learning self-assessment exercises), with space for you to write the definitions for each term. Terms are in boldface type the first time they are explained or described in your textbook and are defined in the Glossary of Key Terms. Definitions can also be found in a medical or standard dictionary.

The second section of your *Study Guide* contains **lecture notes** that will closely follow the PowerPoint slide presentation of your instructor's lecture. The pages are perforated and can be taken out and brought to class. Key points in the lectures are left blank. To promote active listening skills and to reinforce your understanding of the lectures, fill in the key points as they are covered in class. These notes can be used with or without the PowerPoint presentation. Either way, they will be an important study tool for reviewing for your quizzes and examinations.

The third section of your *Study Guide* contains **competency evaluation forms** for procedures in the textbook. Each form has a place for students to complete a self-evaluation, partners to evaluate them, and, finally, for the instructor's evaluation.

CONTENTS

Medicine and Medical Assisting

CHAPTER COMPETENCIES

Review the information in your text that supports the following course objectives.

Learning Objectives

1. Spell and define the key terms

2. Outline a brief history of medicine

3. Identify the key founders of medical science

4. Explain the system of health care in the United States

5. Discuss the typical medical office

6. List medical specialties a medical assistant may encounter

7. List the duties of a medical assistant

8. Describe the desired characteristics of a medical assistant

9. Explain the pathways of education for medical assistants

10. Discuss the importance of program accreditation

11. Name and describe the two nationally recognized accrediting agencies for medical assisting education programs

12. Explain the benefits and avenues of certification for the medical assistant

13. List the benefits of membership in a professional organization

14. Identify members of the health care team

15. List settings in which medical assistants may be employed

CHAPTER OUTLINE

CHAPTER OUTLINE	NOTES
History of Medicine	
Ancient Medical History	
Modern Medical History	
Recent Medical History	
The American Health Care System	
The Medical Office	
Medical Specialties	
The Medical Assisting Profession	
What Is a Medical Assistant?	
Duties of a Medical Assistant	
Administrative Duties	
Clinical Duties	
Laboratory Duties	

CHAPTER OUTLINE   *continued* | NOTES

Characteristics of a Professional Medical Assistant	
Members of the Health Care Team	
Physicians	
Physician Assistants	
Nurses	
Nurse Practitioners	
Allied Health Professionals	
The History of Medical Assisting	
Medical Assisting Education	
Medical Assisting Program Accreditation	
The Commission on Accreditation of Allied Health Education Programs	
The Accrediting Bureau of Health Education Schools	
Medical Assisting Certification	
Certified Medical Assistant	
Registered Medical Assistant	
Medical Assisting and Related Allied Health Associations	
Association Membership	
American Association of Medical Assistants	
American Medical Technologists	
Professional Coder Associations	
The American Health Information Management Association	
American Association of Medical Transcription	
Employment Opportunities	

LEARNING SELF-ASSESSMENT EXERCISES

Key Terms

Define the following key terms:

accreditation _____

administrative _____

caduceus _____

certification _____

clinical _____

cloning _____

continuing education units _____

externship _____

inpatient _____

laboratory _____

medical assistant _____

multidisciplinary _____

multiskilled health professional _____

outpatient _____

recertification _____

role delineation chart _____

specialty _____

Matching

Match the description in part 1 with the individual in part 2.

PART 1

_____ 1. First public health officer

_____ 2. Father of Experimental Physiology

_____ 3. Father of Anatomy

_____ 4. Father of Scientific Surgery

_____ 5. Discovered smallpox vaccine

_____ 6. Discovered penicillin

_____ 7. Applied antiseptics to wounds

PART 2

a. Lister

b. Fleming

c. Hunter

d. Vesalius

e. Jenner

f. Galen

g. Moses

Skill Drills

1. List two benefits of certification.

_____

_____

2. List four benefits of membership in a professional organization.

_____

_____

_____

_____

3. List three settings in which medical assistants may be employed.

_____

_____

_____

4. List six duties of a medical assistant.

_____

_____

_____

_____

_____

_____

5. Identify six members of the health care team.

_____

_____

_____

_____

_____

_____

Multiple Choice

1. The earliest recorded evidence of medical history dates to
   a. Moses
   b. The Greeks
   c. The Romans
   d. The Egyptians

2. Supplemental iron was recognized as a treatment for anemia by the
   a. Greeks
   b. Romans
   c. Chinese
   d. Arabs

3. What society made great strides in public health, including the provision of a clean water supply and sewers and an emphasis on personal cleanliness?
   a. Roman
   b. Chinese
   c. Arab
   d. Greek

4. After what year were only graduates of an accredited school of medical assisting allowed to sit for certification examinations for the AAMA?
   a. 1997
   b. 1998
   c. 1999
   d. 2000

5. A group of specialized people who are brought together to meet the needs of the patient is called
   a. Multiskilled
   b. Multifaceted
   c. Multidisciplinary
   d. Multitrained

6. Few advances were made in medicine during which period?
   a. 700 to 900 A.D
   b. 400 to 1400 A.D
   c. 100 to 800 A.D
   d. 800 to 1000 A.D

7. The discovery of what vaccine opened the door to an emphasis on prevention of disease rather than simply trying to cure preventable illnesses?
   a. Smallpox
   b. Cowpox
   c. Puerperal fever
   d. Typhoid

Critical Thinking Practice

1. Explain the four pathways of education for medical assistants.

_____

_____

_____

_____

2. Describe four characteristics of a medical assistant and explain how they relate to professional performance.

_____

_____

_____

_____

2

Law and Ethics

CHAPTER COMPETENCIES

Review the information in your text that supports the following course objectives.

Learning Objectives

1. Spell and define the key terms

2. Identify the two branches of the American legal system

3. List the elements and types of contractual agreements and describe the difference in implied and expressed contracts

4. List four items that must be included in a contract termination or withdrawal letter

5. List six items that must be included in an informed consent form and explain who may sign consent forms

6. List five legally required disclosures that must be reported to specified authorities

7. Describe the purpose of the Self-Determination Act

8. Describe the four elements that must be proven in a medical legal suit

9. Describe four possible defenses against litigation for the medical professional

10. Explain the theory of respondeat superior, or law of agency, and how it applies to the medical assistant

11. List ways that a medical assistant can assist in the prevention of a medical malpractice suit

12. Outline the laws regarding employment and safety issues in the medical office

13. List the requirements of the Americans with Disabilities Act relating to the medical office

14. Differentiate between legal issues and ethical issues

15. List the seven American Medical Association principles of ethics

16. List the five ethical principles of ethical and moral conduct outlined by the American Association of Medical Assistants

17. List 10 opinions of the American Medical Association's Council pertaining to administrative office procedures

CHAPTER OUTLINE	NOTES
The American Legal System	
Sources of Law	
Branches of the Law	
Public Law	
Private or Civil Law	
The Rise in Medical Legal Cases	
Physician–Patient Relationship	

CHAPTER OUTLINE *continued*	NOTES
Rights and Responsibilities of the Patient and Physician	
Contracts	
Implied Contracts	
Expressed Contracts	
Termination or Withdrawal of the Contract	
Consent	
Implied Consent	
Informed or Expressed Consent	
Refusal of Consent	
Releasing Medical Information	
Legally Required Disclosures	
Vital Statistics	
Medical Examiner's Reports	
Infectious or Communicable Diseases	
National Childhood Vaccine Injury Act of 1986	
Abuse, Neglect, or Maltreatment	
Violent Injuries	
Other Reports	
Specific Laws and Statutes That Apply to Health Professionals	
Medical Practice Acts	
Licensure, Certification, and Registration	
Controlled Substances Act	
Good Samaritan Act	
Basis of Medical Law	
Tort Law	
Negligence and Malpractice (Unintentional Torts)	
Duty	
Dereliction of Duty	
Direct Cause	
Damage	
Jury Awards	
Intentional Torts	
Assault and Battery	
Duress	
Invasion of Privacy	

CHAPTER OUTLINE   *continued* | NOTES

Defamation of Character	
Fraud	
Tort of Outrage	
Undue Influence	
The Litigation Process	
Defenses to Professional Liability Suits	
Medical Records	
Statute of Limitations	
Assumption of Risk	
Res Judicata	
Contributory Negligence	
Comparative Negligence	
Immunity	
Defense for the Medical Assistant	
Respondeat Superior or Law of Agency	
Employment and Safety Laws	
Civil Rights Act of 1964, Title VII	
Sexual Harassment	
Americans with Disabilities Act	
Occupational Safety and Health Act	
Other Legal Considerations	
Medical Ethics	
American Medical Association (AMA) Code of Ethics	
Medical Assistant's Role in Ethics	
Patient Advocacy	
Patient Confidentiality	
Honesty	
American Association of Medical Assistants (AAMA) Code of Ethics	
Principles	
Bioethics	
American Medical Association (AMA) Council on Ethical and Judicial Affairs	
Social Policy Issues	
Allocation of Resources	
Clinical Investigations and Research	
Obstetric Dilemmas	

CHAPTER OUTLINE *continued*	NOTES
Organ Transplantation	
Withholding or Withdrawing Treatment	
Professional and Ethical Conduct and Behavior	
Ethical Issues in Office Management	

LEARNING SELF-ASSESSMENT EXERCISES

Key Terms

Define the following key terms:

abandonment _____

advance directive _____

age of majority _____

appeal _____

artificial insemination _____

assault _____

battery _____

bench trial _____

bioethics _____

blood-borne pathogens _____

breach _____

censure _____

certification _____

civil law _____

coerce _____

common law _____

comparative negligence _____

confidentiality _____

consent _____

consideration _____

contract _____

contributory negligence _____

cross-examination _____

damages _____

defamation of character _____

defendant _____

depositions _____

direct examination _____

durable power of attorney _____

duress _____

emancipated minor _____

ethics _____

expert witness _____

expressed consent _____

expressed contracts _____

fee splitting _____

fraud _____

implied consent _____

implied contracts _____

informed consent _____

intentional tort _____

legally required disclosure _____

libel _____

licensure _____

litigation _____

locum tenens _____

malpractice _____

negligence _____

noncompliant _____

plaintiff _____

precedents _____

protocol _____

registered _____

res ipsa loquitur _____

res judicata _____

respondeat superior _____

slander _____

stare decisis _____

statute of limitations _____

statutes _____

tort _____

unintentional tort _____

verdict _____

Matching

Match the definition in part 1 with the correct term in part 2.

PART 1

_____ 1. Identifies what physician may or may not do; fees to charge

_____ 2. Uses Percival and Hippocrates as foundation for ethical standards

_____ 3. Hospital conduct and charitable work

_____ 4. Focuses on rights of patients and physician's moral conduct

_____ 5. Formal discharge

_____ 6. Temporary removal of privileges

_____ 7. Verbal or written reprimand

PART 2

a. Censure

b. Hammurabi

c. Suspension

d. AMA

e. Percival

f. Hippocrates

g. Expulsion

Skill Drills

1. List the seven American Medical Association principles of ethics.

_____

_____

_____

_____

_____

2. List the five ethical principles stated by the American Association of Medical Assistants.

_____

_____

_____

_____

3. List 10 opinions of the AMA's Council pertaining to administrative office procedures.

_____

_____

_____

_____

_____

_____

_____

_____

_____

_____

Multiple Choice

1. Your primary responsibility as a medical assistant is to
   a. Follow physicians' orders
   b. Honor patients' requests
   c. Be a patient advocate.
   d. All of the above

2. Patient information may be released by permission of the
   a. Physician
   b. Patient
   c. Spouse
   d. Medical assistant

3. The mark of a true professional is a person's
   a. Level of education
   b. Salary
   c. Ability to admit mistakes
   d. Ability to problem solve

4. The steps to examining ethical dilemmas
   a. Depend on the issues
   b. Remain the same
   c. Are made by the physician regardless of the issues
   d. Are made by the patient

5. The medical assistant's responsibility regarding unethical behavior is to
   a. Ignore it if not personally involved
   b. Report it if a patient is involved
   c. Report it regardless of who is involved
   d. Report it to the physician

6. The opinions that the Council on Ethical and Judicial Affairs of the American Medical Association holds on medical and bioethical issues are
   a. The law
   b. Guidelines
   c. Rules only
   d. Revised yearly

7. According to the AMA, priority care is given to the person or persons who
a. Have insurance
b. Are the youngest
c. Are the oldest
d. Will receive the greatest long-term benefit

Critical Thinking Practice

1. Describe the difference between legal issues and ethical issues. Give an example of each.

_____
_____
_____
_____

2. Describe the difference between medical ethics and bioethics.

_____
_____
_____
_____

3. Describe the four steps that you can use to resolve an ethical dilemma.

_____
_____
_____
_____

4. Describe the opinions of the American Medical Association Council on Ethical and Judicial Affairs on social policy issues.

_____
_____
_____
_____

Matching

Match the definition in part 1 with the correct legal term in part 2.

PART 1

_____ 1. Previous decision stands

_____ 2. The thing has been decided

_____ 3. Let the master answer

_____ 4. Not having control over the mind or intellect

_____ 5. Under penalty you shall take with you

_____ 6. A court order requiring the recipient to appear

_____ 7. The thing speaks for itself

PART 2

a. Non compos mentis

b. Subpoena duces tecum

c. Respondeat superior

d. Stare decisis

e. Res ipsa loquitur

f. Res judicata

g. Subpoena

Skill Drills

1. List four items that must be included in a contract.

_____

_____

_____

_____

2. List six items that must be included in an informed consent form.

_____

_____

_____

_____

_____

_____

3. List five incidents that must be reported to specified authorities.

_____

_____

_____

_____

_____

4. List five ways a medical assistant can help prevent a medical law suit.

_____

_____

_____

_____

_____

Multiple Choice

1. Common law principles are based on the theory of
   a. Stare decisis
   b. Res judicata
   c. Litigation
   d. Statute of limitations

2. The two main branches of the legal system are
   a. Criminal and administrative law
   b. Constitutional and international law
   c. Public and private law
   d. Commercial and tort law

3. Reasons for the escalation of medical malpractice cases include
   a. Unrealistic patient expectations
   b. Economic factors
   c. Scientific advances
   d. All of the above

4. What component or components do all contractual agreements have?
   a. Offer
   b. Consideration

c. Durable power of attorney
   d. *a* and *b* only

5. Patients have the right to
   a. Obtain copies of their own medical records
   b. Refuse treatment
   c. Expect continuity of care
   d. All of the above

6. Minors may sign a consent form when
   a. They are 16 years old
   b. They become sexually active
   c. They request treatment for a communicable disease
   d. None of the above

7. Each state has laws pertaining to which deaths must be reported to the medical examiner's office. Generally, these include
   a. The death of anyone over 65 years old
   b. Deaths from unknown causes
   c. Deaths from terminal illnesses
   d. Any death occurring in a hospital

8. A physician's license may be revoked or suspended for various reasons, such as
   a. Refusing to see new patients
   b. Fraud
   c. Fee splitting
   d. *b* and *c* only

9. A narcotic inventory record must be kept for
   a. 4 to 6 years
   c. 5 to 7 years
   b. 2 to 3 years
   d. 10 years

10. COBRA is a Medicare law designed to
    a. Act as an advance directive
    b. Be a durable power of attorney
    c. Prevent patient dumping
    d. None of the above

Critical Thinking Practice

1. Describe the purpose of the Self-Determination Act.

_____

_____

_____

_____

2. What are intentional torts? Give four examples.

_____

_____

_____

_____

3. Explain the theory of respondeat superior and describe how it applies to the medical assistant.

_____

_____

_____

_____

4. A patient asks your opinion of a particular pediatrician's treatment of a certain illness and then tells you that she does not care for that physician's bedside manner. You know that the pediatrician is not well liked by his office staff because he is impatient and hard to get along with. How do you respond to this patient's question and statement so as to remain professional and to avoid defamation of character?

_____

_____

_____

_____

Patient Education

1. An elderly patient being seen preoperatively in the medical office tells you that she has heard others talk about filling out advance directives, but she doesn't know what that means. How do you explain advance directives to this patient?

_____

_____

_____

3
Fundamental Communication Skills

CHAPTER COMPETENCIES

Review the information in your text that supports the following course objectives.

Learning Objectives

1. Spell and define the key terms

2. List two major forms of communication

3. Explain how various components of communication can affect the meaning of verbal messages

4. Define active listening

5. List and describe the six interviewing techniques

6. Give an example of how cultural differences may affect communication

7. Discuss how to handle communication problems caused by language barriers

8. List two methods that you can use to promote communication among hearing-, sight-, and speech-impaired patients

9. List five actions that you can take to improve communication with a child

10. Discuss how to handle an angry or distressed patient

11. Discuss your role in communicating with a grieving patient or family member

12. Discuss the key elements of interdisciplinary communication

CHAPTER OUTLINE	NOTES
Basic Communication Flow	
Forms of Communication	
Verbal Communication	
Nonverbal Communication	
Active Listening	
Interview Techniques	
Reflecting	
Paraphrasing or Restatement	
Asking for Examples or Clarification	
Asking Open-Ended Questions	
Summarizing	
Allowing Silences	

CHAPTER OUTLINE *continued*	NOTES
Factors Affecting Communication	
Cultural Differences	
Stereotyping and Biased Opinions	
Language Barriers	
Special Communication Challenges	
Hearing-Impaired Patients	
Sight-Impaired Patients	
Speech Impairments	
Mental Health Illnesses	
Angry or Distressed Patients	
Children	
Communicating With a Grieving Patient or Family Member	
Establishing Positive Patient Relationships	
Proper Form of Address	
Professional Distance	
Teaching Patients	
Professional Communication	
Communicating With Peers	
Communicating With Physicians	
Communicating With Other Facilities	

LEARNING SELF-ASSESSMENT EXERCISES

Key Terms

Define the following key terms:

anacusis _____

bias _____

clarification _____

cultures _____

demeanor _____

discrimination _____

dysphasia _____

dysphonia _____

feedback _____

grief _____

messages _____

mourning _____

nonlanguage _____

paralanguage _____

paraphrasing _____

presbyacusis _____

reflecting _____

stereotyping _____

summarizing _____

therapeutic _____

Matching

Match the definition in part 1 with the correct term in part 2.

PART 1

_____ 1. Facial expressions, gestures

_____ 2. Physical space tolerated by humans

_____ 3. Laughing, sobbing, sighing

_____ 4. Voice quality, pitch, tone

_____ 5. Verification of understanding

_____ 6. Organization of complex information

_____ 7. Restatement of exactly what patient says

PART 2

a. Paraphrasing

b. Kinesics

c. Summarization

d. Proxemics

e. Paralanguage

f. Nonlanguage

g. Reflection

Skill Drills

1. List the four basic components of oral communication.

_____
_____
_____
_____

2. Explain what it means to listen actively.

_____
_____
_____
_____

3. Identify and explain the five stages of grief.

_____
_____
_____
_____

4. List four ways to avoid breaching confidentiality in the medical office.

_____
_____
_____

5. Define professional distance and explain why it is important.

_____

_____

_____

_____

Multiple Choice

1. The more accurate reflection of a person's true feelings and attitudes are demonstrated in
   a. Verbal communication
   b. Nonverbal communication
   c. Written communication
   d. All of the above

2. The limit of personal space is generally considered to be a
   a. 5-foot radius
   b. 10-foot radius
   c. 3-foot radius
   d. 1-foot radius

3. "It sounds as if . . ." is an example of which type of interviewing technique?
   a. Reflection
   b. Restatement
   c. Paraphrasing
   d. Paralanguage

4. "You were saying . . ." is an example of which type of interviewing technique?
   a. Reflection
   b. Restatement
   c. Paraphrasing
   d. Paralanguage

5. Periods of silence can
   a. Be beneficial
   b. Be natural parts of conversation
   c. Offer time for reflection
   d. All of the above

6. Factors leading to miscommunication are
   a. Language barriers
   b. Distractions
   c. Requests for feedback
   d. *a* and *b* only

7. An effective way of communicating with non–English speaking patients is
   a. Raising your voice
   b. Using commonly understood slang
   c. Speaking only to an interpreter
   d. Using simple phrases and speaking slowly

8. To communicate with patients who are hearing-impaired, you must
   a. Raise your voice pitch
   b. Raise your voice level
   c. Talk face to face
   d. None of the above

9. To facilitate communication with children, it is important to
   a. Use proper medical terms
   b. Use eye-level contact
   c. Avoid involving the parent
   d. Discourage play

Critical Thinking Practice

1. Explain how various components of communication can affect the meaning of verbal messages.

_____

_____

_____

_____

Mrs. Smith is a 78-year-old woman with a history of gallstones. She is seeing Dr. Jones for the first time. The medical assistant approaches Mrs. Smith in a friendly manner, saying, "All right, sweetie, it's your turn," and puts her arm around her to guide her to a room. After the interview, the medical assistant leaves the room and calls to the receptionist, telling her that the gallbladder has arrived and has been roomed.

2. Explain what message or messages may have been conveyed to Mrs. Smith by the medical assistant.

_____

_____

_____

_____

3. How could the approach been improved?

_____

_____

_____

_____

Mr. Rivera's wife died a year ago. Since that time, Mr. Rivera has stopped seeing friends and participating in social activities. He visits the cemetery several times a week. Mr. Rivera has an appointment with Dr. Lee to discuss his feelings of depression and sadness. He wonders if he will ever feel any differently.

4. Are Mr. Rivera's feelings normal? Explain your answer.

_____

_____

_____

_____

5. Identify the steps in the grieving process.

_____

_____

_____

_____

Charting Documentation

1. With regard to question 24, write a narrative chart note describing your interaction with the patient.

Date   **Time**

_____

_____

_____

_____

Patient Education

1. Johnny is 5 years old and will be entering kindergarten in September. He is seeing Dr. Smith for his kindergarten physical. He will be receiving several immunizations. His mother tells him not to be afraid, as the shots will not hurt. She apologizes to the medical assistant when Johnny starts to cry. How can you teach Johnny's mother about his reactions?

_____

_____

_____

_____

4

Patient Education

CHAPTER COMPETENCIES

Review the information in your text that supports the following course objectives.

Learning Objectives

1. Spell and define the key terms

2. Explain the medical assistant's role in patient education

3. Define the five steps in the patient education process

4. Identify five conditions that are needed for patient education to occur

5. Explain Maslow's hierarchy of human needs

6. List five factors that may hinder patient education and at least two methods to compensate for each of these factors

7. Discuss five preventive medicine guidelines that you should teach your patients

8. Explain the kinds of information that should be included in patient teaching about medication therapy

9. Identify the components of a healthy diet and explain how to use a food guide pyramid

10. Explain the importance of teaching range-of-motion exercises to patients

11. Explain your role in teaching patients about alternative medicine therapies

12. List and explain relaxation techniques that you can teach patients to help with stress management

13. List three national organizations that can help patients with smoking cessation

14. Identify a national organization that can assist patients with treating alcoholism

15. Describe how to prepare a teaching plan

16. List potential sources of patient education materials

CHAPTER OUTLINE | NOTES

The Patient Education Process	
Assessment	
Planning	
Implementation	
Evaluation	
Documentation	
Conditions Needed for Patient Education	
Maslow's Hierarchy of Needs	
Environment	
Equipment	
Knowledge	
Resources	

CHAPTER OUTLINE *continued*	NOTES
Factors That Can Hinder Education	
Existing Illnesses	
Communication Barriers	
Age	
Educational Background	
Physical Impairments	
Other Factors	
Teaching Specific Health Care Topics	
Preventive Medicine	
Medications	
Nutrition	
The Food Guide Pyramid	
Dietary Guidelines	
Exercise	
Alternative Medicine	
Acupuncture	
Acupressure	
Hypnosis	
Yoga	
Herbal Supplements	
Stress Management	
Positive and Negative Stress	
Relaxation Techniques	
Smoking Cessation	
Substance Abuse	
Patient Teaching Plans	
Developing a Plan	
Selecting and Adapting Teaching Material	
Developing Your Own Material	

LEARNING SELF-ASSESSMENT EXERCISES

Key Terms

Define the following key terms:

alternative _____

assessment _____

carbohydrates _____

coping mechanisms _____

detoxification _____

documentation _____

evaluation _____

implementation _____

learning objectives _____

noncompliance _____

nutrition _____

placebo _____

planning _____

psychomotor _____

range-of-motion _____

stress _____

Skill Drills

1. List five factors that may facilitate patient learning.

_____

_____

_____

_____

_____

2. List five factors that may hinder patient learning.

_____

_____

_____

_____

_____

3. List four sources of patient education materials.

_____

_____

_____

_____

Multiple Choice

1. To educate patients effectively, a medical assistant must
   a. Involve patients
   b. Have a doctor's order
   c. Establish goals
   d. *a* and *c*

2. Teaching demonstrations can fail if they are
   a. Specific to the patient
   b. In a group setting
   c. Unrealistic
   d. None of the above

3. Evaluation of patient teaching
   a. Is not necessary
   b. Occurs only once
   c. Is an ongoing process
   d. Is done by the patient

4. A medical assistant who discovers that a patient is not compliant with goals of an educational plan should *first*
   a. Tell the physician
   b. Reevaluate the assessment
   c. Check for understanding
   d. Document in the chart

5. Documentation of patient teaching includes all of the following *except*
   a. Teaching aids
   b. Phone conversations
   c. Written information
   d. Laboratory values

6. The third step in patient education is
   a. Implementation
   b. Planning
   c. Evaluation
   d. Assessment

7. Which of the following must take place before learning can be achieved?
   a. Motivation of the patient
   b. Perception of need by the patient
   c. Educational plan
   d. *a* and *b*

Critical Thinking Practice

1. Explain the difference between a learning goal and a learning objective. Give an example of each.

_____

_____

_____

_____

2. Explain Maslow's hierarchy of needs. Give an example of each.

_____

_____

_____

_____

3. Describe how a patient who according to Maslow has reached self-actualization would approach health care.

_____

_____

_____

Patient Education

1. Mr. Applebaum is a 68-year-old diabetic who must learn to give himself insulin injections. He is nervous and afraid that the medication will not control his blood sugar. Describe four factors the medical assistant should consider that would promote learning.

_____

_____

_____

_____

Charting Documentation

1. With regard to the patient teaching scenario, give an example of a chart note that you might write following your patient teaching.

Date   **Time**

_____

_____

_____

_____

Matching

Match the definition in part 1 with the correct term in part 2.

PART 1

_____ 1. Most frequently abused drug

_____ 2. Impairs short-term memory

_____ 3. Reaches brain in 6 seconds

_____ 4. Stimulates central nervous system

_____ 5. Has same effect as cocaine

_____ 6. Causes physical and psychological dependence

_____ 7. LSD, PCP, mescaline, and peyote

PART 2

a. Nicotine

b. Alcohol

c. Hallucinogens

d. Cocaine and crack cocaine

e. Depressants and barbiturates

f. Marijuana and hashish

g. Stimulants and amphetamines

Skill Drills

1. Identify three factors to consider when designing a medication therapy teaching tool for a patient.

_____

_____

_____

2. List five main factors that play important roles in health.

_____

_____

_____

_____

_____

3. Identify five components of a healthy diet.

_____

_____

_____

_____

_____

4. Identify and explain five relaxation techniques.

_____

_____

_____

_____

_____

Multiple Choice

1. Nutrition is the study not only of what people eat but of
   a. How food is grown
   b. The effect of exercise on the body
   c. How the body uses food
   d. None of the above

2. In addition to identifying five food groups, the food pyramid
   a. Shows pictures of food
   b. Calculates caloric values
   c. Shows sample menus
   d. Shows maximum servings

3. Dietary guidelines are intended to improve our diet and
   a. Are government guidelines
   b. Include only items in the food pyramid
   c. Are the law
   d. None of the above

4. The role of the medical assistant with regard to physician-ordered diets is
   a. To assist in the selection of the diet
   b. To count the calories
   c. To provide patient information
   d. All of the above

5. Which factor should *not* be considered when sending patients home with a preprinted diet?
   a. Financial circumstances
   b. Religion
   c. Patient's age
   d. None of the above

6. An excellent source of information on exercise is
   a. The American Heart Association
   b. U.S. Exercise
   c. The American Red Cross Association
   d. The physician

7. Exercise can help relieve stress, maintain healthy body weight, and increase circulation and muscle tone if
   a. The heart rate exceeds 100 beats per minute
   b. It is done daily
   c. It is supervised by a physician
   d. None of the above

Critical Thinking Practice

Mrs. Greene, aged 67, had a stroke 3 weeks ago and now has left hemiparesis. She is home from the hospital. Dr. Smith would like her husband to help her begin performing daily range-of-motion exercises.

1. Explain the purpose of range-of-motion exercises to Mr. Greene.

_____

_____

_____

_____

2. Describe range-of-motion exercises to Mr. and Mrs. Greene.

_____

_____

_____

_____

3. Describe the difference between positive and negative stress. Give an example of each.

_____

_____

_____

_____

4. Mr. Alexander is the president of a large manufacturing company. He is seeing Dr. Smith for frequent headaches. Dr. Smith has diagnosed the headaches as stress induced and has recommended that Mr. Alexander develop some coping mechanisms to reduce the stress in his life. As Mr. Alexander leaves the office, he questions the medical assistant about ways he can comply with Dr. Smith's recommendations. What strategies can you offer Mr. Alexander?

_____

_____

_____

_____

Charting Documentation

1. With regard to question 37, write a narrative chart note describing your interaction with the patient.

Date   **Time**

_____

_____

_____

Patient Education

1. Mrs. Jones is taking four medications to control her hypertension and arthritis. She also takes an occasional antacid for indigestion. At a routine visit she tells the medical assistant that she is having difficulty taking all of the medication because she feels she is *always* taking pills and is not sure they are doing any good. How can you teach Mrs. Jones about her medication schedule? What critical factors should be considered before you begin a discussion with Mrs. Jones?

_____

_____

_____

5

The First Contact: Telephone and Reception

CHAPTER COMPETENCIES

Review the information in your text that supports the following course objectives.

Learning Objectives

1. Spell and define the key terms

2. Explain the importance of displaying a professional image to all patients

3. List six duties of the medical office receptionist

4. List four sources from which messages can be retrieved

5. Discuss various steps that can be taken to promote good ergonomics

6. Describe the basic guidelines for waiting room environments

7. Describe the proper method for maintaining infection control standards in the waiting room

8. Discuss the five basic guidelines for telephone use

9. Describe the types of incoming telephone calls received by the medical office

10. Describe how to triage incoming calls

11. Discuss how to identify and handle callers with medical emergencies

12. List the information that should be given to an emergency medical service dispatcher

13. Describe the types of telephone services and special features

CHAPTER OUTLINE	NOTES
Professional Image	
Importance of a Good Attitude	
The Medical Assistant as a Role Model	
Courtesy and Diplomacy in the Medical Office	
First Impressions	
Reception	
Definition of a Receptionist	
Duties and Responsibilities of the Receptionist	
Prepare the Office	
Retrieve Messages	
Prepare the Charts	
Welcome Patients and Visitors	
Register and Orient Patients	
Manage Waiting Time	

CHAPTER OUTLINE *continued*	NOTES
Ergonomics Concerns for the Receptionist	
The Waiting Room Environment	
General Guidelines for Waiting Rooms	
Guidelines for Pediatric Waiting Rooms	
Americans with Disabilities Act Requirements	
Infection Control Issues	
The End of the Patient Visit	
Telephone	
Importance of the Telephone in the Medical Office	
Basic Guidelines for Telephone Use	
Diction	
Pronunciation	
Expression	
Listening	
Courtesy	
Routine Incoming Calls	
Appointments	
Billing Inquires	
Diagnostic Test Results	
Routine and Satisfactory Progress Reports	
Test Results	
Unsatisfactory Progress Reports and Test Results	
Prescription Refills	
Other Calls	
Challenging Incoming Calls	
Unidentified Callers	
Irate Patients	
Medical Emergencies	
Triaging Incoming Calls	
Taking Messages	
Outgoing Calls	
General Guidelines for Outgoing Calls	
Calling Emergency Medical Services	
Services and Special Features	
Telecommunication Relay Systems	

LEARNING SELF-ASSESSMENT EXERCISES

Key Terms

Define the following key terms:

attitude _____

closed captioning _____

diction _____

diplomacy _____

emergency medical service (EMS) _____

ergonomic _____

receptionist _____

teletypewriter (TTY) _____

triage _____

Matching

Match the phrase in part 1 with its association in part 2.

PART I

_____ 1. Acting as a role model

_____ 2. Speak clearly

_____ 3. Positive expression

_____ 4. Listen attentively

_____ 5. Well-managed waiting time

_____ 6. Fundamental to successful human relations

_____ 7. Patient information not divulged

_____ 8. Acceptance of the patient as a unique
          individual

PART 2

a. Personal appearance

b. Confidentiality

c. Nonjudgmental

d. Courtesy and diplomacy

e. Conversation focused

f. Pronunciation

g. Keep patient informed

h. Friendly attitude

Skill Drills

1. List seven duties of the medical office receptionist.

_____

_____

_____

_____

_____

_____

_____

2. Describe the eleven types of incoming calls received by the medical office.

_____

_____

_____

_____

_____

_____

_____

_____

_____

_____

3. List the six items of information necessary to document a telephone message.

_____

_____

_____

_____

_____

_____

4. Identify six of the thirteen items that are found on a patient registration form.

_____

_____

_____

_____

_____

_____

Multiple Choice

5. How you feel influences how you act; therefore
   a. Attitude shapes behavior
   b. Behavior shapes attitude
   c. Feelings do not affect attitude
   d. None of the above

6. Which of the following items of jewelry should not be worn by the medical professional?
   a. Small stud earrings
   b. Wedding rings
   c. Dangling earrings
   d. All of the above

7. Each morning the medical receptionist should
   a. Make coffee
   b. Review the appointment schedule
   c. Prepare charts
   d. *b* and *c* only

8. The patient registration may be completed
   a. During the interview with the patient
   b. After the patient leaves
   c. Over the telephone
   d. None of the above

9. Office policies and procedures may include
   a. How the bill will be paid
   b. When the bill will be paid
   c. Who will pay the bill
   d. *a* and *b* only

10. Preferred medical office color schemes are
    a. Primary colors
    b. Muted colors
    c. Bright colors
    d. Dark colors

11. The use of sofas in a medical office is
   a. Comfortable
   b. Preferred over chairs
   c. Not recommended
   d. Esthetically pleasing

12. The preferred subjects for artwork for a medical office are
   a. Abstract
   b. Floral
   c. Landscapes
   d. *b* and *c* only

13. Most pediatricians' offices have
   a. A children's play area
   b. One large waiting area
   c. Separate areas for sick and well children
   d. *a* and *c* only

14. When speaking on the phone, *never*
   a. Chew gum
   b. Prop the headset on your shoulder
   c. Speak rapidly
   d. All of the above

Critical Thinking Practice

You receive a call from a patient who complains of being short of breath.

1. What questions will you ask this patient to determine whether this is an emergency?

_____

_____

_____

_____

2. What information will you ask for first?

_____

_____

_____

_____

3. Describe the different types of telephone services and special features that are available for medical offices.

_____

_____

_____

_____

4. In reviewing your tickler file, you discover that it is time to schedule a follow-up appointment for Mrs. Smith. You place an outgoing call to the patient. Explain the procedure or procedures you will use in making this call and patient appointment.

_____

_____

_____

_____

Charting Documentation

Using the information from question 26, write a narrative chart note describing your interaction with the patient.

Date   **Time**

_____

_____

_____

_____

6

Managing Appointments

CHAPTER COMPETENCIES

Review the information in your text that supports the following course objectives.

Learning Objectives

1. Spell and define the key terms

2. Describe the various systems for scheduling patient office visits, including manual and computerized scheduling

3. Identify the factors that affect appointment scheduling

4. Explain guidelines for scheduling appointments for new patients and return visits

5. List three ways to remind patients about appointments

6. Describe how to triage patient emergencies, acutely ill patients, and walk-in patients

7. Describe how to handle late patients and patients who miss their appointments

8. Explain what to do if the physician is delayed

9. Describe how to handle appointment cancellations made by the office or by the patient

10. Schedule an appointment for a new patient

11. Schedule a return appointment

12. Schedule a referral following third-party guidelines

CHAPTER OUTLINE	NOTES
Appointment Scheduling Systems	
Manual Appointment Scheduling	
The Appointment Book	
Establishing a Matrix	
Computerized Appointment Scheduling	
Types of Scheduling	
Structured Appointments	
Clustering	
Wave and Modified Wave	
Fixed Scheduling	
Streaming	
Double Booking	
Flexible Hours	
Open Hours	

CHAPTER OUTLINE *continued*

	NOTES
Factors That Affect Scheduling	
Patients' Needs	
Providers' Preferences and Needs	
Physical Facilities	
Scheduling Guidelines	
New Patients	
Established Patients	
Preparing a Daily or Weekly Schedule	
Patient Reminders	
Appointment Cards	
Telephone Reminders	
Mailed Reminder Cards	
Adapting the Schedule	
Emergencies	
Patients Who Are Acutely Ill	
Walk-in Patients	
Late Patients	
Physician Delays	
Missed Appointments	
Cancellations	
Cancellations by the Office	
Cancellations by the Patient	
Making Appointments for Patients in Other Facilities	
Referrals and Consultations	
Diagnostic Testing	
Surgery	
When the Appointment Schedule Does Not Work	

LEARNING SELF-ASSESSMENT EXERCISES

Key Terms

Define the following key terms:

acute _____

buffer _____

chronic _____

clustering _____

constellation of symptoms _____

consultation _____

double booking _____

matrix _____

precertification _____

providers _____

referral _____

STAT _____

streaming _____

tickler file _____

wave scheduling system _____

Matching

Match the definition in part 1 with the correct term in part 2.

PART I

_____ 1. Each patient assigned a time

_____ 2. Greater range of appointment times available

_____ 3. Patients taken in order of arrival

_____ 4. More than one patient scheduled in a single time slot

_____ 5. Several patients scheduled in the first half hour and none in the second half-hour

PART 2

a. Double booking

b. Scheduled appointments

c. Wave scheduling

d. Open scheduling

e. Flexible hours

Skill Drills

1. List three ways to remind patients about appointments.

_____

_____

_____

2. Identify three factors that affect appointment scheduling.

_____

_____

_____

3. Identify three ways to remind patients of an appointment.

_____

_____

_____

Multiple Choice

1. Sign-in sheets are
   a. Used by many offices
   b. Legal documents
   c. Subject to subpoena
   d. All of the above

2. Before using the appointment book, you have to set up a
   a. Tickler file
   b. Matrix
   c. Staff schedule
   d. Color code system

3. Computerized scheduling
   a. Saves time
   b. Is time consuming
   c. Is difficult to learn
   d. None of the above

4. Before scheduling an appointment, you should
   a. Talk to the physician
   b. Ask about special transportation
   c. Know whether the patient has seen someone else for the condition
   d. All of the above

5. Office visitors other than patients include
   a. Other physicians
   b. Sales representatives
   c. Personal friends
   d. All of the above

6. Open time slots should be scheduled for any problems that arise. These slots are called
   a. Open time
   b. Flexible time
   c. Open blocks
   d. Flexible blocks

7. The issue of patient confidentiality *must* be considered in which of the following circumstances?
   a. Office sign-in sheets
   b. Home message machines
   c. Postcard appointment reminders
   d. All of the above

8. When making a series of appointments for a patient, it is helpful to
   a. Schedule appointments on the same day of the week
   b. Schedule appointments at the same time of day
   c. Give the patient a card for each visit
   d. *a* and *b* only

9. Preprinted appointment cards should
   a. Never be used
   b. Be used for annual examinations
   c. Include the reason for the visit
   d. Be used for all appointments

10. Patients who are more than 15 minutes late are
    a. Always rescheduled
    b. Always seen immediately
    c. Asked to explain
    d. Informed that they may have to wait

Critical Thinking Practice

1. Compare and contrast guidelines for scheduling appointments for new patients and return visits.

_____

_____

_____

_____

2. Dr. Wong calls at 11:30 A.M. to say that he is delayed at the hospital and expects to be in the office by 2:30 P.M. Two patients are waiting in the office and three are on the schedule for 1:30 to 2:30 P.M. Describe how you will handle this delay and how you will handle the patients waiting to be seen.

_____

_____

_____

3. Dr. Walters calls in ill and asks you to cancel her first morning appointment. You call Mrs. Steel and inform her of the situation. Write a script of your conversation with this patient.

_____

_____

_____

_____

Charting Documentation

1. With regard to question 21, write a narrative chart note describing your interaction with the patient.

Date   **Time**

_____

_____

_____

_____

7

Written Communications

CHAPTER COMPETENCIES

Review the information in your text that supports the following course objectives.

Learning Objectives

1. Spell and define the key terms

2. Discuss the basic guidelines for grammar, punctuation, and spelling

3. Describe six key guidelines for medical writing

4. Discuss the eleven key components of a business letter

5. Describe the three steps to writing a business letter

6. Describe the process of writing a memorandum

7. Discuss the various mailing options

8. Identify the types of incoming written communication seen in a physician's office

9. List the items that must be included in an agenda

10. Identify the items that must be included when typing minutes

Performance Objectives

1. Write a business letter

2. Write a memorandum

3. Address and send written communication

4. Open and sort mail

CHAPTER OUTLINE	NOTES
Professional Writing	
Basic Grammar and Punctuation Guidelines	
Basic Spelling Guidelines	
Guidelines for Medical Writing	
Accuracy	
Spelling	
Capitalization	
Abbreviations and Symbols	
Plural and Possessive	
Numbers	
Letter Development	
Components of a Letter	
Letter Formats	
Full Block	

CHAPTER OUTLINE *continued*

	NOTES
Block	
Semiblock	
Writing a Business Letter	
Preparation	
Composition	
Editing	
Types of Business Letters	
Memorandum Development	
Components of a Memorandum	
Sending Written Communication	
Facsimile Machines	
Electronic Mail	
United States Postal Service	
Addressing Envelopes	
Affixing Postage	
USPS Mailing Options	
USPS Special Services	
Other Delivery Options	
Receiving and Handling Incoming Mail	
Types of Incoming Mail	
Opening and Sorting Mail	
Annotation	
Composing Agendas and Minutes	

LEARNING SELF-ASSESSMENT EXERCISES

Key Terms

Define the following key terms:

agenda _____

annotation _____

BiCaps _____

block _____

enclosure _____

font _____

full block _____

intercaps _____

margin _____

memorandum _____

proofread _____

salutation _____

semiblock _____

template _____

Matching

Match the definition in part 1 with the correct term in part 2.

PART 1

_____ 1. Greeting of the letter

_____ 2. Something included with a letter

_____ 3. Conclusion of the letter

_____ 4. Indication of who dictated the letter and who wrote it

_____ 5. Most formal format and most commonly used for professional letters

_____ 6. Same as block except first sentence of each paragraph is indented five spaces

_____ 7. Date, subject line, closing, and signature flush with the right margin

PART 2

a. Full block

b. Closing

c. Block

d. Enclosure

e. Identification line

f. Salutation

g. Semiblock

Skill Drills

1. Name the six types of mailing options.

_____

_____

_____

_____

_____

_____

2. Name the 12 types of incoming written communication seen in the physician's office.

_____

_____

_____

_____

_____

_____

_____

_____

_____

_____

_____

_____

3. Name the nine items that must be included in minutes.

_____

_____

_____

_____

_____

_____

_____

_____

_____

4. Name the five items that must be included in an agenda.

_____

_____

_____

_____

_____

Multiple Choice

1. In letters to a physician, the salutation should
   a. Always be in capital letters
   b. Begin with Dr."
   c. Be written out with the word Doctor"
   d. Never use the first name

2. Which of the following items *can* be abbreviated in an inside address?
   a. City
   b. Town
   c. Business title
   d. State

3. The subject line of a letter is
   a. Placed five spaces below the inside address
   b. Mandatory
   c. Used to highlight the intent of a letter
   d. None of the above

4. Which of the following is *not* a step in writing a professional business letter?
   a. Mailing status
   b. Preparation
   c. Editing
   d. Composition

5. Facsimile machines allow transmission of
   a. Orders
   b. Test results
   c. Prescriptions
   d. All of the above

6. Electronic mail, or e-mail, allows for what type of communication?
   a. Computer to computer
   b. Computer to physician
   c. Physician to computer
   d. Physician to physician

7. The standard business envelope (No. 10) is
   a. 4 × 5 inches
   b. 3.5 × 5 inches
   c. 4 × 5.5 inches
   d. 4.25 × 9.5 inches

8. Which type of mailing option should be used to ensure the delivery of a letter or package by noon the next day?
   a. Priority mail
   b. Express mail
   c. First class mail
   d. Top priority mail

9. Carbon copies of letters are usually sent to
   a. The patient
   b. Managers
   c. The individual who requested that the given information be provided
   d. *b* and *c* only

10. Computer spell checks should be used
    a. With caution
    b. Only once
    c. To check grammar
    d. None of the above

Critical Thinking Practice

1. The office manager has asked you to write an interoffice memorandum to explain the new policy regarding vacation scheduling. Describe the process of memorandum development.

_____

_____

_____

_____

2. Dr. Smith has asked you to assume responsibility for transcribing physical examination reports for the office. This is a new task for you. Discuss the transcription process, including the skills necessary to transcribe accurately and the basic parts of a transcription machine and their functions.

_____

_____

_____

_____

3. Dr. Adams has asked you to type a letter to Dr. Smith, an associate of Dr. Adams, to request Mrs. Jones' medical records. Dr. Adams would also like to know whether Dr. Smith considers Mrs. Jones an acceptable candidate for a new drug study for patients with chronic hypertension. As you prepare to compose this letter, you may envision yourself speaking to Dr. Smith. Explain how this would benefit composing this letter. Be specific.

_____

_____

_____

_____

4. The goal of composition of a letter is **clear, concise,** and **accurate** writing. Give an example of an **unclear** statement, a **wordy** statement, and an **inaccurate** statement. Next to each example **rewrite the messages** properly.

Unclear _____

_____

_____

_____

Wordy _____

_____

_____

_____

_____

Inaccurate _____

_____

_____

_____

_____

8

Medical Records and Record Management

CHAPTER COMPETENCIES

Review the information in your text that supports the following course objectives.

Learning Objectives

1. Spell and define the key terms

2. Describe standard and electronic medical record systems

3. Explain the process for releasing medical records to third-party payers and individual patients

4. List and explain the EMR guidelines established to protect computerized records

5. List the standard information included in medical records

6. Identify and describe the types of formats used for documenting patient information in outpatient settings

7. Explain how to make an entry in a patient's medical record, using abbreviations when appropriate

8. Explain how to make a correction in a standard and electronic medical record

9. Identify the various ways medical records can be stored

10. Compare and contrast the differences between alphabetic and numeric filing systems and give an example of each

11. Explain the purpose of the Health Insurance Portability and Accountability Act

Performance Objective

1. Prepare and file a medical record file folder

CHAPTER OUTLINE	NOTES
Standard Medical Records	
Contents of the Medical Record	
Electronic Medical Records	
Electronic Medical Record Security	
Other Technologies for Medical Record Maintenance	
Medical Record Organization	
Provider Encounters	
Narrative Format	
SOAP Format	
POMR Format	

CHAPTER OUTLINE *continued*	NOTES
Documentation Forms	
Medical History Forms	
Flow Sheets	
Progress Notes	
Medical Record Entries	
Charting Communications With Patients	
Additions to Medical Records	
Workers' Compensation Records	
Medical Record Preparation	
Filing Procedures	
Filing Systems	
Alphabetic Filing	
Numeric Filing	
Other Filing Systems	
Classifying Medical Records	
Inactive Record Storage	
Storing Active Medical Records	
Record Retention	
Releasing Medical Records	
Releasing Records to Patients	
Reporting Obligations	

LEARNING SELF-ASSESSMENT EXERCISES

Key Terms

Define the following key terms:

alphabetic filing _____

chief complaint _____

chronological order _____

cross-reference _____

demographic data _____

electronic medical records (EMR) _____

flow sheet _____

medical history forms _____

microfiche _____

microfilm _____

narrative _____

numeric filing _____

present illness _____

problem-oriented medical record (POMR) _____

reverse chronological order _____

SOAP _____

subject filing _____

workers' compensation _____

Matching

Match the definition in part 1 with the correct term in part 2.

PART 1

_____ 1. Uses digits to file records

_____ 2. Way to organize material

_____ 3. List of patients and matching numeric code

_____ 4. Use of letters to file records

_____ 5. Use of dates to file records

_____ 6. Use of topics to file

PART 2

a. Subject filing

b. Numeric filing

c. Filing system

d. Alphabetic filing

e. Cross-reference

f. Chronological filing

Skill Drills

1. Identify the four ways that medical records can be stored.

_____
_____
_____
_____

2. List the 14 standard topics of information included in a medical record.

_____
_____
_____
_____
_____
_____
_____
_____
_____
_____
_____
_____
_____
_____
_____
_____

3. No matter how the records are stored, make sure that the information meets the following six criteria.

_____

_____

_____

_____

_____

_____

Multiple Choice

1. In source-oriented medical records, all similar categories or sources of information are grouped together. Among such categories are
   a. Physician orders
   b. Progress notes
   c. Radiographic results
   d. *a* and *b* only

2. Problem-oriented medical records are divided into four components. An example of primary components is
   a. Databases
   b. Treatment plans
   c. Progress notes
   d. All of the above

3. The oldest and least structured documentation form is
   a. Focus charting
   b. PIE charting
   c. Narrative charting
   d. SOAP charting

4. The term PIE stands for
   a. Problem, implementation, evaluation
   b. Prognosis, intervention, evaluation
   c. Plan, intervention, evaluation
   d. Procedure, implementation, evaluation

5. No matter what form is used for documentation, you must always include

   a. The date and time
   b. The procedure performed
   c. Your signature
   d. All of the above

6. All additions to the medical record (laboratory, radiography, consultations) should be
   a. Checked for spelling
   b. Initialed by the medical assistant
   c. Initialed by the physician
   d. None of the above

7. Workers' compensation cases are kept open
   a. For 2 years from the last date of treatment
   b. For 2 years from the initial date of treatment
   c. According to office protocol
   d. According to the employer's protocol

8. The golden rule refers to
   a. Legal documentation
   b. Abbreviation rules
   c. The principle that if it is not documented, it was not done
   d. Filing procedures

9. With the *terminal digit filing system*, the groups of numbers are read from
   a. The end first
   b. From right to left
   c. From left to right
   d. *a* and *b*

Critical Thinking Practice

1. ABC Insurance Company has sent a written request for a copy of Mr. Johnson's medical records. Explain what information has to be included in the request for records *and* how you will process this request, including the guidelines for charging the insurance company for this type of processing.

_____

_____

_____

_____

2. Compare and contrast alphabetic and numeric filing systems; give an example of each.

_____

_____

_____

_____

Patient Education

1. Ms. Winters is 17 years old and still lives with her parents. She has been a patient of Dr. Wahlgren for many years. She comes into the office and asks you for a copy of her medical records. How do you respond?

_____

_____

_____

_____

9

Transcription

CHAPTER COMPETENCIES

Review the information in your text that supports the following course objectives.

Learning Objectives

1. Explain the role of the medical assistant in performing medical transcription

2. Explain the roles of the JCAHO and HIPAA on medical transcription

3. List the various reports generated in inpatient and outpatient medical facilities

4. List the rules of medical transcription as outlined by the AAMT

5. Discuss the various medical transcription systems

Performance Objectives

1. Transcribe various medical reports from taped dictation

2. Use proper punctuation, grammar, and spelling

CHAPTER OUTLINE	NOTES
Medical Transcription	
The Transcription Process	
Off-site Transcription	
Report Formatting	
Types of Medical Reports	
History and Physical Examination Reports	
Consultation Reports	
Progress Reports	
SOAP Notes	
Hospital Reports	
Operative Report	
Pathology Report	
Autopsy Report	
Radiology Report	
Discharge Summary	
Transcription Rules	
Abbreviations	
Capitalization	

CHAPTER OUTLINE *continued*	NOTES
Numbers	
Punctuation	
Apostrophes	
Commas	
Semicolons	
Colons	
Periods	
Quotation Marks	
Slash Marks	
Hyphens	
Grammar	
Spelling	
Transcription Systems	
Traditional Tape Dictation Systems	
Digital Systems	
Voice Recognition Systems	
Transcription With Word Processing Software	

LEARNING SELF-ASSESSMENT EXERCISES

Key Terms

Define the following key terms:

analogue _____

digital _____

transcription _____

Matching

Match the description in part 1 with the correct term in part 2.

PART 1

_____ 1. Typing a previously dictated message

_____ 2. Controls play, rewind, and fast forward

_____ 3. Used between items in a series

_____ 4. Used after headings

_____ 5. To show titles of articles, short stories, subdi-
visions, and so on

PART 2

a. Foot pedal

b. Colon

c. Quotation marks

d. Comma

e. Transcription

Skill Drills

1. List the personal qualities needed to transcribe well.

_____

_____

_____

_____

2. List the five requirements of a professional document.

_____

_____

_____

_____

_____

3. What is JCAHO?

_____

_____

4. List JCAHO's two requirements regarding history and physical examination reports.

_____

_____

Multiple Choice

1. When one provider refers a patient to a specialist, what does the consulting physician prepare to report the findings of the encounter?
   a. Outpatient procedural code
   b. Consultation report
   c. Progress report
   d. None of the above

2. Entries in the medical record must be
   a. Neat and in red ink
   b. In chronological order
   c. Progress sheets
   d. Can be on sticky notes

3. Information that cannot be detected or measured is
   a. Chief complaint data
   b. Objective data
   c. History data
   d. Subjective data

4. The patient's appearance, vital signs, rashes, and the results of a urinalysis are all
   a. Chief complaint data
   b. Objective data
   c. History data
   d. Subjective data

5. Hospital reports include all of the following _except_
   a. Consultation reports
   b. Discharge summaries
   c. Pathology reports
   d. Chief complaints

6. Which report outlines the findings of gross and microscopic examinations performed on organs and tissue samples?
   a. Autopsy report
   b. Pathology report
   c. History report
   d. Biopsy report

7. Which of the following is a concise report of the reason for a patient's admission, tests performed, treatments given, results of those treatments and tests, and the condition of the patient when being moved to another facility?
   a. Autopsy report
   b. Discharge summary
   c. Transfer summary
   d. History report

8. Every licensed medical facility is required to keep a list of approved abbreviations that should be updated yearly.
   a. True
   b. False

9. For balance and clarity a zero should be added
   a. Before and after a decimal
   b. Before a decimal
   c. After a decimal
   d. Neither; the number should be spelled out

10. One of the most important skills necessary to be an efficient and productive transcriptionist is the ability to
   a. Speak clearly
   b. Type 120 words per minute
   c. Do more that one transcription at a time
   d. Punctuate without direction

Critical Thinking Practice

1. Define SOAP and state why the SOAP format for documentation is so vital to the medical record.

_____
_____
_____
_____

2. Using the punctuation rules of transcription and given a transcribed report, edit the report for possible errors.

_____
_____
_____
_____

3. List and state the use of each part of a transcription machine.

_____
_____
_____
_____
_____
_____

10

Computer Applications in the Medical Office

CHAPTER COMPETENCIES

Review the information in your text that supports the following course objectives.

Learning Objectives

1. Spell and define the key words

2. Identify the basic computer components

3. Explain the basics of connecting to the Internet

4. Discuss the safety concerns for online searching

5. Describe how to use a search engine

6. List sites that can be used by professionals and sites geared for patients

7. Describe the benefits of an intranet and explain how it differs from the Internet

8. Describe the various types of clinical software that might be used in a physician's office

9. Describe the various types of administrative software that might be used in a physician's office

10. Describe the benefits of a handheld computer

11. Describe the considerations for purchasing a computer

12. Describe various training options

13. Discuss the ethics related to computer access

Performance Objectives

1. Search a given topic on the Internet

2. Conduct a basic literary search

CHAPTER OUTLINE

CHAPTER OUTLINE	NOTES
The Computer	
Hardware	
Peripherals	
Care and Maintenance of the System and Equipment	
Internet Basics	
Getting Started and Connected	
Security	
Viruses	
Downloading Information	
Working Offline	
Electronic Mail	
Access	
Composing Messages	

CHAPTER OUTLINE *continued*

CHAPTER OUTLINE *continued*	NOTES
Address Books	
Attachments	
Opening Electronic Mail	
Medical Applications of the Internet	
Search Engines	
Professional Medical Sites	
Literary Searches	
Health-Related Calculators	
Insurance-Related Sites	
Patient Teaching Issues Regarding the Internet	
Buying Medications Online	
Financial Assistance for Medications	
Medical Records	
Medical Record Forms	
Injury Prevention	
Intranet	
Medical Software Applications	
Clinical Applications	
Administrative Applications	
Paging System Software	
PowerPoint	
Meeting Maker	
Handheld Computers	
Purchasing a Computer	
Training Options	
Computer Ethics	

SELF-ASSESSMENT LEARNING EXERCISES

Key Terms

Define the following key terms:

cookies _____

downloading _____

encryption _____

Ethernet _____

Internet _____

intranet _____

literary search _____

search engine _____

surfing _____

virtual _____

virus _____

Matching

Match the definition in part 1 with the correct term in part 2.

PART 1

_____ 1. Start a computer

_____ 2. A single character

_____ 3. 1 million characters

_____ 4. Where computer stores programs

_____ 5. Gets information on and off diskette

_____ 6. Printed computer data

_____ 7. Another name for diskette

_____ 8. Another name for central processing unit

_____ 9. Computer breakdown

PART 2

a. Microprocessor

b. Floppy disk

c. Megabyte

d. Crash

e. Disk drive

f. Boot

g. Byte

h. Hard copy

i. Hard drive

Skill Drills

1. List the four categories of computer components.

_____

_____

_____

_____

2. List five maintenance regimens.

_____

_____

_____

_____

_____

3. List *two* types of administrative software for each of the following:

   a. Desktop publishing

   _____

   _____

   b. Graphics

   _____

   _____

   c. Spreadsheets

   _____

   _____

   d. Word processing

   _____

   _____

4. List five types of clinical application software.

   _____

   _____

   _____

   _____

   _____

Multiple Choice

1. A fiberglass board that contains the PCU, memory, expansion slots, and many other pieces of circuitry is a
   a. Microprocessor
   b. Motherboard
   c. Directory
   d. Mainframe

2. The read-only memory chip, the permanent memory inside the computer, is called
   a. ROM
   b. RAM
   c. PCU
   d. VDT

3. The main memory, primary memory, or short-term memory is contained in a set of silicon chips called
   a. ROM
   b. RAM
   c. PCU
   d. VDT

4. An example of a special function key is
   a. Alt
   b. Ctrl
   c. Insert
   d. All of the above

5. The display unit of a computer that resembles a television is the
   a. Visual display terminal
   b. Monitor
   c. Modem
   d. *a* and *b* only

6. The location at which data will be entered into the computer is identified by a flashing line called a
   a. Cursor
   b. Login
   c. Password
   d. None of the above

7. A directory that can be further broken down is called a
   a. Backup
   b. Second set
   c. Secondary category
   d. Subdirectory

8. A freestanding device that is used to control the cursor on a display screen is called a
   a. Login
   b. Modem
   c. Mouse
   d. Indicator

9. A communication device that connects a computer to the standard telephone system is a
   a. Modem
   b. Monitor
   c. Terminal
   d. Cable

10. The special code used to access a computer is referred to as a
   a. Database
   b. Login
   c. Password
   d. None of the above

Critical Thinking Practice

1. Compare and contrast the advantages and disadvantages of automating the front office.

_____

_____

_____

_____

2. As the administrative medical assistant, you have been asked to research types of computers and software packages for purchase for the office. Explain what considerations you should explore and make suggestions for both administrative and clinical software.

_____

_____

_____

_____

3. Computer automation is new to your office, and the staff is unsure how to use software applications. What training options will you use to help them feel more comfortable with basic computer use and various software applications?

_____

_____

_____

_____

11

Quality Improvement and Risk Management

CHAPTER COMPETENCIES

Review the information in your text that supports the following course objectives.

Learning Objectives

1. Spell and define the key terms

2. List four regulatory agencies that require medical office settings to have quality improvement programs

3. Describe the accreditation process of the Joint Commission on Accreditation of Healthcare Organizations

4. Describe the intent of the Clinical Laboratory Improvement Amendments Act

5. Describe the intent of the Health Insurance Portability and Accountability Act

6. Describe the steps to developing a quality improvement program

7. List five guidelines for completing incident reports

8. Explain how quality improvement programs and risk management work together in a medical office to improve overall patient care and employee needs.

Performance Objective

1. Complete an incident report

CHAPTER OUTLINE	NOTES
Quality Improvement Programs in the Medical Office Setting	
Regulatory Agencies	
Joint Commission on Accreditation of Healthcare Organizations (JCAHO)	
Occupational Safety and Health Administration	
Centers for Medicare & Medicaid Services	
State Health Departments	
Developing a Quality Improvement Program	
Seven Steps for a Successful Program	
Risk Management	
Incident Reports	
When to Complete an Incident Report	
Information Included on an Incident Report	

CHAPTER OUTLINE *continued*	NOTES
Guidelines for Completing an Incident Report	
Trending Incident Reports	
Putting It All Together: A Case Review	

LEARNING SELF-ASSESSMENT EXERCISES

Key Terms

Define the following key terms:

Centers for Medicare & Medicaid Services _____

Clinical Laboratory Improvement Amendments Act _____

expected threshold _____

incident reports _____

Health Insurance Portability and Accountability Act _____

Joint Commission on Accreditation of Healthcare Organizations _____

Occupational Safety and Health Administration _____

outcomes _____

quality improvement _____

sentinel event _____

task force _____

Matching

Match the definition in part 1 with the correct term in part 2.

PART 1

_____ 1. Assures the community that an organization has met basic practice standards

_____ 2. A second survey

_____ 3. Numerical goal

_____ 4. Occurred for unknown reasons

_____ 5. Joint Commission's quality improvement standards

_____ 6. Correct test and procedures done

_____ 7. Action or treatment effective

PART 2

a. Efficacy

b. Threshold

c. IOP

d. Accreditation

e. Appropriateness

f. Focus survey

g. Idiopathic

Skill Drills

1. List the three regulatory agencies that require medical office settings to have quality improvement plans.

_____

_____

_____

2. List six health care settings for which JCAHO presently sets standards and evaluates care.

_____

_____

_____

_____

_____

_____

3. Identify the seven steps in the process of acquiring JCAHO accreditation.

_____

_____

_____

_____

_____

_____

_____

4. Give five resources that may be used to obtain suggestions for improving care.

_____

_____

_____

_____

_____

Multiple Choice

1. The period for which JCAHO accreditation is valid is
   a. 5 years
   b. 2 years
   c. 3 years
   d. 4 years

2. The primary focus of IOP standards is for the organization to
   a. Do the right thing
   b. Do the right thing well
   c. Conduct a survey well
   d. *a* and *b*.

3. OSHA compliance is
   a. Not voluntary
   b. Voluntary
   c. Subject to review
   d. Required for facilities with 50 or more employees

4. Examples of quality improvement (QI) committees include
   a. Critical care
   b. Patient education
   c. Nursing services
   d. All of the above

5. How many elements do QI monitoring plans have?
   a. Four
   b. Five
   c. Three
   d. Six

6. Under risk management, risk factors for patients and employees are
   a. Safety concerns
   b. Financial accountability
   c. Liability concerns
   d. *a* and *c*

7. Incident reports are sometimes referred to as
   a. An employer liability
   b. A patient liability
   c. Occurrence reports
   d. Administrative reports

8. Incident reports should be completed within
   a. 12 hours
   b. 24 hours
   c. 48 hours
   d. 72 hours

9. Documentation in the patient's chart that an incident report has been completed is
   a. Always done
   b. Done only if the patient is injured
   c. Done on advisement of insurance company
   d. Never done

10. Patient care settings for which JCAHO is responsible include
    a. Ambulatory care
    b. Inpatient care
    c. Outpatient care
    d. All of the above

Critical Thinking Practice

1. An elderly patient slipped and fell in the waiting room. What type of report will you fill out, and what guidelines will you follow?

_____

_____

_____

_____

2. You are a newly hired administrative medical assistant, and the physician has asked you to develop a QI program for the practice. How will you set up a successful program?

_____

_____

_____

_____

3. There are many newly hired employees in your clinic, and you need to explain how quality improvement programs and risk management work together to improve overall patient care and employee needs. What will you tell this group?

_____

_____

_____

_____

_____

12

Management of the Medical Office Team

CHAPTER OUTLINE *continued*	NOTES
Policy and Procedures Manuals	
Tips for Writing Personnel Manuals	
Developing Promotional Materials	
Financial Concerns	
Budgets	
Payroll	
Petty Cash	
Maintenance and Inventory of Supplies	
Service Contracts	
Inventory	
Education	
Staff Education	
Patient Education	
Manager Education	
Legal Issues Regarding Office Management	
Americans with Disabilities Act	
Sexual Harassment	
Family and Medical Leave Act	
Other Legal Considerations	

LEARNING SELF-ASSESSMENT EXERCISES

Key Terms

Define the following key terms:

Americans with Disabilities Act _____

budget _____

compliance officer _____

Family and Medical Leave Act _____

job description _____

mission statement _____

organizational chart _____

policy _____

procedure _____

Matching

Match the definition in part 1 with the correct term in part 2.

PART 1

_____ 1. Up to 12 weeks (unpaid) leave to meet family needs

_____ 2. Contains specific rules and regulations regarding laboratory safety

_____ 3. Federal agency that sets standards for employee safety

_____ 4. Private organization that sets standards for health care administration

_____ 5. Regulations designed to meet the needs of people with physical and mental disabilities

_____ 6. Logical system to keep track of supplies

_____ 7. Large outlays of money for equipment, property management, and building maintenance

PART 2

a. Capital budget

b. Inventory

c. ADA

d. OSHA

e. Family and Medical Leave Act

f. CLIA

g. JCAHO

Skill Drills

1. List the seven responsibilities of the medical office manager.

_____

_____

_____

_____

_____

_____

_____

2. List the seven types of policies and procedures that should be included in a medical office's policy and procedures manual.

_____

_____

_____

_____

_____

_____

_____

3. List five types of promotional material that a medical office may distribute.

_____

_____

_____

_____

4. Identify three ways that a manager can communicate with medical office staff.

_____

_____

_____

Multiple Choice

1. Staff meetings should
   a. Never be canceled
   b. Never be canceled except in an emergency
   c. Be canceled if there is no quorum
   d. Be canceled if the manager is not present

2. Staffing issues
   a. Take most of the office manager's time
   b. Are delegated to line staff
   c. Are the prerogative of the physician
   d. None of the above

3. Job descriptions
   a. Are written by employees only
   b. Can be written with help of employees
   c. Are never given to employees
   d. Are signed by the manager only

4. Which of the following topics is *not appropriate* on a job application?
   a. Years of experience
   b. Last employer
   c. Schools attended
   d. Physical or mental disabilities

5. Disciplinary actions may be
   a. Written
   b. Verbal
   c. Recorded in the employee's file
   d. All of the above

6. The primary goal of scheduling is to meet the needs of the
   a. Office
   b. Employees
   c. Manager
   d. Patients

7. Requests for time off should
   a. Always be granted
   b. Be in writing
   c. Be received by a given date
   d. All of the above

8. All policies and procedures should be
   a. Signed annually
   b. Reviewed annually
   c. Written annually
   d. *a* and *b* only

9. A practice's mission statement can be
   a. Included in the policy and procedures manual
   b. Framed and placed in the waiting room
   c. Printed in patient instruction booklets
   d. All of the above

10. Developing and writing a budget is done with instructions from
    a. The manager only
    b. The financial officer
    c. The physician
    d. *b* and *c* only

Critical Thinking Practice

1. Dr. Abrams has asked you, the senior medical assistant, to assume the responsibility for staffing the office. What are the major issues to be considered? Identify one major focus for each issue.

_____

_____

_____

_____

2. Miss Young is a new medical assistant in the office. You have been asked to orient her to the operations of the clinic. One of the first items of discussion should be the organizational structure of the office. What will you explain to Miss Young when you describe the organizational structure?

_____

_____

_____

3. Mrs. Jones is the office manager for a six-physician group orthopedic practice. The budget for this practice is large and complex, as there are two clinic sites for the practice and a staff of 30 individuals. Discuss three financial concerns that the medical office manager must be capable of addressing to maintain control of the budget.

_____

_____

_____

_____

4. Legal issues are an area of responsibility of the medical office manager. Discuss four legal issues for the manager that involve employees and/or regulations governing the medical practice.

_____

_____

_____

_____

_____

13 Credit and Collections

CHAPTER COMPETENCIES

Review the information in your text that supports the following course objectives.

Learning Objectives

1. Spell and define the key terms
2. Explain the physician fee schedule
3. Discuss forms of payment
4. Explain the legal considerations in extending credit

5. Discuss the legal implications of credit collection
6. Describe three methods of debt collection

Performance Objectives

1. Use an aging schedule
2. Write a collection letter

CHAPTER OUTLINE	NOTES
Fees	
Fee Schedules	
Discussing Fees in Advance	
Forms of Payment	
Payment by Insurance Companies	
Adjusting Fees	
Credit	
Extending Credit	
Legal Considerations	
Collections	
Legal Considerations	
Collecting a Debt	
Monthly Billings	
Aging Accounts	
Collecting Overdue Accounts	
Collection Alternatives	

LEARNING SELF-ASSESSMENT EXERCISES

Key Terms

Define the following key terms:

adjustment _____

aging schedule _____

collections _____

credit _____

installment _____

participating provider _____

patient co-payment _____

professional courtesy _____

write-off _____

Matching

Match the definition in part 1 with the correct term in part 2.

PART I

_____ 1. List of unpaid accounts

_____ 2. Allowable unpaid balance on bill

_____ 3. Cancellation of an unpaid debt

_____ 4. Health care professionals are charged a
           reduced rate

_____ 5. Changes in a posted account

_____ 6. Acquiring funds that are due

PART 2

a. Professional courtesy

b. Aging schedule

c. Write-off

d. Sliding scale fees

e. Adjustments

f. Credit

Skill Drills

1. Describe three methods of debt collection.

_____

_____

_____

2. Identify three forms of payment for services.

_____

_____

_____

3. Identify five practices that a debt collector *may not* use to collect a debt from an individual.

_____

_____

_____

_____

Multiple Choice

1. Discussion of fees with a patient should be
   a. Done in advance
   b. Done by the physician
   c. In writing
   d. *a* and *c*

2. The fees for a patient new to the practice should be
   a. Reduced
   b. 50% of the usual fee
   c. Collected at the first visit
   d. 80% of the usual fee

3. The patient's insurance card should
   a. Never be copied
   b. Be put in the chart
   c. Be examined once a year
   d. Be copied and the copy put in the chart

4. Interest that may be charged to a patient account is determined by
   a. The physician
   b. The patient
   c. The insurance company
   d. The law

5. Monthly billing statements may be
   a. All sent at the same time
   b. Divided by alphabet
   c. Mailed at different times
   d. All of the above

6. If a billing cycle is to be changed, you are legally required to notify patients
   a. 3 months prior to the billing change
   b. 2 months prior to the billing change
   c. 1 month prior to the billing change
   d. None of the above

7. Aging of an account is calculated from the
   a. First office visit
   b. First date of billing
   c. Date the appointment is scheduled
   d. Procedure date

8. A practice's billing and collection procedures should be reviewed if the aging report shows what portion of fees are being collected 30 days or more after billing?
   a. 20%
   b. 23%
   c. 40%
   d. 50%

9. Fees paid to a medical practice may be paid for by
   a. A third party
   b. The patient
   c. An insurer
   d. Any of the above

10. When credit cards are accepted by a medical practice, the medical practice agrees to pay the credit card company
    a. 5.2%
    b. 1.8%
    c. 2.3%
    d. 3.1%

Critical Thinking Practice

1. Mrs. Smith is seeing Dr. Jones for the first time and has asked the medical assistant to explain Dr. Jones' fees. Explain to Mrs. Smith how Dr. Jones establishes the fees he charges his patients.

_____

_____

_____

_____

2. Explain the legal considerations in extending credit.

_____

_____

_____

_____

3. Describe the legal implications of credit collections.

_____

_____

_____

_____

_____

14

Bookkeeping and Banking

CHAPTER COMPETENCIES

Review the information in your text that supports the following course objectives.

Learning Objectives

1. Spell and define the key terms

2. Explain the concept of the pegboard bookkeeping system

3. Describe the components of the pegboard system

4. Identify and discuss the special features of the pegboard day sheet

5. Describe the functions of a computer accounting system

6. List the uses and components of computer accounting reports

7. Explain the services and procedures of the bank

Performance Objectives

1. Record financial transactions, such as charges, payments, credits, and adjustments to patient ledger cards

2. Balance a day sheet

3. Complete a bank deposit slip and make a deposit

4. Reconcile a bank statement

5. Write a check

6. Maintain a petty cash account

CHAPTER OUTLINE	NOTES
Daily Bookkeeping	
Manual Accounting	
Pegboard Bookkeeping System	
Day Sheet	
Ledger Cards	
Encounter Forms and Charge Slips	
Posting a Charge	
Posting a Payment	
Posting a Credit	
Posting a Credit Adjustment	
Posting a Debit Adjustment	
Posting to Cash-Paid-Out Section of Day Sheet	
Computer Accounting	
Posting to Computer Accounts	
Computer Accounting Reports	

CHAPTER OUTLINE *continued*

	NOTES
Banking	
Banks and Their Services	
Checking Accounts	
Savings Accounts	
Money Market Accounts	
Bank Fees	
Monthly Service Fees	
Overdraft Protection	
Returned Check Fee	
Types of Checks	
Writing Checks for Accounts Payable	
Receiving Checks and Making Deposits	
Reconciling Bank Statements	
Petty Cash	

LEARNING SELF-ASSESSMENT EXERCISES

Key Terms

Define the following key terms:

accounts payable _____

accounts receivable _____

adjustment _____

balance _____

bookkeeping _____

charge slip _____

credit _____

day sheet _____

debit _____

encounter form _____

ledger card _____

posting _____

returned check fee _____

service charge _____

Matching

Match the definition in part 1 with the correct term in part 2.

PART 1

_____ 1. A book of accounts

_____ 2. Money owed *to* the practice

_____ 3. Money owed *by* the practice

_____ 4. Charge

_____ 5. Payment

_____ 6. Be equal

_____ 7. Indicates name and account number on back of check

_____ 8. Fee charged monthly for using bank account

PART 2

a. Service charge

b. Accounts payable

c. Ledger

d. Credit

e. Accounts receivable

f. Debit

g. Endorse

h. Balance

Skill Drills

1. Describe four major components of the pegboard system.

_____

_____

_____

_____

2. Identify the five special features of a pegboard day sheet.

_____

_____

_____

_____

_____

3. Describe the steps to be taken when balancing a day sheet.

_____

_____

_____

_____

4. List the three primary steps in reconciling a monthly bank statement.

_____

_____

_____

Multiple Choice

1. In a bookkeeping system, things of value relating to the practice are called
   a. Liabilities
   b. Assets
   c. Debits
   d. Credits

2. The amount of capital the physician has invested in the practice is referred to as
   a. Equity
   b. Credits
   c. Assets
   d. Liabilities

3. If an error is made when posting a charge, you
   a. May erase carefully
   b. Write the word "error" in red
   c. Neatly white-out the error
   d. Draw a single line through the error, then rewrite the transaction

4. A ledger card is a legal document and should be kept for
   a. 10 years
   b. 7 years
   c. 5 years
   d. 1 year

5. Overpayments under $5 are
   a. Sent back to the patient
   b. Placed in petty cash
   c. Left on the account as a credit
   d. Deposited in a special overpayment account

6. Computer bookkeeping systems
   a. Operate as expanded calculators
   b. Are faster than pegboards
   c. Easily generate a variety of reports
   d. All of the above

7. An impress account refers to
   a. Petty cash
   b. A special bank account
   c. Computerized software
   d. Insurance funds

8. Ledger cards are filed
   a. By patient number
   b. Under the physician's name
   c. By time order
   d. Alphabetically

9. In bookkeeping, when brackets are used around a number it means
   a. The same as
   b. The opposite of
   c. An error
   d. A deletion

10. Most facilities request that medical offices write off the balance of an account once it is sent to a collection agency, so that
    a. Books always balance
    b. It complies with tax law on accounts receivable
    c. There is better control
    d. None of the above

Critical Thinking Practice

1. Compare and contrast pegboard and computer bookkeeping systems.

_____

_____

_____

_____

2. Explain the concept of the pegboard bookkeeping system.

_____

_____

_____

_____

_____

15

Accounts Payable and Payroll

CHAPTER COMPETENCIES

Review the information in your text that supports the following course objectives.

LEARNING OBJECTIVES

1. Spell and define the key terms

2. Describe the accounting cycle

3. Describe the components of a record-keeping system

4. Explain the process of ordering supplies and paying invoices

5. Discuss the types of payroll records

6. Explain which taxes are withheld from paychecks

Performance Objectives

1. Issue a payroll check, using the pegboard system

2. Calculate the amount of an employee's payroll check for a given pay period

CHAPTER OUTLINE	NOTES
Accounting Cycle	
Record-Keeping Components	
Accounts Payable	
Ordering Goods and Services	
Receiving Supplies	
Paying Invoices	
Manual Payment	
Pegboard Payment	
Computer Payment	
Payroll	
Types of Payroll Systems	
Manual Payroll Systems	
Pegboard Payroll Systems	
Computer Payroll Systems	
Employee Records	
Tax Withholdings	
Payment of Taxes	
W-2 Forms	
Preparation of Reports	
Assisting With Audits	

LEARNING SELF-ASSESSMENT EXERCISES

Key Terms

Define the following key terms:

accounting cycle _____

audit _____

check register _____

check stub _____

FICA _____

federal unemployment tax _____

gross income _____

Internal Revenue Service (IRS) _____

invoice _____

liabilities _____

net pay _____

packing slip _____

payroll _____

payroll journal _____

profit-and-loss statement _____

purchase order _____

summation report _____

withholding _____

Matching

Match the definition in part 1 with the correct term in part 2.

PART 1

_____ 1. Reviews of accounts

_____ 2. Back page of each check register

_____ 3. Amount of money earned before taxes

_____ 4. Pay to employees and taxes

_____ 5. Amount of money earned after taxes

_____ 6. Employer pays this for each employee based on the employee's gross income.

_____ 7. Federal and state taxes removed from employee's paycheck

PART 2

a. Payroll journal

b. Unemployment tax

c. Audit

d. Gross income

e. Net pay

f. Tax withholding

g. Payroll

Skill Drills

1. Describe the two types of accounting cycles.

_____

_____

_____

2. List the four components that should be included in a practice's financial records.

_____

_____

_____

_____

3. Describe the five types of information that should be recorded on a check stub.

_____

_____

_____

_____

_____

4. Computer accounts payable have all of the advantages that a pegboard system offers. List five advantages.

_____

_____

_____

_____

_____

Multiple Choice

1. The Internal Revenue Service examines a business's income statements for the amount of profit and the resulting owed fees
   a. Once per year
   b. Twice per year
   c. Four times per year
   d. None of the above

2. Records such as receipts should be retained for
   a. 5 years
   b. 7 years
   c. 10 years
   d. 2 years

3. It is preferable to pay for supplies by
   a. Check
   b. Cash
   c. Credit card
   d. *a* and *c*

4. A purchase order lists
   a. Supplies ordered
   b. Supply order numbers
   c. Previous purchases
   d. *a* and *b*

5. Bills can be paid
   a. Daily
   b. Weekly
   c. Biweekly
   d. All of the above

6. Corrections on facility checks
   a. May never be done
   b. May be carefully erased
   c. May be crossed out
   d. May be done carefully using Wite-Out

7. Computerized financial data should be recorded
   a. On the hard drive
   b. On a floppy disk
   c. On hard copy
   d. All of the above

8. Biweekly payroll checks are issued
   a. 52 times per year
   b. 26 times per year
   c. 12 times per year
   d. 24 times per year

9. The federally mandated taxes are
   a. Social Security
   b. Medicare
   c. Federal income tax
   d. All of the above

10. The compilation of a business's financial records is called
    a. Bookkeeping
    b. Accounting
    c. Ledger management
    d. Database tracking

Critical Thinking Practice

1. You are a newly hired administrative assistant responsible for ordering supplies. Explain all of the things you will need to consider to make sure you are getting quality supplies at a reasonable cost.

_____

_____

_____

_____

2. A large order of supplies has been delivered to your office. How can you be sure that you have received all of the items that were ordered?

_____

_____

_____

_____

3. Compare and contrast the manual payroll system with the pegboard payroll system.

_____

_____

_____

_____

16

Health Insurance

CHAPTER COMPETENCIES

Review the information in your text that supports the following course objectives.

Learning Objectives

1. Spell and define the key terms
2. Describe group, individual, and government-sponsored (public) health benefits and explain the differences between them
3. Explain the differences between Medicare and Medicaid
4. List the information required on a medical claim form and explain why each piece of information is needed
5. Name two legal issues affecting claims submissions
6. Explain how managed care programs work
7. Explain the differences between health maintenance organizations, preferred provider organizations, and physician hospital organizations

Performance Objective

1. Fill out a CMS-1500 claim form

CHAPTER OUTLINE	NOTES
Health Benefits Plans	
Group Health Benefits	
Individual Health Benefits	
Government-Sponsored (Public) Health Benefits	
Medicare	
Medicaid	
TRICARE/CHAMPVA	
Managed Care	
Health Maintenance Organizations	
Preferred Provider Organizations	
Physician Hospital Organizations	
Other Managed Care Programs	
The Future of Managed Care	
Workers' Compensation	
Filing Claims	
Electronic Claims Submission	
Explanation of Benefits	
Policies in the Practice	

LEARNING SELF-ASSESSMENT EXERCISES

Key Terms

Define the following key terms:

assignment of benefits _____

balance billing _____

birthday rule _____

capitation _____

carrier _____

claims _____

claims administrator _____

coinsurance _____

coordination of benefits _____

co-payments _____

crossover claim _____

deductible _____

dependent _____

eligibility _____

employee _____

explanation of benefits (EOB) _____

fee-for-service _____

fee schedule _____

group member _____

health maintenance organization (HMO) _____

independent practice association (IPA) _____

insurance _____

insured _____

managed care _____

Medicare _____

peer review organization _____

physician hospital organization _____

plan maximum _____

preexisting condition _____

preferred provider organization (PPO) _____

third-party administrator _____

unbundling _____

usual, customary, and reasonable (UCR) _____

utilization review _____

Matching

Match the definition in part 1 with the correct term in part 2.

PART 1

_____ 1. Provide medical care for the elderly

_____ 2. Medical program for uniformed services

_____ 3. Government-sponsored program providing health care to low-income individuals

_____ 4. Covers medical expenses for work-related injury or illness

_____ 5. Program administered by the area Veterans Administration

_____ 6. Kaiser Permanente Health Plan

_____ 7. Nongroup physicians organized into entities

PART 2

a. Workers' compensation

b. IPA

c. Medicare

d. HMO

e. CHAMPUS

f. CHAMPVA

g. Medicaid

Skill Drills

1. Explain the differences between Medicare and Medicaid.

_____
_____
_____
_____
_____
_____
_____

2. List 10 of the 33 items of information required on a medical claim form and explain why each piece of information is needed.

_____
_____
_____
_____
_____
_____
_____
_____
_____
_____
_____

3. Name two legal issues affecting claims submission.

_____
_____

4. List the six areas of health care covered by Medicaid.

_____

_____

_____

_____

_____

_____

Multiple Choice

1. Medicaid patients receive a new ID card
   a. Once every 3 months
   b. Once a month
   c. Once a year
   d. Once every 6 weeks

2. Health benefits are commonly referred to as
   a. Insurance
   b. Plans
   c. Insured
   d. Assets

3. Medicare provides benefits for all of the following individuals *except*
   a. Persons with end-stage renal disease
   b. Elderly persons age 65 or older
   c. All injured persons
   d. Disabled persons who have been receiving Social Security benefits for 24 months

4. Persons who are entitled to Social Security
   a. Are automatically enrolled in Medicare Part A
   b. Are automatically enrolled in Medicare Part B
   c. Are automatically enrolled in Medicare Parts A and B
   d. Are not automatically enrolled in Medicare

5. After the deductible has been met, what percentage of the approved charges does Medicare reimburse to the physician?
   a. 70
   b. 80
   c. 90
   d. 20

6. Medicare will accept original claims (no copies) filed on a
   a. CMS-1500
   b. CMA 1500
   c. CSM 1500
   d. HPCA 1500

7. When a patient gives written authorization for an insurance plan to reimburse the physician for billed charges, the patient has
   a. Relinquished benefits
   b. Determined benefits
   c. Assigned benefits
   d. The money sent to himself or herself, not the physician

8. Claims that are submitted electronically
   a. Are more accurate than others
   b. Are not rejected
   c. Cannot be corrected online
   d. Reduce the reimbursement cycle

9. Managed care programs often have a gatekeeper provision. A gatekeeper is
   a. A primary care physician
   b. A specialty physician
   c. A referring physician
   d. Any of the above

10. Balance billing is
    a. Illegal
    b. Practiced by HMOs
    c. Prohibited by managed care
    d. Practiced by IPS HMOs

Critical Thinking Practice

1. Explain how managed care programs work.

_____

_____

_____

_____

2. Describe group, individual, and government-sponsored (public) health benefits and explain the differences between each.

_____

_____

_____

_____

3. Explain the differences between HMOs, PPOs, and physician hospital organizations.

_____

_____

_____

_____

4. A patient may be covered by more than one health plan, such as by an employer while being a dependent on a spouse's plan. With regard to this situation, identify the primary plan and explain coordination of benefits.

_____

_____

_____

_____

Patient Education

1. Mrs. Smith is moving out of the area and is seeing Dr. Jones, her private practice physician, for the last time. After the move, Mrs. Smith will have to choose a new physician. Mrs. Smith has the choice of a HMO or a PPO. Mrs. Smith approaches Dr. Jones' medical assistant and asks her to explain the difference. How can you teach Mrs. Smith about the differences between a HMO and a PPO?

_____

_____

_____

_____

_____

17

Diagnostic Coding

CHAPTER COMPETENCIES

Review the information in your text that supports the following course objectives.

Learning Objectives

1. Spell and define the key terms

2. Name and describe the coding system used to describe diseases, injuries, and other reasons for encounters with a medical provider

3. Give four examples of how diagnostic coding is used

4. Describe the relationship between coding and reimbursement

5. Explain the format of the ICD-9-CM

6. List the steps in identifying a proper code

7. Name common errors in outpatient diagnostic coding

CHAPTER OUTLINE

	NOTES
Diagnostic Coding	
Inpatient Versus Outpatient Coding	
ICD-9-CM: The Code Book	
Volume 1: Tabular List of Diseases	
Supplementary Classifications	
Volume 2: Alphabetic Index to Diseases	
Volume 3: Inpatient Coding	
Locating the Appropriate Code	
Using ICD-9-CM Conventions	
Main Term	
Fourth and Fifth Digits	
Primary Codes	
When More Than One Code Is Used	
Late Effects	
Coding Suspected Conditions	
Documentation Requirements	
The Future of Diagnostic Coding: *International Classification of Diseases, Tenth Revision*	

LEARNING SELF-ASSESSMENT EXERCISES

Key Terms

Define the following key terms:

advance beneficiary notice _____

audits _____

conventions _____

cross-reference _____

E-codes _____

eponym _____

etiology _____

inpatient _____

International Classification of Diseases, Ninth Revision, Clinical Modification _____

late effects _____

main terms _____

medical necessity _____

outpatient _____

primary diagnosis _____

service _____

specificity _____

V-codes _____

Matching

Match the definition in part 1 with the correct term in part 2.

PART 1

_____ 1. The assignment of a number to a verbal state-
         ment or description

_____ 2. Used to report services and procedures

_____ 3. Ensures payment of treatments and proce-
         dures likely to be denied by Medicare

_____ 4. Alphabetic Index to Diseases

_____ 5. Include general notes using specific terms,
         cross-references, abbreviations, punctuation
         marks, symbols, typeface, and format

PART 2

a. Volume 2

b. Conventions

c. ABN

d. Coding

e. CPT

Skill Drills

1. List five reasons medical information is standardized by coding systems.

_____

_____

_____

_____

_____

2. Summarize the CMS Diagnostic Coding Guidelines.

_____

_____

_____

_____

3. Compare and contrast inpatient and outpatient coding.

_____

_____

_____

_____

4. Discuss the purpose of the CMS-1500 and state the other name for this form.

_____

_____

_____

_____

Multiple Choice

1. Which organization developed the ICD-9-CM statistical classification system?
   a. WHO
   b. CDC
   c. OSHA
   d. NCHS

2. Where can you purchase updates and addenda for ICD-9-CM coding books?
   a. AMA
   b. Local medical society
   c. Coding book publisher
   d. CMS

3. How many sections does the alphabetic index of the ICD-9-CM have?
   a. Six
   b. Three
   c. Four
   d. Ten

4. What is used to justify physician services, whether those services are provided in the hospital or the office?
   a. Volume 1
   b. Volume 2
   c. Volume 3
   d. Volumes 1 and 2

5. The daily visits the physician makes to the inpatient are billed and coded by
   a. The hospital
   b. The physician's office
   c. Medicare
   d. CMS

6. To become an expert coder you need general knowledge in all the following areas *except*
   a. Anatomy and physiology
   b. Medical terminology
   c. Pharmacology
   d. Using the code books

7. E-codes, which range from E800 to E999, are used to classify external causes of
   a. Injuries
   b. Diseases
   c. Poisonings
   d. *a* and *c* only

8. What is used to code live-born infants according to type of birth?
   a. E-codes
   b. B-codes
   c. V-codes
   d. E/M-codes

9. Which is organized by main terms printed in boldface type?
   a. Volume 1, section 2
   b. Volume 3, section 3
   c. Volume 2, section 1
   d. Volume 1, section 2

10. The patient's chief complaint or the reason the patient sought medical attention is
    a. The preliminary diagnosis
    b. The working diagnosis
    c. Listed last on the CMS-1500
    d. The primary diagnosis

Critical Thinking Practice

1. At a medical office staff meeting, you are asked to explain the relationship between coding and reimbursement. What can you tell this group?

_____

_____

_____

_____

2. What event in a medical office could trigger a chart audit? Discuss how this could be avoided.

_____

_____

_____

_____

3. List three key points to the future of diagnostic coding.

_____

_____

_____

_____

18

Outpatient Procedural Coding

CHAPTER COMPETENCIES

Review the information in your text that supports the following course objectives.

Learning Objectives

1. Spell and define the key terms

2. Explain the format of Current Procedural Terminology (CPT-4) and its use

3. Explain the Healthcare Common Procedure Coding System (HCPCS) and level 2 and 3 codes

4. Explain what diagnostic related groups (DRGs) are and how they are used to determine Medicare payments

5. Discuss the goals of resource-based relative value system (RBRVS)

6. Describe the relationship between coding and reimbursement

CHAPTER OUTLINE

CHAPTER OUTLINE	NOTES
Physician's Current Procedural Terminology	
Reading Descriptors	
Guidelines	
Unlisted Procedures and Special Reports	
Evaluation and Management Codes	
Anesthesia Codes	
Surgery Codes	
Unstarred Codes	
Starred Codes	
Integumentary System	
Repairs	
Cast Reapplication	
Multiple Procedures Furnished on the Same Day	
Radiology Codes	
Pathology and Laboratory Codes	
Medicine Codes	
CPT-4 Modifiers	

CHAPTER OUTLINE *continued*	NOTES
Healthcare Common Procedure Coding System	
HCPCS Level 1 Codes	
HCPCS Level 2 Codes: National Codes	
HCPCS Level 3 Codes: Local Codes	
Reimbursement	
Diagnostic Related Groups	
Resource-Based Relative Value Scale	
Fraud and Coding	

LEARNING SELF-ASSESSMENT EXERCISES

Key Terms

Define the following key terms:

Current Procedural Terminology _____

descriptor _____

diagnostic related group _____

Healthcare Common Procedure Coding System _____

key component _____

modifiers _____

outlier _____

procedure _____

resource-based relative value scale _____

upcoding _____

Matching

Match the definition in part 1 with the correct term in part 2.

PART 1

_____ 1. Congress decided to use CPT-4 to code all physicians' procedures and services for Medicare patients

_____ 2. CPT-4 is divided into this many major sections

_____ 3. A copy of the procedure must be submitted with the claim when the code is this

_____ 4. Five-digit numbers that begin with 9

_____ 5. Classifications of histories and physical examinations

PART 2

a. Unlisted

b. Six

c. 1980

d. Four

e. E/M

Skill Drills

1. State the importance of key components in CPT coding.

_____

_____

_____

_____

2. What must the physician do to qualify for a decision-making level for an established patient? For a new patient?

_____

_____

_____

_____

3. State the two types of modifiers.

_____

_____

4. State the significance of the asterisk (*) in surgical codes.

_____

_____

_____

_____

5. Why do you have to pay special attention when coding automated multichannel tests?

_____

_____

_____

_____

Multiple Choice

1. What organization established CPT coding?
   a. American Heart Association
   b. American Physicians Association
   c. American Association of Medical Assistants
   d. American Medical Association

2. CPT-4 coding allows insurance companies to do all of the following *except*
   a. Communicate easily with one another
   b. Speed claims processing
   c. Specify what the physician will be paid
   d. Compare reimbursement amounts

3. What five-digit numbers begin with 9?
   a. E/M codes
   b. Pathology and laboratory codes
   c. Surgery codes
   d. All CPT codes

4. Which of the following is not a classification of histories and physicals?
   a. Problem focused
   b. Counseling
   c. Expanded problem focused
   d. Detailed

5. What do codes that begin with 0 designate?
   a. Anesthesia
   b. Emergency
   c. Radiology
   d. Surgery

6. What do codes that begin with 8 designate?
   a. Pathology and laboratory
   b. Radiology
   c. Emergency
   d. Medicines

7. Cardiac diagnostic testing is covered under which section of the CPT codes?
   a. E/M codes
   b. Medicine codes
   c. History and physicals
   d. Surgery

8. A list of all CPT modifiers is found in
   a. Appendix B
   b. Appendix E
   c. Appendix C
   d. Appendix A

9. HCPCS is the acronym for
   a. Health Care Plans Control Services
   b. Health Care Physicians Centralized Services
   c. Health Care Procedure Control Systems
   d. Healthcare Common Procedure Coding System

10. Categories into which inpatients are placed according to similarity of their diagnoses, treatment, and length of hospital stay are
    a. Diagnostic related groups
    b. Diagnostic rules governing hospital stays
    c. Diagnostic procedures and treatment plans
    d. Diagnostic plans and follow-up of hospital admissions

Critical Thinking Practice

1. You are a medical assistant working in a family practice. The medical assistant who usually does the coding is on maternity leave. You have been assigned to take that position for 6 months. After 2 months you realize that many Medicare claims have been overcoded. What do you do? What might happen to this physician if this continues to occur?

_____

_____

_____

_____

2. How often does the CPT code book have to be replaced? What are the possible consequences if it is not replaced as indicated?

_____

_____

_____

_____

19

Medical Asepsis and Infection Control

CHAPTER COMPETENCIES

Review the information in your text that supports the following course objectives.

Learning Objectives

Upon successfully completing this chapter, you will be able to:

1. Spell and define key terms.

2. Describe conditions that promote the growth of microorganisms.

3. Explain the components of the infectious process cycle.

4. List the various ways microbes are transmitted.

5. Compare the effectiveness in reducing or destroying microorganisms using the four levels of infection control.

6. Describe the procedures for cleaning, handling, and disposing of biohazardous waste in the medical office.

7. Explain the concept of medical asepsis.

8. Discuss risk management procedures required by the Occupational Safety and Health Administration guidelines for the medical office.

9. List the required components of an exposure control plan.

10. Explain the importance of following Standard Precautions in the medical office.

11. Identify various personal protective equipment (PPE) items.

12. Describe circumstances when PPE items would be appropriately worn by the medical assistant.

13. Explain the facts pertaining to the transmission and prevention of the Hepatitis B virus and the Human Immunodeficiency Virus in the medical office.

14. Describe how to avoid becoming infected with the Hepatitis B and Human Immunodeficiency viruses.

Performance Objectives

Upon successfully completing this chapter, you will be able to:

1. Perform a medical aseptic handwashing procedure (Procedure 19-1).

2. Remove and discard contaminated personal protective equipment appropriately (Procedure 19-2).

3. Clean and decontaminate biohazardous spills (Procedure 19-3).

CHAPTER OUTLINE	NOTES
Microorganisms, Pathogens, and Normal Flora	
Conditions That Favor the Growth of Pathogens	
The Infection Cycle	
Modes of Transmission	
Principles of Infection Control	
Medical Asepsis	

CHAPTER OUTLINE   *continued*

	NOTES
Levels of Infection Control	
Sanitation	
Disinfection	
Occupational Safety and Health Administration Guidelines for the Medical Office	
Exposure Risk Factors and the Exposure Control Plan	
Standard Precautions	
Personal Protective Equipment	
Handling Environmental Contamination	
Disposing of Infectious Waste	
Hepatitis B and Human Immunodeficiency Viruses	

LEARNING SELF-ASSESSMENT EXERCISES

Key Terms

Define the following key terms:

aerobe _____

anaerobe _____

asymptomatic _____

bactericidal _____

biohazard _____

carrier _____

disease _____

disinfection _____

exposure control plan _____

exposure risk factors _____

germicide _____

immunization _____

infection _____

medical asepsis _____

microorganisms _____

normal flora _____

OSHA _____

pathogens _____

personal protective equipment _____

postexposure testing _____

resident flora _____

resistance _____

spore _____

sanitation _____

sanitization _____

standard precautions _____

sterilization _____

transient flora _____

vector _____

viable _____

virulent _____

Matching

Match the term in Part 1 with the correct definition in Part 2.

PART 1

_____ 1. Asymptomatic

_____ 2. Carrier

_____ 3. Medical asepsis

_____ 4. Microorganisms

_____ 5. OSHA

_____ 6. Use of topics to file

_____ 7. Pathogens

PART 2

a. Subject filing

b. Without any symptoms

c. A person infected with a microorganism

d. Microscopic living organisms

e. Removal or destruction of microorganisms

f. Occupational Safety and Health Administration

g. Disease-causing microorganisms

Skill Drills

1. List six of the body's natural defense systems.

   a. _____

   b. _____

   c. _____

   d. _____

   e. _____

   f. _____

2. List six conditions that microorganisms require for growth and reproduction.

   a. _____

   b. _____

   c. _____

   d. _____

   e. _____

   f. _____

3. Identify the five links in the chain of the infection cycle.

   a. _____

   b. _____

   c. _____

   d. _____

   e. _____

Multiple Choice

1. What is the cornerstone of infection control?
   a. Understanding and practicing medical asepsis
   b. Educating patients about the transmission of disease
   c. Handwashing
   d. Following policies of the medical facility where you work

2. Disease-producing microorganisms are referred to as pathogens and are classified into groups. Which of the following is not a group of pathogens?
   a. Bacteria or viruses
   b. Fungi
   c. Leukocytes
   d. Protozoa

3. Decreased resistance in a host is one condition that may allow transient flora to become pathogenic. Which of the following is least likely to be a factor in lowering a person's resistance to disease?
   a. Age (particularly the elderly)
   b. Chemotherapy (anticancer drugs)
   c. Experiencing an unusual amount of stress
   d. Low serum potassium and high serum sodium

4. One link in the infection cycle is the mode of transmission. Which of the following are examples of direct transmission?
   a. Inhaling infected droplets (from another person's cough or sneeze)
   b. Intimate contact with an infected person
   c. Sharing eating utensils
   d. *a* and *b*

5. Indirect transmission is another mode of spreading disease. Which of the following is not an example of indirect contact?
   a. Sharing eating or drinking utensils
   b. Disease-carrying insects
   c. Kissing an infected person
   d. Contact with a contaminated but inanimate object

6. This chapter gives a statistic about how many infectious carriers a medical assistant may work with in a clinical setting. What is that statistic?
   a. One infectious carrier for every 10 known infected patients
   b. Five infectious carriers for every 10 known infected patients
   c. Five infectious carriers for every one known infected patient
   d. Two infectious carriers for every two known infected patients

7. Handwashing is one element of medical asepsis. Read the following list, and identify when you need to wash your hands.
   a. Before and after every patient contact
   b. Before and after putting on examination gloves
   c. Before and after every work break
   d. All of the above

8. Which of the following is the highest level of infection control?
   a. Sanitation
   b. Sterilization
   c. Disinfection
   d. Chemical immersion

9. Which of the following is not a category of disinfection?
   a. Ultramaximum
   b. Low
   c. High
   d. Intermediate

10. Intermediate-level disinfection kills all but one of the following. Identify the exception.
    a. Spores
    b. Viruses
    c. Fungi
    d. *Mycobacterium tuberculosis*

Critical Thinking Practice

1. A middle-aged man comes into the clinic with symptoms of low-grade fever and a productive cough that has lasted several weeks. The doctor orders a chest x-ray to aid in diagnosis. After the patient goes to the radiology department, you clean the room for the next patient. What level of disinfection will you use? What common household chemical will serve the purpose? If you have the chemical, but it is not diluted, how much water would you add to 1/2 cup of the chemical?

_____

_____

_____

_____

_____

2. Every medical facility must have a written exposure control plan to help avoid coming into contact with biohazardous materials and to teach employees what to do in the event an exposure occurs. What equipment or medical preparation will you implement to protect yourself in the clinical setting?

_____

_____

_____

_____

_____

Patient Education

1. One of your patients expresses concern about what happens to contaminated needles and other supplies that are generated in your clinic. What can you tell the patient about infectious waste disposal? (Summarize to 2-3 short paragraphs.)

_____

_____

_____

_____

_____

_____

_____

_____

_____

_____

20

Medical History and Patient Assessment

CHAPTER COMPETENCIES

Review the information in your text that supports the following course objectives:

Learning Objectives

Upon successfully completing this chapter, you will be able to:

1. Spell and define key terms.

2. Give examples of the type of information included in each section of the medical history.

3. Identify guidelines for conducting a patient interview.

4. Explain the difference between a sign and symptom and give examples of each.

5. Compare the chief complaint and present illness.

6. Discuss open-ended and closed-ended questions and explain when to use each type during the patient interview.

Performance Objectives

Upon successfully completing this chapter, you will be able to:

1. Interview a patient using appropriate communication techniques (Procedures 20-1 and 20-2).

2. Correctly complete the various sections of the medical history form (Procedure 20-1).

3. Accurately document a chief complaint and present illness (Procedure 20-2).

CHAPTER OUTLINE	NOTES
The Medical History	
Methods of Collecting Information	
Elements of the Medical History	
Conducting the Patient Interview	
Preparing for the Interview	
Introducing Yourself	
Barriers to Communication	
Assessing the Patient	
Signs and Symptoms	
Chief Complaint and Present Illness	

LEARNING SELF-ASSESSMENT EXERCISES

Key Terms

Define the following key terms:

assessment _____

chief complaint _____

demographic _____

familial disorder _____

hereditary traits _____

HIPAA _____

homeopathic medicine _____

medical history _____

over-the-counter _____

signs _____

symptoms _____

Matching

Match the term in Part 1 with the correct definition in Part 2.

PART 1

_____ 1. Social history

_____ 2. Past history

_____ 3. Family history

_____ 4. Demographics

_____ 5. Chief complaint

_____ 6. "I feel chilled"

PART 2

a. Home address

b. Immunizations

c. Father's cause of death

d. Married

e. Symptom

f. Sore throat

Skill Drills

1. Name and describe six interviewing techniques that help you obtain accurate and pertinent information from the patient.

_____

_____

_____

_____

_____

_____

2. List three ways you can safeguard the patient's confidentiality when you conduct your interview.

_____

_____

_____

3. What six questions could you ask to obtain information about the present illness (PI)?

_____

_____

_____

_____

_____

_____

Multiple Choice

1. You notice that a 4-year-old boy has several bruises on his arms. Where will this be noted in the medical record?
   a. It should be noted so that the doctor will see it.
   b. It should be noted under the present illness.
   c. The medical assistant should speak with the doctor about it.
   d. All of the above

2. Which of the following is not part of the patient's medical history?
   a. Present history
   b. Insurance data
   c. Family history
   d. Social history

3. Childhood illnesses, hospital stays, surgeries, and diagnostic tests are all included in which portion of the medical history?
   a. Chief complaint
   b. Present illness
   c. Review of systems
   d. Past history

4. The medical assistant is responsible for
   a. helping to obtain information for the medical history and assessment.
   b. working cooperatively with the physician to complete the patient medical history.
   c. protecting the patient's privacy during the interview.
   d. All the above

5. Which of the following statements is NOT an open-ended question?
   a. Can you describe the pain?
   b. What did you do to try and relieve the pain?
   c. Does it hurt?
   d. What activities were you involved in when the pain started?

6. Examples of observations about a patient's medical status may include
   a. pale or flushed skin.
   b. personal hygiene.
   c. visual or hearing deficit.
   d. All the above

7. What are appropriate statements to make when you begin a patient interview?
   a. "Good day, Mr. Brown. My name is Paula, and I'm Dr. White's nurse."
   b. "Hello Mr. Green. My name is Paula and I'm a medical assistant. I work with Dr. White."
   c. "I would like to ask you a few questions that will help Dr. White diagnose and treat you appropriately."
   d. only *b* and *c*

8. It is important to review the medical history form before interviewing the patient. Which of the following is not relevant to this type of review?
   a. Spelling errors must be corrected before the interview.
   b. Being familiar with the form will help you be more efficient.
   c. Asking questions out of order disrupts flow of the interview.
   d. Shuffling papers while talking is a distraction.

9. Avoid making judgments about observations when charting because
   a. terminology such as "depressed" or "abused" may be diagnostic.
   b. judgments may be out of the medical assistant scope of practice.
   c. most doctors do not want a medical assistant to do chart documentation.
   d. only *a* and *b*

10. Many factors lead to communication barriers. Which of the following is least likely to contribute to a communication barrier?
    a. Patient unfamiliarity with the English language
    b. Hearing or speech impairment
    c. Cognitive impairment
    d. Visual impairment

11. An example of a closed-ended question would be
    a. What is the reason for your visit?
    b. Did you sleep last night?
    c. Can you describe the pain for me?
    d. Please describe the symptoms you have after eating.

12. Chief complaint (CC) is one statement that describes the signs and symptoms that led the patient to seek medical care and is documented at each visit. Which of the following would not be a CC?
    a. Stumbled and hurt knee yesterday after tripping on a shoelace
    b. Plugged ear since swimming last weekend
    c. Nauseous since eating clam chowder last evening
    d. Several small bruises on lower legs

Critical Thinking Practice

1. Indicate which of the following terms represent a sign or a symptom.

   Flushed -
   Dizzy -
   Unsteady -
   Nauseous -
   Vomiting -
   Hunched -
   Dark urine -
   Burning -
   Ringing in ears -
   Squinting -

2. Review the following and indicate the section of the medical history in which the information should be included and explain why.

   Divorced–
   Patient had a breast reduction in 1985–
   Mother died of influenza at age 70–
   Allergic to tetracycline and morphine–
   Has two children living and in good health–
   Patient is a retired accountant–
   Sister has hypertension and thyroid disease, age 55–

Patient Education

1. While interviewing a patient about his or her chief complaint, you may have an opportunity to teach the patient about various topics. If the patient is a current smoker, what information might you share?

   _____

   _____

   _____

   _____

21

Anthropometric Measurements and Vital Signs

CHAPTER COMPETENCIES

Review the information in your text that supports the following course objectives.

Learning Objectives

Upon successfully completing this chapter, you will be able to:

1. Spell and define key terms.

2. Explain the procedures for measuring a patient's height and weight.

3. Identify and describe the types of thermometers.

4. Compare the procedures for measuring a patient's temperature using the oral, rectal, axillary, and tympanic methods.

5. List the fever process, including the stages of fever.

6. Describe the procedure for measuring a patient's pulse and respiratory rates.

7. Identify the various sites on the body used for palpating a pulse.

8. Define Korotkoff sounds and the five phases of blood pressure.

9. Identify factors that may influence the blood pressure.

10. Explain the factors to consider when choosing the correct blood pressure cuff size.

Performance Objectives

Upon successfully completing this chapter, you will be able to:

1. Measure and record a patient's weight (Procedure 21-1).

2. Measure and record a patient's height (Procedure 21-2).

3. Measure and record a patient's oral temperature using a glass mercury thermometer (Procedure 21-3).

4. Measure and record a patient's rectal temperature using a glass mercury thermometer (Procedure 21-4).

5. Measure and record a patient's axillary temperature using a glass mercury thermometer (Procedure 21-5).

6. Measure and record a patient's temperature using an electronic thermometer (Procedure 21-6).

7. Measure and record a patient's temperature using a tympanic thermometer (Procedure 21-7).

8. Measure and record a patient's radial pulse (Procedure 21-8).

9. Measure and record a patient's respirations (Procedure 21-9).

10. Measure and record a patient's blood pressure (Procedure 21-10).

CHAPTER OUTLINE	NOTES
Anthropometric Measurements	
Weight	
Height	

CHAPTER OUTLINE *continued*	NOTES
Vital Signs	
Temperature	
Pulse	
Respiration	
Blood Pressure	

LEARNING SELF-ASSESSMENT EXERCISES

Key Terms

Define the following key terms:

afebrile _____

aneroid _____

anthropometric _____

baseline _____

calibrated _____

cardiac cycle _____

cardinal signs _____

diastole _____

diaphoresis _____

febrile _____

hyperpyrexia _____

hypertension _____

intermittent _____

palpation _____

postural hypotension _____

pyrexia _____

relapsing fever _____

remittent fever _____

sphygmomanometer _____

sustained fever _____

systole _____

tympanic thermometer _____

Matching

Match the term in Part 1 with the correct definition in Part 2.

PART 1

_____ 1. Diastole

_____ 2. Intermittent

_____ 3. Sustained

_____ 4. Diaphoresis

PART 2

a. Describes a fever that is constant or not fluctuating

b. Profuse sweating

c. The relaxation phase of the cardiac cycle

d. A fever that occurs at intervals

_____ 5. Systole   e. The contraction phase of the cardiac cycle

_____ 6. Anthropometric   f. Pertaining to measurements of the human body

Skill Drills

1. List five types of thermometers.

   a. _____   _____

   b. _____

   c. _____

   d. _____

   e. _____

2. What are eight causes of errors in blood pressure readings?

   a. _____

   b. _____

   c. _____

   d. _____

   e. _____

   f. _____

   g. _____

   h. _____

Multiple Choice

1. Which of the following is not an example of why obtaining patient weights is important?
   a. Some patients are on medication prescribed according to weight.
   b. Some medications are prescribed for patients attempting to gain or lose weight.
   c. Some weight loss may be due to illness.
   d. It is a reality check showing that obese persons need to diet.

2. Which of the following is not true about tympanic temperature, when used accurately?
   a. Gives a reading comparable to PO
   b. Is also called an aural temperature
   c. Is positioned toward the tympanic membrane
   d. Gives a reading comparable to the axillary temperature

3. Fever process is explained by the following statements:
   a. Body temperature is regulated by the hypothalamus.
   b. When the hypothalamus senses the body is too warm, peripheral vasodilation is initiated.
   c. Core body heat is carried to the body surface via circulation, and perspiration increases to cool the body by evaporation.
   d. All of the above

4. Which of the following statements is not accurate?
   a. Fluctuations up or down in body temperature may be due to illness.
   b. Children have higher metabolisms than adults and tend to have higher temperatures than adults.
   c. Temperature of the very young and very old tends to be easily affected by environment.
   d. Exercise does not affect body temperature.

5. Heartbeat (pulse) can be felt at various points on the body where you can press an artery against a bone or other underlying firm surface. Which of the following is not a commonly used location:
   a. carotid, apical, brachial
   b. temporal
   c. popliteal, posttibial, dorsalis pedia
   d. radial, femoral

6. Pulse characteristics include
   a. rate—number of beats per minute.
   b. rhythm—time interval between beats.
   c. volume—strength of force against the heart-beat.
   d. All of the above

7. Volume, the strength or force of the heartbeat, may be described as all but one of the following. Identify the exception.
   a. Soft, bounding
   b. Irregular or regular
   c. Strong or full
   d. Weak, thready

8. Many factors affect the force, speed, and rhythm of the heart. Which of the following does not affect these three factors?
   a. Youth—young children and infants have a faster heart rate than adults
   b. Being an athlete (conditioned)
   c. Age—older adults; decreased myocardial efficiency
   d. Nationality and cultural influence

9. Respiration is controlled by the respiratory center of the brainstem and by feedback from thermosensors in the carotid arteries that monitor the CO_2 content in the blood. The physiology of respiration also includes
   a. inspiration (oxygen brought into lungs).
   b. expiration (expels CO_2).
   c. alveoli of the respiratory tract that absorb O_2.
   d. All of the above

10. The radial artery is most often used to determine pulse rates, and which of the following statements does not apply?
    a. If the pulse is irregular, the apical pulse is the site of choice.
    b. If the pulse is irregular, the doctor should assess the rate.
    c. An irregular rhythm should be counted for a full minute to determine the rate.
    d. A Doppler unit is an appropriate choice to auscultate a pulse.

11. After taking a patient's blood pressure, take the opportunity to educate the patient with high blood pressure. What would you never tell a patient in this situation?
    a. Encourage the patient to keep a log of daily blood pressure readings.
    b. Emphasize that the patient should never stop taking the blood pressure medication without the doctor's permission.
    c. Free-standing blood pressure machines in pharmacies and supermarkets are not always calibrated properly or calibrated on a regular basis. The readings may not be accurate.
    d. Tell the patient that a relative, a registered nurse, may adjust a dose or prescribe a new medication if the doctor is unavailable.

12. A blood pressure that drops suddenly when the patient stands from a sitting or lying position is referred to as **postural hypotension,** or **orthostatic hypotension.** Which symptom is not associated with this condition?
    a. Vertigo
    b. Some patients with postural hypotension may faint.
    c. This may occur as a patient moves from a position of lying down to sitting or standing.
    d. Sudden onset of nausea and vomiting

13. Indicate which of the following factors does not influence blood pressure.
    a. Age, activity
    b. Stress, body position
    c. Height
    d. Medications

Critical Thinking Practice

1. Ms. Green arrived at the office late for her appointment, frantic and explaining that her alarm clock had not gone off. She discovered that her car was almost out of gas, and she had to stop to refuel. Once she got to the clinic, she could not find a parking place in the parking lot and had to park a block down the street. How would you expect these events to affect her vital signs? Explain why.

_____

_____

_____

_____

2. What size cuff would you likely choose for Mrs. Daily, an elderly female patient who is 5 feet, 4 inches tall and weighs approximately 200 pounds? Why?

_____

_____

_____

_____

Patient Education

1. Ms. White, mother of a 6 month old and a 4 year old, would like to purchase a thermometer. She is not sure how to use them or what possible variations may occur in readings. Create a graph for her showing the types of thermometers and temperature comparisons. Include centigrade readings.

_____

_____

_____

_____

22

Assisting With the Physical Examination

CHAPTER COMPETENCIES

Review the information in your text that supports the following course objectives.

Learning Objectives

Upon successfully completing this chapter, you will be able to:

1. Spell and define key terms.

2. Identify and state the use of the basic and specialized instruments and supplies used in the physical examination.

3. Describe the four methods used to examine the patient.

4. List the basic sequence of the physical examination.

5. State your responsibilities before, during, and after the physical examination.

Performance Objective

Upon successfully completing this chapter, you will be able to:

1. Assist the physician with a patient's physical examination (Procedure 22-1).

CHAPTER OUTLINE	NOTES
Basic Instruments and Supplies	
Percussion Hammer	
Tuning Fork	
Nasal Speculum	
Otoscope and Audioscope	
Ophthalmoscope	
Examination Light and Gooseneck Lamp	
Stethoscope	
Penlight or Flashlight	
Instruments and Supplies in Specialized Examinations	
Head Light or Mirror	
Laryngeal Mirror and Laryngoscope	
Vaginal Speculum	
Lubricant	
Anoscope, Proctoscope, Sigmoidoscope	

CHAPTER OUTLINE *continued*	NOTES
Examination Techniques	
Inspection	
Palpation	
Percussion	
Auscultation	
Responsibilities of the Medical Assistants	
Room Preparation	
Patient Preparation	
Assisting the Physician	
Post-examination Duties	
Physical Examination Format	
Head and Neck	
Eyes and Ears	
Nose and Sinuses	
Mouth and Throat	
Chest, Breasts, and Abdomen	
Genitalia and Rectum	
Legs	
Reflexes	
Posture, Gait, Coordination, Balance, and Strength	
General Health Guidelines and Checkups	

LEARNING SELF-ASSESSMENT EXERCISES

Key Terms

Define the following key terms:

applicator _____

asymmetry _____

auscultation _____

Babinski reflex _____

baseline _____

bimanual _____

bruit _____

cerumen _____

diagnosis _____

extraocular _____

gait _____

hernia _____

inguinal _____

inspection _____

lubricant _____

manipulation _____

nasal septum _____

occult _____

palpation _____

Papanicolaou (Pap) test or smear _____

percussion _____

peripheral _____

PERRLA _____

range of motion (ROM) _____

rectovaginal _____

sclera _____

speculum _____

symmetry _____

transillumination _____

tympanic membrane _____

Matching

Match the term in Part 1 with the correct definition in Part 2

PART 1

_____ 1. Gait

_____ 2. Inguinal

_____ 3. Inspection

_____ 4. Lubricant

_____ 5. Manipulation

_____ 6. Nasal septum

PART 2

a. The skillful use of the hands in diagnostic procedures

b. The act or process of inspecting; visual examination

c. Pertaining to the regions of the groin

d. An agent that reduces friction between parts

e. The manner or style of walking

f. The wall or partition dividing the nostrils

Skill Drills

1. List the seven examination positions and the area of the body that will be examined.

    a. _____

    b. _____

    c. _____

    d. _____

    e. _____

    f. _____

    g. _____

2. List nine instruments that are commonly used during a physical examination.

    a. _____

    b. _____

c. _____

d. _____

e. _____

f. _____

g. _____

h. _____

i. _____

3. List six instruments that are commonly used in specialized examinations.

a. _____

b. _____

c. _____

d. _____

e. _____

f. _____

Multiple Choice

1. What is the purpose of the obturator, which is part of an anoscope, proctoscope, and rigid sigmoidoscope?
   a. It houses a small light bulb for better visualization of the intestine.
   b. It has a rounded tip that allows the instrument to be easily inserted into the rectum.
   c. It has a telescoping ability and lengthens the scope.
   d. It is a magnifying lens that enhances visualization.

2. What are the benefits of a flexible sigmoidoscope versus a rigid sigmoidoscope?
   a. Smaller diameter and less discomfort
   b. Greater depth during examination
   c. Better visualization of the intestinal mucosa
   d. All of the above

3. What are the four basic techniques used by the physician during a physical examination?
   a. Inspection, flexion, percussion, visualization
   b. Inspection, palpation, regression, diagnosis
   c. Inspection, palpation, percussion, auscultation
   d. Inspection, palpation, percussion, reflexion

4. Which of the following is not usually a responsibility of the medical assistant working in a medical facility?
   a. Cleaning examination rooms between patients
   b. Keeping the room stocked with necessary supplies
   c. Making sure that batteries in equipment are checked daily and replaced as needed.
   d. Taking home used gowns and drapes to wash, dry, and return the next workday

5. What may be the medical assistant's responsibility before the physician sees a patient?
   a. Obtaining and recording the patient's history or chief complaint
   b. Taking vital signs and obtaining appropriate mensurations
   c. Providing patients with a beverage while they wait for the doctor
   d. *a* and *b*

6. Which of the following would be appropriate for the medical assistant when the physician is doing a patient examination?
   a. Assisting the patient into appropriate positions and providing a drape as needed
   b. Assessing the patient's expressions and level of anxiety
   c. Offering the patient support and reassurance
   d. All of the above

7. When is the first Pap smear recommended for women?
   a. Between the ages of 18 and 20 and annually thereafter
   b. At age 21 and annually thereafter
   c. After the age of 20, but not later than age 24
   d. Whenever the woman becomes sexually active

8. How often is a tetanus booster recommended?
   a. Every 5 years
   b. Before entering college and every 8 years thereafter
   c. Every 10 years, or sooner if the patient has an open wound
   d. Each doctor has a personal preference and will order it as needed.

9. How often is a mammogram recommended for women?
   a. A baseline between ages 35 and 40 and every 2 years until age 50 (annually thereafter)
   b. At age 21 and every 2 years until age 40 (annually thereafter)
   c. A baseline at age 25 and annually thereafter
   d. A baseline at age 30 and every 2 years thereafter

10. A patient in the supine position
    a. is lying down and looking toward the ceiling.
    b. is lying down and looking toward the floor.
    c. is lying down and looking toward the wall.
    d. is sitting and looking toward the floor.

11. Why is it important for a woman between the ages of 20 and 40 to perform a self-examination of her breasts monthly?
    a. Cancers are more likely to be cured if detected early.
    b. By checking monthly, the woman becomes very familiar with her breasts and can more readily detect changes.
    c. Abnormal lumps may occur without prior symptoms such as pain or tenderness.
    d. All of the above

12. Mr. Smith has come to the clinic with symptoms of a sinus infection. What instruments will you make sure are available for the doctor?
    a. Glove, tongue blade, penlight or ophthalmoscope
    b. Glove, tongue blade, nasal swab
    c. Tongue blade, penlight or ophthalmoscope, tuning fork
    d. Tongue blade, glove, nasal swab

Critical Thinking Practice

1. Mrs. Grayson, age 80, has come in for her annual physical. Though she is mentally "sharp as a tack," she has arthritis and must walk with two canes. What information will you obtain and what preparation will you do before the doctor comes to the room?

_____

_____

_____

_____

2. Sometimes patients are embarrassed about why they come to see the doctor. The medical assistant rooms a patient of the opposite gender. When the medical assistant asks the reason for the visit, the patient looks uncomfortable and says, "It's kind of personal." What would you do?

_____

_____

_____

_____

Patient Education

1. Miss Kirk, almost 18 years old, has come in for her annual physical. You obtain her vital signs and instruct her to obtain a urine sample and then return to the room to disrobe and gown. She appears nervous, and you ask if she has any questions or concerns. She tells you she has never had a Pap smear before. Explain the procedure to her in a way that will help reduce her anxiety.

_____

_____

_____

_____

23

Surgical Instruments and Sterilization

CHAPTER COMPETENCIES

Review the information in your text that supports the following course objectives.

Learning Objectives

Upon successfully completing this chapter, you will be able to:

1. Spell and define key terms.

2. Describe several methods of sterilization.

3. Categorize surgical instruments based on use and identify each by its characteristics.

4. Identify surgical instruments specific to designated specialties.

5. State the difference between reusable and disposable instruments.

6. Explain the procedure for storing supplies, instruments, and equipment.

7. Describe the necessity and procedure for maintaining documents and records of maintenance for instruments and equipment.

Performance Objectives

Upon successfully completing this chapter, you will be able to:

1. Sanitize equipment and instruments (Procedure 23-1).

2. Properly wrap instruments in preparation for sterilization in an autoclave (Procedure 23-2).

3. Operate an autoclave while observing for pressure, time, and temperature determined by the items being sterilized (Procedure 23-3).

CHAPTER OUTLINE	NOTES
Principles and Practices of Sterile Asepsis	
Sterilization	
Surgical Instruments	
Forceps	
Scissors	
Scalpels and Blades	
Towel Clamps	
Probes and Directors	
Retractors	
Care and Handling of Surgical Instruments	
Storage and Record Keeping	
Maintaining Surgical Supplies	

LEARNING SELF-ASSESSMENT EXERCISES

Key Terms

Define the following key terms:

autoclave _____

disinfection _____

ethylene oxide _____

forceps _____

hemostat _____

needle holder _____

obturator _____

OSHA _____

ratchet _____

sanitation _____

sanitize _____

scalpel _____

scissors _____

serration _____

sound _____

sterilization _____

Matching

Match the instrument in Part 1 with its common use in Part 2.

PART 1

_____ 1. Straight scissors

_____ 2. Curved scissors

_____ 3. Thumb forceps

_____ 4. Probe or director

_____ 5. Retractor

_____ 6. Kelly clamp

PART 2

a. Holding open layers of tissue, exposing the areas beneath

b. Curved or straight forceps or hemostat for grasping vessels or tissue, etc.

c. Cutting deep or delicate tissue and cutting sutures

d. Dissecting superficial and delicate tissues

e. Probing depth and direction of an operative area

f. Grasping tissue for dissecting or suturing

Skill Drills

1. List six instruments used in obstetrics and gynecology practice and briefly state the use of each.

   a. _____

   b. _____

   c. _____

   d. _____

   e. _____

   f. _____

2. What six items should be included on a sterilization record?

   a. _____

   b. _____

c. _____

d. _____

e. _____

f. _____

Multiple Choice

1. The practice of sterile asepsis is also known as
   a. medical asepsis.
   b. sterile technique.
   c. clinical asepsis.
   d. hospital asepsis.

2. Some medical facilities expect medical assistants to be familiar with all but one of the following. Identify the exception.
   a. Many types of surgical instruments
   b. Use of disinfection and sterilization techniques
   c. Principles and practices of surgical technique
   d. Maintenance and repair of autoclave equipment

3. Identify the correct order of disinfection and sterilization practices.
   a. Sterilization, sanitation, disinfection
   b. Sanitation, disinfection, sterilization
   c. Disinfection, sanitization, sterilization
   d. None of the above

4. Sterilization by autoclave is achieved by which of the following combinations?
   a. Chemical disinfection followed by hot steam
   b. Chemical sanitation and exposure to gas under pressure
   c. Chemical sterilization then dried in the autoclave at high temperature
   d. Proper temperature, pressure, length of time

5. Which one of the following statements is not correct?
   a. Packs sterilized on site are considered sterile for 30 days.
   b. Adequate space between packs is necessary when autoclaving.
   c. Packs should dry before they are removed from the autoclave.
   d. Use of sterilization indicators or tape is optional.

6. Hemostat, Kelly clamp, sterilizer forceps, and needle holder are all part of which instrument group?
   a. Blades
   b. Punches
   c. Forceps
   d. Scissors

7. A scalpel is a very common instrument used in surgical procedures. Which statements are true about the scalpel?
   a. It has a straight handle with detachable, disposable blades.
   b. Disposable scalpels can be purchased and used once before discarding.
   c. Blades come with curved (convex) or straight cutting edges.
   d. All of the above

8. Straight, curved, suture, and bandage are some names of what group of instruments?
   a. Hemostats
   b. Retractors
   c. Scissors
   d. Probes

9. Serrations or teeth, curved or straight blades, ring tips, blunt tips, sharp tips, and ratchets are descriptions that may apply to what group of instruments?
   a. Scissors
   b. Scalpels
   c. Forceps
   d. Retractors

10. The autoclave is commonly used to sterilize all but one of the following. Identify the exception.
    a. Minor surgical instruments
    b. Latex surgical gloves
    c. Surgical bowls and cups
    d. Canisters of gauze sponges

Critical Thinking Practice

1. As you remove minor surgery packs from the autoclave and lay them on the counter, you notice some dampness remaining between them. What will you do? Why?

_____

_____

_____

2. You notice a patient in the waiting room who is coughing frequently and who appears to be very ill. What would you say or do?

_____

_____

_____

Patient Education

1. Dr. Day has just diagnosed a 10-year-old pediatric patient with a viral upper respiratory infection. What information about infection control could you share with the parents of the child that they can practice at home on a regular basis?

_____

_____

_____

24

Assisting With Minor Office Surgery

CHAPTER COMPETENCIES

Review the information in your text that supports the following course objectives.

Learning Objectives

Upon successfully completing this chapter, you will be able to:

1. Spell and define key terms.

2. List your responsibilities before, during, and after minor office surgery.

3. Identify the guidelines for preparing and maintaining sterility of the field and surgical equipment during a minor office procedure.

4. State your responsibility in relation to informed consent and patient preparation.

5. Describe the types of needles and sutures and the uses of each.

6. Explain the purpose of local anesthetics and list three commonly used in the medical office.

7. Describe the various methods of skin closure used in the medical office.

8. Explain your responsibility during surgical specimen collection.

9. Describe the guidelines for applying a sterile dressing.

10. List the types of laser surgery and electro-surgery used in the medical office and explain the precautions for each.

Performance Objectives

Upon successfully completing this chapter, you will be able to:

1. Open sterile surgical packs (Procedure 24-1).

2. Use sterile transfer forceps (Procedure 24-2).

3. Add sterile solution to a sterile field (Procedure 24-3).

4. Perform skin preparation and hair removal (Procedure 24-4).

5. Apply sterile gloves (Procedure 24-5).

6. Apply a sterile dressing (Procedure 24-6).

7. Change an existing sterile dressing (Procedure 24-7).

8. Assist with excisional surgery (Procedure 24-8).

9. Assist with incision and drainage (Procedure 24-9).

10. Remove sutures (Procedure 24-10).

11. Remove staples (Procedure 24-11).

CHAPTER OUTLINE	NOTES
Preparing and Maintaining a Sterile Field	
Sterile Surgical Packs	
Sterile Transfer Forceps	
Adding Peel-back Packages and Pouring Sterile Solutions	

CHAPTER OUTLINE *continued*	**NOTES**
Preparing the Patient for Minor Office Surgery	
Patient Instructions and Consent	
Positioning and Draping	
Preparing the Patient's Skin	
Assisting the Physician	
Local Anesthetics	
Wound Closure	
Specimen Collection	
Electrosurgery	
Laser Surgery	
Postsurgical Procedures	
Sterile Dressings	
Cleaning the Examination Table and Operative Area	
Commonly Performed Office Surgical Procedures	
Excision of a Lesion	
Incision and Drainage	
Assisting with Suture and Staple Removal	

LEARNING SELF-ASSESSMENT EXERCISES

Key Terms

Define the following key terms:

approximate _____

atraumatic _____

bandage _____

cautery _____

coagulate _____

dehiscence _____

dressing _____

electrode _____

fulgurate _____

keratosis _____

lentigines _____

preservative _____

purulent _____

swaged needle _____

traumatic _____

Matching

Match the definition in Part 1 with the correct term in Part 2

PART 1

_____ 1. Open wound

_____ 2. Needle with an eye

_____ 3. Technique to cover sterile field

_____ 4. Domestic needle

_____ 5. Microorganisms absorbed through damp packaging

_____ 6. Swaged needle

PART 2

a. Atraumatic

b. Straight

c. Wicking action

d. Sterile technique

e. Surgical asepsis

f. Traumatic

Skill Drills

1. List the three types of wound healing.

_____

_____

_____

2. What are the three phases of wound healing?

_____

_____

_____

Multiple Choice

1. When preparing a sterile field for minor surgery, you must observe the following guidelines:
   a. Hold all sterile items above waist level.
   b. Do not cough or sneeze over the field.
   c. Always face the sterile field.
   d. All of the above

2. Which of the following items is not necessary to include on a signed consent form for minor surgery?
   a. Patient signature
   b. Date
   c. Blood type
   d. Doctor and witness signatures

3. Which of the following items is not considered contaminated?
   a. A sterile pack that has been splashed by tap water
   b. Sterile surgical supplies dropped into the middle of a sterile field using surgical asepsis
   c. A bottle of sterile irrigating solution with original lid and seal intact
   d. A package whose date reads Nov. 2, 2005, when the actual date is Nov. 5, 2005

4. When preparing a laboratory sample, which of the following is not necessary?
   a. Selecting the proper container with appropriate preservative
   b. Refrigerating the specimen until it can be transported to the laboratory
   c. Holding the container steady to avoid touching the sides while the physician drops the specimen into the preservative
   d. Attaching a label that includes patient's name, date

5. Electrosurgery does not include
   a. electromodularity, modifying large scars so they are less visible.
   b. removal of moles, cysts, warts, and some types of skin cancers.
   c. various tips, such as blades, needles, loops, and balls.
   d. fulguration, which destroys tissue using controlled sparks.

6. Types of wound drainage to observe do not include
   a. purulent.
   b. copious.

c. serous.

d. sanguinous.

7. When documenting the appearance of an infected wound, the following does not need to be noted:

a. Amount of drainage

b. Presence of inflammation

c. Allergies to medication

d. Tenderness during cleansing

8. Surgical instruments are considered sterile when

a. they have been processed in an autoclave at proper temperature, pressure, steam, and time.

b. they are not placed on contaminated surfaces until thoroughly dry after being autoclaved.

c. the sterilization strip inside the package has changed color.

d. All of the above

Critical Thinking Practice

1. A teenage boy received 20 stitches in the emergency room 5 days ago after accidentally hitting his thigh with an axe while chopping kindling. You remove the original dressing of gauze sponges and tape. One end of the incision appears inflamed, and there is purulent drainage on the dressing.

_____

_____

_____

_____

2. A surgical procedure has just been performed in room 3. Another procedure is scheduled in the same room in 10 minutes.

_____

_____

_____

_____

3. A 7-year-old boy has been brought to the office for removal of sutures from his forehead. He is clinging to his mother's hand, trailing a bit behind her as they enter the examination room. How will you cleanse the incision area?

_____

_____

_____

_____

Patient Education

1. A 40-year-old man has had a cyst excised from his lower arm. What do you need to tell him about the signs of bleeding or infection?

_____

_____

_____

_____

25 Pharmacology

CHAPTER COMPETENCIES

Review the information in your text that supports the following course objectives.

Learning Objectives

Upon successfully completing this chapter, you will be able to:

1. Spell and define key terms.

2. Identify chemical, trade, and generic drug names.

3. Name the regulations and branches of government that impact prescription medications and controlled substances.

4. Explain the various drug actions and interactions including pharmacodynamics and pharmacokinetics.

5. Describe the difference between medication side effects and allergies.

6. Name the sources for locating information on pharmacology.

CHAPTER OUTLINE

CHAPTER OUTLINE	NOTES
Medication Names	
Legal Regulations	
Food and Drug Administration	
Drug Enforcement Agency	
Sources of Drugs	
Drug Actions and Interactions	
Pharmacodynamics	
Pharmacokinetics	
Drug Interactions	
Side Effects and Allergies	
Sources of Information	
Prescriptions	

LEARNING SELF-ASSESSMENT EXERCISES

Key Terms

Define the following key terms:

allergy _____

anaphylaxis _____

antagonism _____

chemical name _____

contraindication _____

drug _____

generic name _____

interaction _____

pharmacodynamics _____

pharmacokinetics _____

pharmacology _____

potentiation _____

synergism _____

trade name _____

Matching

Match the term in Part 1A with the correct definition in Part 1B

PART 1A

_____ 1. Adrenergics

_____ 2. Analgesics

_____ 3. Antacids

_____ 4. Anthelmintics

_____ 5. Antianginal agents

_____ 6. Antianxiety agents

_____ 7. Antiarrhythmics

PART 1B

a. Act on subcortical areas of the brain to relieve symptoms of anxiety

b. Kill parasitic worms

c. Mimic the activity of the sympathetic nervous system (adrenaline)

d. Neutralize or reduce the acidity of the stomach

e. Promote vasodilation

f. Reduce or prevent cardiac irregular rhythms

g. Relieve pain

Match the term in Part 2A with the correct definition in Part 2B

PART 2A

_____ 1. Antibiotics

_____ 2. Anticoagulants and thrombolytics

_____ 3. Anticonvulsants

_____ 4. Antidepressants

_____ 5. Antidiarrheals

_____ 6. Antiemetic agents

PART 2B

a. Decrease intestinal peristalsis

b. Destroy, interrupt, or interfere with the growth of microorganisms

c. Prevent nausea and vomiting

d. Prevent the formation of blood clots or dissolve blood clots

e. Reduce the excitability of the brain

f. Prevent or reduce the symptoms of psychological depression

Skill Drills

List the five categories of the Controlled Substance List and give examples of each.

a. _____

b. _____

c. _____

d. _____

e. _____

Multiple Choice

1. When a drug is administered for local effect, all of the following are correct except one. Identify the exception.
   a. The effect is limited to the area where administered.
   b. The drug could be in the form of an ointment.
   c. The drug may be in the form of a lotion.
   d. It would not cause an allergic reaction.

2. Which of the following does not apply to a drug that has a systemic effect?
   a. It is absorbed by blood.
   b. It is transported via the circulatory system to organs and/or tissue.
   c. Administration may be by mouth (po), sublingual (sl), by injection, by inhalation, transdermal, or rectal.
   d. It is administered only by injection.

3. If kidneys are compromised by disease, some medications
   a. may not be properly eliminated from the person's body.
   b. may be contraindicated.
   c. may result in a cumulative effect of the medication resulting in toxicity.
   d. All of the above

4. Drug interactions may cause undesirable reactions in all of the following cases except one. Identify the exception.
   a. Between two or more prescription (Rx) medications
   b. Between medications and ethyl alcohol
   c. Between Rx medications and herbal supplements
   d. When intentionally prescribed to potentiate a desired outcome

5. Why is it important to ask a patient about allergies of any sort?
   a. To avoid placing the patient in contact with any allergen, which may include medication, topical dressings, etc.
   b. Allergic reactions can include uncomfortable symptoms such as itching, hives, wheezing, or dyspnea
   c. Anaphylaxis, a life-threatening allergic reaction, may occur
   d. All of the above

6. Which of the following is an allergic reaction rather than a side effect?
   a. Itching rash on hands and feet
   b. Nausea
   c. Decreased libido
   d. Constipation or diarrhea

7. Identify the item below that is not an over-the-counter medication.
   a. Aspirin
   b. Common cold remedies
   c. Common cough syrup
   d. Morphine

8. Some popular herbal supplements include all but one of the following. Which one is not an herbal supplement?
   a. Gingko biloba
   b. Vitamin C 1000 mg
   c. St. John's wort
   d. Ginseng

9. An adult patient with a temperature of 101°F would benefit from taking which of the following medications?
   a. Antipyretic
   b. Antihypertensive
   c. Antipsychotic
   d. Cardiotonic

10. A patient with exercise-induced asthma would be wise to carry which of the following items?
    a. Antiinflammatory medication
    b. Antianxiety medication
    c. Bronchodilator inhaler
    d. Antacid

11. A patient with symptoms of a low-grade fever, sinus and chest congestion, and nighttime cough may benefit from taking which of the following medications?
    a. Antitussive, expectorant
    b. Antihistamine
    c. Antifungal
    d. Antineoplastic

Critical Thinking Practice

1. Taking herbal supplements is very common in our society. Is it important to ask patients whether or not they use herbal supplements? Why? If they do take them, should the information be documented in the chart? Why?

_____

_____

_____

Patient Education

1. You are obtaining Mr. Null's medical history. When you ask if he has any allergies to medications, he states, "Oh, I had a reaction to sulfa, but that was fifty years ago. It probably doesn't matter anymore." What will you tell Mr. Null about why it is important to always let the doctor know he has a sulfa allergy?

_____

_____

_____

26

Preparing and Administering Medications

CHAPTER COMPETENCIES

Review the information in your text that supports the following course objectives.

Learning Objectives

Upon successfully completing this chapter, you will be able to:

1. Spell and define the key terms.

2. List the safety guidelines for medication administration.

3. Explain the difference between the oral and parenteral routes of medication administration.

4. Describe the parts of a syringe and needle and name the parts that must be kept sterile.

5. Compare the types of injections (intradermal, subcutaneous, and intramuscular) and locate the sites and anatomical landmarks used to determine where each may be administered safely.

6. List the various needle lengths, gauges, and preferred sites for each type of injection.

7. Explain and demonstrate how to calculate adult and child dosages.

8. Identify and list the rights used for medication administration.

9. Discuss when the Z-track method for administering an intramuscular injection is indicated.

10. Describe the procedure for reading an intradermal tuberculosis screening test and explain what is meant by a positive result.

11. Explain the principles for calculating an intravenous fluid rate.

Performance Objectives

Upon successfully completing this chapter, you will be able to:

1. Administer oral medications (Procedure 26-1).

2. Prepare an injection (Procedure 26-2).

3. Administer an intradermal injection (Procedure 26-3).

4. Administer a subcutaneous injection (Procedure 26-4).

5. Administer an intramuscular injection (Procedure 26-5)

6. Administer an intramuscular injection using the Z-track method (Procedure 26-6).

7. Apply transdermal medications (Procedure 26-7).

8. Prepare an intravenous line for medication administration (Procedure 26-8).

CHAPTER OUTLINE	NOTES
Medication Administration Basics	
Safety Guidelines	
Seven Rights for Correct Medication	
Systems of Measurement	

CHAPTER OUTLINE *continued*	NOTES
Routes of Medication Administration	
Oral, Sublingual, and Buccal Routes	
Parenteral Administration	

LEARNING SELF-ASSESSMENT EXERCISES

Key Terms

Define the following key terms:

ampule _____

apothecary system of measurement _____

buccal medication _____

contraindication _____

diluent _____

gauge _____

induration _____

infiltration _____

Mantoux _____

metric system _____

nebulizer _____

ophthalmic medication _____

otic medication _____

parenteral medication _____

sublingual medication _____

topical medication _____

vial _____

Matching

Match the term in Part 1 with the correct definition in Part 2.

PART 1

_____ 1. NPO

_____ 2. HS

_____ 3. NKA

_____ 4. qid

_____ 5. SL

_____ 6. P.O., p.o.

PART 2

a. No known allergies

b. Four times a day

c. Sublingual

d. Nothing by mouth

e. By mouth

f. Hour of sleep/bedtime

Skill Drills

1. List the seven rights for correct medication administration.

   a. _____

   b. _____

c. _____

d. _____

e. _____

f. _____

g. _____

2. Read the 21 safety guidelines for administering medications. List the first 10 below.

a. _____

b. _____

c. _____

d. _____

e. _____

f. _____

g. _____

h. _____

i. _____

j. _____

Multiple Choice

1. Before administering medications, you should be familiar with all but one of the following. Identify the exception.
   a. The medication ordered
   b. Procedures for safe and accurate administration
   c. Method of administration
   d. The physician's DEA number

2. Prefixes micro-, milli-, centi-, deci-, and kilo- are associated with
   a. the apothecary system.
   b. the metric system.
   c. the household measuring system.
   d. Chinese herbalists.

3. In calculating adult doses, you must remember
   a. that errors in calculation could prove fatal.
   b. that two methods for calculating are the ratio method and the formula method.
   c. that measurements must be in the same system (preferably metric).
   d. All of the above

4. The most accurate method for calculating pediatric doses is by body surface area (BSA). Which of the following statements are accurate?
   a. A nomogram estimates BSA according to height and weight.
   b. The result is expressed in square meters.
   c. The total head circumference equals BSA divided by 10.
   d. Lines for height and weight intersect to give the BSA.

5. Which of the following is an advantage in taking medications by the oral route?
   a. Patients with nausea and vomiting cannot keep the medicine down.

   b. Patients who are npo by doctor's orders prior to diagnostic testing or surgery cannot take oral medications.
   c. Oral medications can be formulated in a time-release or sustained-release dose.
   d. They are slow to take effect.

6. Use of the sublingual and buccal routes to administration medication requires specific instructions. Which of the following is not recommended?
   a. The drug is dissolved by saliva and absorbed through the oral mucosa.
   b. Do not eat or drink until the medication is completely absorbed.
   c. If the taste is intolerable, chew and swish, then swallow.
   d. The medication is not intended to be swallowed.

7. When a powdered drug is reconstituted in a multiple-dose vial, which of the following need not be written on the label?
   a. Date of reconstitution
   b. Initials of person reconstituting
   c. Diluent used
   d. Prescribing doctor's initials

8. Needles and syringes come in a variety of sizes and are selected for injections on the bases of the type of injection and the size of the patient. Which statement is not correct?
   a. A 5-mL or 10-mL syringe is often used for irrigation of a small wound.
   b. A tuberculin syringe is usually 1 mL with 100 calibration lines, each representing 0.01 mL.
   c. A 25-gauge 5/8″ needle is commonly used to inject subcutaneously
   d. Insulin may be given with a 1-mL tuberculin syringe.

9. Intradermal injections such as tuberculin antigen serum for allergy testing are administered into the dermal layer of skin. Which of the following statements is not accurate?
   a. The needle tip and lumen will be slightly visible under the skin.
   b. The needle is inserted at a 10–15° angle.
   c. Recommended sites include the posterior forearm and across the stomach.
   d. A small bubble, known as a wheal, will be raised in the skin surface when the solution is injected.

10. Subcutaneous injections are
    a. given into the fatty layer of tissue below the skin.
    b. injected holding the needle at a 45° angle to the skin.
    c. Subcutaneous injection sites are ideal for drugs that should not be absorbed as rapidly as intramuscular or intravenous injections.
    d. All of the above

Critical Thinking Practice

1. Mr. Kerry comes into the clinic for his tetanus booster of 0.5 mL. This is an intramuscular injection. Mr. Kerry is 6 feet tall and weighs 225 lb. What size syringe and needle will you choose and why?

_____

_____

_____

2. The doctor orders 120 drops (gtt) of an expectorant cough syrup every 6 hours for a patient. The drug label gives instructions in teaspoons. How many teaspoons should you administer? Include your calculations in this answer.

_____

_____

_____

Patient Education

1. The doctor has prescribed a transdermal hormone patch for Mrs. Brown. He asks you to instruct her on application, using a pharmaceutical sample of the product. What will you tell her?

_____

_____

_____

27

Diagnostic Imaging

CHAPTER OUTLINE *continued*	NOTES
The Medical Assistant's Role in Radiological Procedures	
Patient Education	
Assisting with Examinations	
Handling and Storing Radiographic Films	
Transfer of Radiographic Information	
Teleradiology	

LEARNING SELF-ASSESSMENT EXERCISES

Key Terms

Define the following key terms:

cassette _____

contrast medium _____

film _____

fluoroscopy _____

magnetic resonance imaging _____

nuclear medicine _____

radiograph _____

radiography _____

radiologist _____

radiology _____

radiolucent _____

radionuclide _____

radiopaque _____

teleradiology _____

tomography _____

ultrasound _____

x-rays _____

Matching

Match the term in Part 1 with the correct definition in Part 2.

PART I

_____ 1. PTCA

_____ 2. Vascular stents

_____ 3. Teleradiology

_____ 4. Supine

_____ 5. Prone

_____ 6. Recumbent

PART 2

a. Balloon angioplasty

b. Lying on the back

c. Lying down in any position

d. Lying face downward

e. Radiology over a great distance

f. Maintain lumen patency

Skill Drills

1. List five safety guidelines to be followed to protect patients when they are to have radiography.

_____

_____

_____

_____

2. List six safety precautions the radiology staff is supposed to follow.

_____

_____

_____

_____

Multiple Choice

1. Which of the following statements is not true about radiography?
   a. Production of x-rays occurs within a part of the machine called the tube.
   b. High-voltage electricity applied to the tube results in x-ray production.
   c. X-rays exit the tube in hundreds of miniscule beams.
   d. X-rays exit the tube in many small beams.

2. Which of the following statements is not correct about radiology?
   a. Many work with computers to produce digital images.
   b. Images are formed on x-ray film as rays pass through, or are absorbed by, body tissues.
   c. Fluoroscopic units can visualizing motion within the body.
   d. Though bone is dense, x-rays have no problem passing through it to form a high-quality image.

3. Many clinics and other health care facilities provide diagnostic imaging services on an outpatient basis. Which statement is inaccurate?
   a. Because medical assistants work under the supervision of the physician, the physician can legally train the medical assistant on the job to take and develop radiographs.
   b. In some states, medical assistants are permitted to take and process simple radiographs, such as bone or chest radiographs.
   c. Some states require that medical assistants attend an approved course and take a written examination before they are allowed to take and develop radiographs.

   d. Maintaining a reference file and storing radiographs may be part of a medical assistant's duties in a small medical clinic.

4. Instructing the patient about examination sequencing is very important because
   a. simple noninvasive diagnostics are done before more complex invasive tests.
   b. contrast media, such as barium, should be used for an upper GI series before a lower GI series because of the time it takes to evacuate the barium from the body.
   c. the patient may not understand the consequences of not following instructions, including having to repeat the test or procedure.
   d. All of the above

5. Which statement is not accurate about routine radiographic examinations?
   a. Most require little or no preexamination preparation by the patient.
   b. They are primarily done to view bone structure or abnormalities.
   c. They are most readily accepted by patients.
   d. They are risk free for any group of patients.

6. Which of the following statements is not true about mammography?
   a. It is an important screening tool for breast cancer.
   b. Needle localization studies may be performed to obtain cell samples.
   c. Only women benefit from having a mammogram.
   d. The frequency of having a mammogram depends on age and a personal and family history of breast cancer.

7. Which statement is not accurate about contrast media used for radiographic examinations?
   a. It helps to evaluate structure and function.
   b. It may be introduced several ways to enhance particular anatomical structures.
   c. Radiopaque contrast helps differentiate body structures that may otherwise be superimposed over each other
   d. One chemical form of contrast media is used for all studies.

8. Nuclear medicine involves injection of small amounts of radionuclides (radioactive material with a short half-life). Which statement is not accurate?
   a. It is illegal in some states because of the use of radioactive material.
   b. Positron emission tomography (PET) produces detailed sectional images of the body's physiological process.
   c. Common nuclear imaging studies include those of the thyroid, brain, and kidneys.

   d. Contrast is designed to concentrate in specific areas of the body.

9. Magnetic resonance imagining (MRI)
   a. uses a combination of high to intense magnetic fields, radio waves, and computer analysis to create cross-sectional images of the body.
   b. results depend on the chemical makeup of the body.
   c. may be used for a variety of studies including central nervous system (CNS) and joint structure.
   d. All of the above

10. Radiation therapy is used to treat cancer. Which statement is not accurate about radiation therapy?
    a. Treatment follows a precise regimen of therapy.
    b. Treatment does not cause side effects like many of the chemotherapy drugs.
    c. It is sometimes used in conjunction with surgery or chemotherapy.
    d. The radiation is intense enough to destroy cancer cells.

Critical Thinking Practice

1. Patients are often anxious about going through diagnostic testing. What are some reasons for this and how may the medical assistant affect the patients' emotional response?

_____

_____

_____

2. Mrs. Kay had several radiographic and contrast media studies over the past 5 years. She is now moving to another state and wants to know how to get copies of the films and reports to her new physician. What will you tell her about transferring these records?

_____

_____

_____

Patient Education

1. Ms. Amarillo, a 25-year-old patient, phones the clinic. She has never had a mammogram and asks you about the guidelines. What are the current American Cancer Society recommendations for mammography?

_____

_____

_____

28

Medical Office Emergencies

CHAPTER COMPETENCIES

Review the information in your text that supports the following course objectives.

Learning Objectives

Upon successfully completing this chapter, you will be able to:

1. Spell and define the key terms.

2. Describe the role of the medical assistant in an emergency before the ambulance arrives.

3. Identify the five types of shock and the management of each.

4. Describe how burns are classified and managed.

5. Explain the management of allergic reactions.

6. Describe the management of poisoning and the role of the poison control center.

7. List the three types of hyperthermic emergencies and the treatment for each type.

8. Discuss the treatment of hypothermia.

9. Describe the role of the medical assistant in managing psychiatric emergencies.

CHAPTER OUTLINE

CHAPTER OUTLINE	NOTES
Medical Office Emergency Procedures	
Emergency Action Plan	
Emergency Medical Kit	
The Emergency Medical Services System	
Patient Assessment	
Recognizing the Emergency	
The Primary Assessment	
The Secondary Assessment	
Types of Emergencies	
Shock	
Bleeding	
Burns	
Musculoskeletal Injuries	
Cardiovascular Emergencies	
Neurological Emergencies	
Allergic and Anaphylactic Reactions	
Poisoning	

CHAPTER OUTLINE   NOTES

Heat- and Cold-Related Emergencies

Behavioral and Psychiatric Emergencies

LEARNING SELF-ASSESSMENT EXERCISES

Key Terms

Define the following key terms:

allergen _____

anaphylactic shock _____

cardiogenic shock _____

contusion _____

ecchymosis _____

full-thickness burn _____

heat cramps _____

heat stroke _____

hematoma _____

hyperthermia _____

hypothermia _____

hypovolemic shock _____

infarction _____

ischemia _____

melena _____

neurogenic shock _____

partial-thickness burn _____

seizure _____

septic shock _____

shock _____

splint _____

superficial burn _____

Matching

Match the term in Part 1 with the correct definition in Part 2.

PART 1

_____ 1. Ischemia

_____ 2. Hypothermia

_____ 3. Shock

_____ 4. Hematoma

_____ 5. Full-thickness burn

_____ 6. Superficial burn

PART 2

a. A decrease in oxygen to tissues

b. Lack of oxygen to individual cells of the body

c. Burn that has destroyed all skin layers

d. Below-normal body temperature

e. A blood clot that forms at an injury site

f. A burn that is limited to the epidermal layer of the skin

Skill Drills

1. Documentation is always important. In the event of a medical emergency, name at least seven things that need to be documented about the patient.

_____

_____

_____

_____

_____

_____

_____

2. To gain an accurate impression during the secondary assessment, what four areas are assessed? Give examples from each area.

_____

_____

_____

_____

Multiple Choice

1. Emergency medical care, when properly performed, can make a difference in several situations. Which statement is irrelevant to emergency medical attention.
   a. It can mean the difference between life and death.
   b. It can make the difference between rapid recovery and long hospitalization.
   c. It can make a difference between temporary or permanent disability.
   d. It can mean a difference between a good diagnosis and a misdiagnosis.

2. An emergency situation can occur anywhere and to anyone. What emergencies should medical personnel be prepared to handle in a medical clinic setting?
   a. Cardiac emergency, such as cardiac arrhythmia
   b. Respiratory emergency, such as anaphylaxis
   c. Hemorrhaging, such as miscarriage
   d. All of the above

3. An emergency medical kit should be kept in each medical facility. Which one of the following statements has little importance regarding emergency supplies?
   a. Contents of the kit should be checked regularly for completeness and outdates.
   b. Supplies are purchased on the basis of brand name.
   c. When supplies are used they should be promptly replaced.
   d. Supplies are based on the medical specialty of the facility.

4. Which of the following statements is not accurate?
   a. Guardians of minors must be contacted before any emergency treatment.
   b. Do not assume that the obvious injuries are the only ones present.
   c. Look for causes of the injury; they may provide clues to the extent of injury.
   d. Primary objectives are to identify and correct life-threatening problems.

5. Primary assessment of the patient includes responsiveness, airway, breathing, and circulation. What is the least likely reason for lack of responsiveness?
   a. Head trauma
   b. Electric shock
   c. Sleeping
   d. Cardiac arrest

6. An unconscious patient in a supine position may have partial or total airway obstruction. Why?
   a. Swallowed gum
   b. Air bubble swallowed while drinking water
   c. The tongue fell back into the oropharynx
   d. Small mouth and oversize tongue for the space

7. Checking circulation is an important part of patient assessment. What are some ways that circulation may be evaluated besides counting the pulse?
   a. Evaluate perfusion by checking the temperature and moisture of the skin.

b. Observe the color of the skin and capillary filling in nail beds.
c. Count the respirations.
d. *a and b*

8. Following the primary and secondary assessment of a patient receiving emergency care, a physician does a head-to-toe physical examination. He or she will examine the arms and legs, looking for specific things. Identify the item that is least important during this examination.
a. Moles with irregular margins
b. Swelling
c. Deformity
d. Tenderness

9. The physician checks for sensation by
a. using a safety pin or other tool to determine patient response to pain.
b. having the patient squeeze each of the doctor's hands as hard as possible.
c. using the tuning fork next to each of the patient's ears.
d. having the patient push each foot against the doctor's hands as hard as possible.

10. Blunt object trauma to the body may cause injury. Some of these injuries are closed wounds. Which of the following are symptoms of closed wounds?
a. Bleeding within a confined area or a contusion
b. Swelling at the site
c. A black-and-blue mark, called an ecchymosis
d. All of the above

11. Anaphylaxis is a life-threatening allergic reaction. Which of the following is not a sign or symptom of an allergic reaction?
a. Cough or wheeze
b. Pale and/or moist skin
c. Abdominal cramps
d. Rash, hives, or wheals

12. Exposure to toxins in the home or workplace is increasing. When a parent arrives at the clinic with a child who has ingested a household chemical (i.e., chemical cleaner or medications), what steps will you take?
a. Obtain the weight and age of the child.
b. Ask the name of the substance and the approximate amount ingested.
c. Obtain any previous history of chemical exposure.
d. *a and b*

Critical Thinking Practice

1. One of the clinic patients has had a seizure. The patient's sister phones your clinic to report the incident and to ask for advice. She reports that her brother, the patient, is now "awake, but very tired." What patient history information will you need to report the episode to the doctor?

_____

_____

_____

_____

2. Mrs. Clay, one of the clinic patients, phones to report that her daughter and grandson are on their way to the clinic. Her grandson is allergic to bee stings. He was stung by a yellow jacket about 5 minutes ago. She estimates that they will arrive at the clinic within the next 5–10 minutes. What would you do to prepare for their arrival?

_____

_____

_____

_____

Patient Education

1. One of your patients is planning a backpacking trip up one of the local mountain trails. He is going with a small group and wants to be prepared for emergencies. It is late October, and the patient asks you for advice about treating hypothermia. What will you say? What additional resources might you suggest?

_____

_____

_____

_____

29

Dermatology

CHAPTER COMPETENCIES

Review the information in your text that supports the following course objectives.

Learning Objectives

Upon successfully completing this chapter, you will be able to:

1. Spell and define the key terms.

2. Describe common skin disorders.

3. Explain common diagnostic procedures.

4. Prepare the patient for examination of the integument.

5. Assist the physician with examination of the integument.

6. Explain the difference between bandages and dressings and give the purpose of each.

7. Identify the guidelines for applying bandages.

Performance Objectives

Upon successfully completing this chapter, you will be able to:

1. Apply a warm or cold compress. (Procedure 29-1).

2. Assist with therapeutic soaks. (Procedure 29-2).

3. Apply a tubular gauze bandage. (Procedure 29-3).

CHAPTER OUTLINE

CHAPTER OUTLINE	NOTES
Common Disorders of the Integumentary System	
Skin Infections	
Inflammatory Reactions	
Disorders of Wound Healing	
Disorders Caused by Pressure	
Alopecia	
Disorders of Pigmentation	
Skin Cancers	
Diagnostic Procedures	
Physical Examination of the Skin	
Wound Cultures	
Skin Biopsy	
Urine Melanin	
Wood's Light Analysis	
Bandaging	
Types of Bandages	
Bandage Application Guidelines	

LEARNING SELF-ASSESSMENT EXERCISES

Key Terms

Define the following key terms:

abscess _____

alopecia _____

bandage _____

benign tumor _____

bulla _____

carbuncle _____

cellulitis _____

comedo _____

cyst _____

dermatitis _____

dermatophytosis _____

dressing _____

eczema _____

erythema _____

exudate _____

fissure _____

folliculitis _____

furuncle _____

herpes simplex _____

herpes zoster _____

impetigo _____

macule _____

malignant tumor _____

neoplasm _____

nodule _____

papilloma _____

papilloma virus _____

papule _____

pediculosis _____

pruritus _____

psoriasis _____

pustule _____

seborrhea _____

Staphylococcus _____

Streptococcus _____

urticaria _____

verruca _____

vesicle _____

wheal _____

Wood's light _____

Matching

Match the term in Part 1 with the correct definition in Part 2.

PART 1	PART 2
_____ 1. Verruca	a. A vesicle that is filled with pus
_____ 2. Urticaria	b. Itching
_____ 3. Pustule	c. A wart
_____ 4. Pruritus	d. A blackhead
_____ 5. Benign	e. Hives
_____ 6. Bulla	f. Redness of the skin
_____ 7. Papilloma	g. A benign skin tumor
_____ 8. Exudate	h. A large blister or vesicle
_____ 9. Comedo	i. A tumor that is not malignant
_____ 10. Erythema	j. Drainage

Skill Drills

1. List six types of fungal infections and where they are most commonly found.

   a. _____

   b. _____

   c. _____

   d. _____

   e. _____

   f. _____

2. Name four uses for bandages.

   a. _____

   b. _____

   c. _____

   d. _____

3. Name seven uses of a dressing.

   a. _____

   b. _____

   c. _____

   d. _____

   e. _____

   f. _____

   g. _____

Multiple Choice

1. The integumentary system, skin, is the largest organ of the body. Which of the following are true about skin?
   a. Can indicate a person's state of wellness
   b. Helps maintain homeostasis
   c. Protects underlying tissues and organs
   d. Layers thicken and become tougher with age

2. Which of the following statements about skin infections is not true?
   a. Skin disorders may be manifested by lesions or other abnormalities.
   b. Lesions may be primary or secondary.
   c. Gloves need to be worn by the person doing the examination.
   d. Skin infections are most common in the elderly.

3. Impetigo is a bacterial infection that
   a. is most common on face or neck.
   b. is not contagious.
   c. is most common in children.
   d. includes macules, vesicles, bulla, and pustules.

4. Treatment of impetigo involves
   a. washing the area two to three times a day followed by application of topical antibiotics.
   b. cleaning with alcohol sponges twice a day followed by application of topical antibiotics.
   c. washing towels, washcloths, and bed linens daily.
   d. oral antibiotics for severe cases.

5. Folliculitis, furuncle, and carbuncle
   a. are caused by staphylococci.
   b. develop one or more pus sacs.
   c. are treated by use of antibiotics (topical and/or systemic, depending on the diagnosis).
   d. All of the above

6. Sometimes a preexisting infected wound such as a cut or animal or insect bite will cause infection to move into the surrounding tissue. Which statement is not accurate?
   a. Systemic antibiotics are not usually advised.
   b. The infection is called cellulites.
   c. The area becomes red, hot, and edematous.
   d. If not treated, underlying tissue will be destroyed or an abscess will form.

7. Which of the following is not correct about herpes simplex?
   a. The causative agent is herpes simplex virus type 2.
   b. Lesions usually occur on the lips, mouth, face, and nose.

   c. Small vesicles erupt, leave a painful ulcer, and then crust over.
   d. Factors that precipitate an outbreak include stress, trauma, fatigue, sun exposure, menstruation, and upper respiratory infection.

8. Herpes zoster, or shingles is caused by the same virus that causes chickenpox. Which statement is not accurate about herpes zoster?
   a. This virus may be transmitted by sexual contact, and it is believed the virus may stay dormant in the nervous system for years.
   c. When reactivated, the virus spreads down the length of a nerve to the skin.
   d. A bank of lesions may appear, most commonly on the face, back, and chest.
   e. Narcotic analgesics are appropriate to use because of the severe pain associated with an outbreak of shingles.

9. Eczema is an inflammatory skin disorder. Which statement is not accurate about eczema?
   a. It only involves the epidermal layer of skin.
   b. It is more common in adults than in children.
   c. It is characterized by itching and lesions.
   d. The condition is chronic, with periods of remission and exacerbation.

10. Decubitus ulcers are also called pressure sores. Which statements are accurate about decubitus ulcers?
    a. Bedridden and wheelchair-bound patients are at risk for decubitus ulcers.
    b. Decubiti are graded or staged according to the degree of tissue involvement.
    c. Pressure impairs blood, oxygen, and nutritional supply to an area, resulting in a lesion.
    d. All of the above

Critical Thinking Practice

1. Alopecia, or baldness, may occur from physical trauma, systemic disease, bacteria, and other factors. Based on your own experience, what do you think some of the emotional challenges may be for men, women, or children when they lose all their hair? How can you, as a medical assistant, support these individuals?

_____

_____

_____

_____

2. A patient phones the medical office to arrange an appointment. He states that his barber recommended that he see the doctor because of an irregular red patch of nodules on his scalp. This may be a type of cancer. What kind of cancer does the description fit? Why is it important to have it evaluated?

_____

_____

_____

_____

Patient Education

1. The mother of a teenager phones and reports that her son has symptoms of athlete's foot. She would like to know how to treat it. This also gives the medical assistant time to educate the mother about how to prevent the spread of tinea pedis. What will you say?

_____

_____

_____

_____

30

Orthopedics

CHAPTER COMPETENCIES

Review the information in your text that supports the following course objectives.

Learning Objectives

Upon successfully completing this chapter, you will be able to:

1. Spell and define the key terms.

2. List and describe disorders of the musculoskeletal system.

3. Compare the different types of fractures.

4. Identify and explain diagnostic procedures of the musculoskeletal system.

5. Describe the various types of ambulatory aids.

6. Discuss the role of the medical assistant in caring for the patient with a musculoskeletal system disorder.

Performance Objectives

Upon successfully completing this chapter, you will be able to:

1. Apply a triangular arm sling (Procedure 30-1).

2. Apply cold packs (Procedure 30-2).

3. Use a hot water bottle or commercial hot pack (Procedure 30-3).

4. Measure a patient for axillary crutches (Procedure 30-4).

5. Instruct a patient in various crutch gaits (Procedure 30-5).

CHAPTER OUTLINE

	NOTES
The Musculoskeletal System and Common Disorders	
Sprains and Strains	
Dislocations	
Fractures	
Bursitis	
Arthritis	
Tendonitis	
Fibromyalgia	
Spine Disorders	
Abnormal Spinal Curvatures	
Herniated Intervertebral Disk	
Disorders of the Upper Extremities	
Rotator Cuff Injury	
Adhesive Capsulitis, or Frozen Shoulder	
Lateral Epicondylitis, or Tennis Elbow	

CHAPTER OUTLINE   *continued*

	NOTES
Carpal Tunnel Syndrome	
Dupuytren Contracture	
Disorders of the Lower Extremities	
Chondromalacia Patellae	
Plantar Fasciitis	
Gout	
Muscular Dystrophy	
Osteoporosis	
Bone Tumors	
Common Diagnostic Procedures	
Physical Examination	
Diagnostic Studies	
The Role of the Medical Assistant	
Warm and Cold Applications	
Ambulatory Assist Devices	

LEARNING SELF-ASSESSMENT EXERCISES

Key Terms

Define the following key terms:

ankylosing spondylitis _____

arthrogram _____

arthroplasty _____

arthroscopy _____

bursae _____

callus _____

contracture _____

contusion _____

electromyography _____

embolus _____

goniometer _____

iontophoresis _____

kyphosis _____

lordosis _____

phonophoresis _____

prosthesis _____

reduction _____

scoliosis _____

Matching

Match the definition in Part 1 with the correct term in Part 2.

PART 1

_____ 1. Light, water resistant, durable

_____ 2. Enables an amputee to resume functional
activities

_____ 3. Caused by wear and tear on the weight-
bearing joints

_____ 4. Still disease

_____ 5. Fibromyalgia

_____ 6. Plantar fascitis

PART 2

a. Degenerative joint disease (DJD)

b. Rheumatoid arthritis in children

c. Multiple, often nonspecific symptoms including
pain, fatigue, muscle stiffness

d. Fiberglass cast

e. Frequent cause of foot pain

f. Prosthesis

Skill Drills

1. List seven types of casts and tell how each is used.

a. _____

b. _____

c. _____

d. _____

e. _____

f. _____

g. _____

2. List the 12 types of fractures.

a. _____

b. _____

c. _____

d. _____

e. _____

f. _____

g. _____

h. _____

i. _____

j. _____

k. _____

l. _____

Multiple Choice

1. The most common disorders of the musculoskeletal
group include all but
a. sprains and dislocations.
b. fractures and joint disruption.
c. degeneration.
d. temporomandibular joint fusion.

2. Damage to a muscle, ligament, or tendon fibers
may result in
a. swelling.
b. inflammation.
c. joint instability.
d. All of the above

3. Dislocation of a joint (luxation) is not caused by
a. trauma.
b. disease.
c. congenital factors.
d. exercise.

4. Subluxation is a partial dislocation in which the
bone is pulled out of the socket. This will not occur
in
a. shoulders.
b. elbows and fingers.
c. the temporal joint.
d. hips and ankles.

5. All fractures have the symptom of pain in common. Other symptoms, depending on the location of the injury, may include
   a. pressure.
   b. limited movement.
   c. deformity.
   d. All of the above

6. Fractures of the shoulder joint are serious injuries. Which statement does not apply?
   a. Immobilization is necessary for healing.
   b. Scar tissue may develop.
   c. Loss of motion and function may occur.
   d. Physical therapy will include range of motion to a moderate level of pain.

7. Rheumatoid arthritis is a systemic autoimmune disease that usually begins
   a. in non-weight-bearing joints.
   b. only in the elderly.
   c. in the hips.
   d. with sudden onset of pain.

8. Which of the following does not apply to treatment for bursitis?
   a. Antiinflammatory medications
   b. Rest
   c. Heat or cold
   d. Exercise with therapy putty

9. Disorders of the upper extremities do not include which of the following?
   a. Rotator cuff tear
   b. Frozen shoulder
   c. Lateral epicondylitis
   d. Patellar deviation

10. Symptoms of carpal tunnel syndrome may include
    a. edema of the hand and fingers.
    b. night pain that wakes the patient.
    c. numbness in thumb and middle and index finger.
    d. *b* and c

Critical Thinking Practice

1. Carpal tunnel syndrome (CTS) is caused by repetitive motion. What professions can you think of that put individuals at risk for developing CTS? Can you think of ways these various people may reduce the risk of developing severe symptoms?

_____

_____

_____

_____

2. It is not uncommon for elderly patients to fall and break a femur. What are some of the special concerns raised by a fractured femur in this age group?

_____

_____

_____

_____

Patient Education

1. Mr. Silver comes into the clinic for a preemployment physical. He will be working at a warehouse where he will be responsible for lifting and moving boxes of various weight and size. The doctor asks you to give Mr. Silver some information on prevention of back strain. What will you tell him?

_____

_____

_____

_____

31

Ophthalmology and Otolaryngology

CHAPTER COMPETENCIES

Review the information in your text that supports the following course objectives.

Learning Objectives

Upon successfully completing this chapter, you will be able to:

1. Spell and define the key terms.

2. List and define disorders associated with the eye, ear, nose, and throat.

3. Identify diagnostic procedures commonly performed on the eye, ear, nose, and throat.

4. Describe patient education procedures associated with the eye, ear, nose, and throat.

Performance Objectives

Upon successfully completing this chapter, you will be able to:

1. Measure distance visual acuity with a Snellen chart (Procedure 31-1).

2. Measure color perception with an Ishihara color plate book (Procedure 31-2).

3. Instill eye medication (Procedure 31-3).

4. Irrigate the eye (Procedure 31-4).

5. Administer an audiometric hearing test (Procedure 31-5).

6. Irrigate the ear (Procedure 31-6).

7. Instill ear medication (Procedure 31-7).

8. Instill nasal medication (Procedure 31-9).

9. Take a sample for a throat culture (Procedure 31-9).

CHAPTER OUTLINE

CHAPTER OUTLINE	NOTES
Common Disorders of the Eye	
Cataract	
Sty, or Hordeolum	
Conjunctivitis	
Corneal Ulcer	
Retinopathy	
Glaucoma	
Refractive Errors	
Strabismus	
Color Deficit	

CHAPTER OUTLINE *continued*	NOTES
Diagnostic Studies of the Eye	
Visual Acuity Testing	
Color Deficit Testing	
Tonometry and Gonioscopy	
Therapeutic Procedures for the Eye	
Instilling Eye Medications	
Common Disorders of the Ear	
Ceruminosis	
Conductive and Perceptual Hearing Loss	
Ménière's Disease	
Otitis Externa	
Otitis Media	
Otosclerosis	
Diagnostic Studies of the Ear	
Visual Examination	
Audiometry and Tympanometry	
Tuning Fork Tests	
Therapeutic Procedures for the Ear	
Irrigations and Instillations	
Common Disorders of the Nose and Throat	
Allergic Rhinitis	
Epistaxis	
Nasal Polyps	
Sinusitis	
Pharyngitis and Tonsillitis	
Laryngitis	
Diagnostic Studies of the Nose and Throat	
Visual Inspection	
Therapeutic Procedures for the Nose and Throat	
Throat Culture	

LEARNING SELF-ASSESSMENT EXERCISES

Key Terms

Define the following key terms:

astigmatism _____

cerumen _____

decibel (db) _____

fluorescein angiography _____

hyperopia _____

intraocular pressure _____

myopia _____

myringotomy _____

ophthalmologist _____

ophthalmoscope _____

optician _____

optometrist _____

otolaryngologist _____

otoscope _____

presbycusis _____

presbyopia _____

refraction _____

retinal degeneration _____

tinnitus _____

tonometry _____

upper respiratory infection (URI) _____

Matching

Match the term in Part 1 with the correct definition in Part 2.

PART 1

1. Centralis

2. Presbyopia

3. Myopia

4. Presbycusis

5. Intraocular pressure

6. Hyperopia

7. Astigmatism

PART 2

a. The area of greatest visual acuity

b. A type of farsightedness associated with aging

c. Farsightedness

d. Pressure within the eyeball

e. Loss of hearing associated with aging

f. Nearsightedness

g. Unfocused refraction of light rays on the retina

Skill Drills

1. List seven causes of corneal ulcer.

   a. _____

   b. _____

   c. _____

   d. _____

   e. _____

   f. _____

   g. _____

2. List nine common disorders of the eye.

a. _____

b. _____

c. _____

d. _____

e. _____

f. _____

g. _____

h. _____

i. _____

Multiple Choice

1. Four types of strabismus do not include one of the following options. Identify the exception.
   a. Esotropic
   b. Pretropic
   c. Hypotropic
   d. Hypertropic

2. Diagnostic studies of the eye do not include
   a. color deviant testing.
   b. visual acuity testing.
   c. tonometry.
   d. gonioscopy.

3. Common disorders of the ear include
   a. Ménière's disease.
   b. otitis media and externa.
   c. otosclerosis.
   d. All of the above

4. Which of the following does not represent professionalism in a clinical practice?
   a. Demonstrating initiative and responsibility
   b. Prioritizing and performing multiple tasks
   c. Displaying a professional manner and image
   d. Focusing on your own work and expecting co-workers to be just as independent

5. All of the following statements are true about color deficit except one. Identify the exception.
   a. Red, green, or blue perception may be absent or impaired.
   b. Color deficit is more common among women than men.
   c. It may be chemically induced from damage to the cones.
   d. Color deficit has no cure.

6. Common disorders of the nose and throat include all but one of the following. Identify the exception.
   a. Allergic rhinitis
   b. Pharyngitis
   c. Ceruminosis
   d. Epistaxis

7. Visual examination of the interior of the eye may reveal
   a. vascular and hypertensive conditions.
   b. problems with intraocular blood vessels.
   c. injury to the retina.
   d. All of the above

8. Ophthalmic medications and drops are instilled in the eyes for several reasons. Identify the one that is incorrect.
   a. To treat infections or irritations
   b. To apply anesthetic for treatment or testing
   c. To dilate the pupil for the Ishihara test
   d. To irrigate the eye to remove a foreign object

9. Symptoms of otitis media include all but one of the following. Identify the exception.
   a. Low-grade pain
   b. Fever of varying degrees
   c. Mild-to-moderate hearing loss
   d. Infants may be fussy and pull at their ear.

10. Ear irrigations are performed for all but one of the following reasons. Identify the exception.
    a. Improve conductive hearing
    b. Relieve pain
    c. Remove debris or foreign objects
    d. Apply medication solutions

Critical Thinking Practice

1. Colleen is the mother of a 6-month-old boy. She calls the clinic to report that the baby has had a recent runny nose and cough. Last night he was awake and crying most of the night. He has a 99.2° axillary temperature. She tried to put him down with a bottle, which usually helps him sleep, but he would not be comforted last night. "He just

keeps crying and pulling his ear." Does the infant need to be seen today? Based on this recent medical history, what factors, including the infant's age, may have contributed to the present symptoms and possible diagnosis?

_____

_____

_____

_____

2. Symptoms of allergic rhinitis may be so bothersome that allergy testing is recommended. Allergy testing and treatment involves exposure to allergens in minute doses to desensitize the immune reaction. Sensitivity to allergens will vary from person to person. During allergy testing, minute amounts of several allergens may be applied by scratch test or intradermal injection. What allergic reactions would you expect to occur during allergy testing or allergy desensitization? Why are patients not supposed to take antihistamines before being tested for allergies?

_____

_____

_____

_____

Patient Education

1. Dave is a 52-year-old patient at your clinic. He has come in today for a blood pressure check and to renew a prescription for his antihypertensive medication. He also mentions having had a slight nosebleed 2 weeks ago. This is an opportunity for patient teaching. What will you tell him?

_____

_____

_____

_____

32

Pulmonary Medicine

CHAPTER COMPETENCIES

Review the information in your text that supports the following course objectives.

Learning Objectives

Upon successfully completing this chapter, you will be able to:

1. Spell and define the key terms.

2. Identify the primary defense mechanisms of the respiratory system.

3. List and describe disorders of the respiratory system.

4. Explain various diagnostic procedures of the respiratory system.

5. Describe the physician's examination of the respiratory system.

6. Discuss the role of the medical assistant with regard to various diagnostic and therapeutic procedures.

Performance Objectives

Upon successfully completing this chapter, you will be able to:

1. Collect a sputum specimen for culture or cytological examination (Procedure 32-1).

2. Instruct a patient in the use of the peak flowmeter (Procedure 32-2).

3. Administer a nebulized breathing treatment (Procedure 32-3).

4. Perform a pulmonary function test (Procedure 32-4).

CHAPTER OUTLINE	NOTES
Common Respiratory Disorders	
Upper Respiratory Disorders	
Lower Respiratory Disorders	
Common Cancers of the Respiratory System	
Common Diagnostic and Therapeutic Procedures	
Physical Examination of the Respiratory System	
Sputum Culture and Cytology	
Chest Radiography	
Bronchoscopy	
Pulmonary Function Tests	
Arterial Blood Gases	

LEARNING SELF-ASSESSMENT EXERCISES

Key Terms

Define the following key terms:

atelectasis _____

chronic obstructive pulmonary disease (COPD) _____

dyspnea _____

forced expiratory volume (FEV) _____

hemoptysis _____

laryngectomy _____

palliative _____

status asthmaticus _____

thoracentesis _____

tidal volume _____

tracheostomy _____

Matching

Match the term in Part 1 with the correct definition in Part 2.

PART 1

_____ 1. Nebulizer

_____ 2. Tuberculosis

_____ 3. Bronchoscopy

_____ 4. Pulse oximetry

_____ 5. Diagnostic method for evaluating lung disorders

_____ 6. COPD

PART 2

a. Delivery system for a fine mist of bronchodilator to reach the lungs

b. Direct visualization of the trachea and bronchi

c. Wheezing, dyspnea, chronic cough

d. Peak flow meter

e. Percentage of oxygen saturation on capillary blood cells

f. Productive cough, night sweats, malaise, weight loss

Skill Drills

1. List four parts of the traditional chest examination.

   a. _____

   b. _____

   c. _____

   d. _____

2. List the eight defenses of the respiratory system.

   a. _____

   b. _____

   c. _____

   d. _____

   e. _____

f. _____

g. _____

h. _____

Multiple Choice

1. Abnormal breath sounds that may be heard without the use of a stethoscope are
   a. stridor.
   b. wheeze.
   c. stertorous.
   d. All of the above

2. Which one of the following is not an effect of smoking on the airway?
   a. Irritates airway
   b. Increases mucous production
   c. Anesthetizes cilia
   d. Causes tuberculosis

3. In some cases, patients use a rescue inhaler to prevent asthma attacks because
   a. it is recommended by the American Asthma Association.
   b. it expedites delivery of the inhaler used on a daily basis.
   c. asthma sometimes cannot be controlled by the usual daily regimen.
   d. it is part of CPR protocol for asthmatic patients.

4. The respiratory system provides the body with oxygen that all cells need to perform designated functions such as
   a. eliminating carbon dioxide.
   b. eliminating water.
   c. working closely with the cardiovascular system to deliver oxygen to every cell.
   d. All of the above

5. Most common problems of the upper respiratory tract do not include which of the following?
   a. Deep vein thrombosis
   b. Pharyngitis and tonsillitis
   c. Acute rhinitis and sinusitis
   d. Laryngitis

6. Diseases of the lower respiratory tract may be more acute. Circle the one that does not apply.
   a. Asthma
   b. Emphysema
   c. Acute rhinitis
   d. Chronic bronchitis

7. COPD refers to a combination of two diseases. They are
   a. Emphysema and acute bronchitis
   b. Asthma and acute bronchitis
   c. Emphysema and asthma
   d. None of the above

8. Which of the following does not apply to bacterial pneumonia?
   a. Is more sudden and severe in onset
   b. Presents with fever, cough, and chills
   c. Tends to be localized to one lobe or area of the lung
   d. Onset is slow and increases in severity

9. Asthma is a reversible inflammatory process manifested by all but one of the following. Identify the exception.
   a. Constriction of the striated muscle lining the airways
   b. Swelling of the mucous membranes of the airways
   c. Increased mucus production with productive cough
   d. Constriction of the smooth muscle lining the airways and bronchospasm

10. A patient having an asthma attack will present with all the following but one. Identify the exception.
    a. Dyspnea
    b. Cough and wheeze
    c. Cyanosis
    d. Hyperpnea

Critical Thinking Practice

1. Once a patient is diagnosed with COPD, it is usually not reversible. What special challenges may exist for the patient? Why is it not advisable to tell the patient "everything will be all right"?

_____

_____

_____

2. Dr. Taylor believes that Mr. Gray has tuberculosis. Why is it important to teach the patient how to obtain an adequate specimen? When is the best time to obtain one and why?

_____

_____

_____

_____

Patient Education

1. What suggestions would you make to improve the quality of life for a patient with COPD?

_____

_____

_____

_____

33

Cardiology

CHAPTER COMPETENCIES

Review the information in your text that supports the following course objectives.

Learning Objectives

Upon successfully completing this chapter, you will be able to:

1. Spell and define the key terms.

2. List and describe common cardiovascular disorders.

3. Identify and explain common cardiovascular procedures and tests.

4. Describe the role and responsibilities of the medical assistant during cardiovascular examinations and procedures.

5. Discuss the information recorded on a basic 12-lead electrocardiogram.

6. Explain the purpose of a Holter monitor.

Performance Objectives

Upon successfully completing this chapter, you will be able to:

1. Perform a basic 12-lead electrocardiogram (Procedure 33-1).

2. Apply a Holter monitor for a 24-hour test (Procedure 33-2).

CHAPTER OUTLINE	NOTES
Common Cardiovascular Disorders	
Disorders of the Heart	
Carditis	
Congestive Heart Failure	
Myocardial Infarction	
Cardiac Arrhythmia	
Congenital and Valvular Heart Disease	
Disorders of the Blood Vessels	
Atherosclerosis	
Hypertension	
Varicose Veins	
Venous Thrombosis and Pulmonary Embolism	
Cerebrovascular Accident	
Aneurysm	
Anemia	

CHAPTER OUTLINE *continued*	**NOTES**
Common Diagnostic and Therapeutic Procedures	
Physical Examination of the Cardiovascular System	
Electrocardiogram	
Holter Monitor	
Chest Radiography	
Cardiac Stress Test	
Echocardiography	
Cardiac Catheterization and Coronary Arteriography	

LEARNING SELF-ASSESSMENT EXERCISES

Key Terms

Define the following key terms:

aneurysm _____

angina pectoris _____

artifact _____

atherosclerosis _____

bradycardia _____

cardiomegaly _____

cardiomyopathy _____

cerebrovascular accident (CVA) _____

congestive heart failure _____

coronary artery bypass graft _____

electrocardiography _____

endocarditis _____

lead _____

myocardial infarction (MI) _____

myocarditis _____

palpitations _____

percutaneous transluminal coronary angioplasty (PTCA) _____

pericarditis _____

tachycardia _____

transient ischemic attack (TIA) _____

Matching

Match the term in Part 1 with the correct definition in Part 2.

PART 1

_____ 1. TIA

_____ 2. Pericarditis

PART 2

a. An inflammation of the sac that covers the heart

b. A heart rate of more than 100 beats per minute

_____ 3. Cardiomegaly

_____ 4. Bradycardia

_____ 5. Aneurysm

_____ 6. Tachycardia

_____ 7. Murmur

_____ 8. Vasodilator

_____ 9. Anticoagulant

_____ 10. Aortic stenosis

c. An acute episode of reduced blood flow within the cardiovascular system (a result of narrowing of an artery, emboli, or vasospasm)

d. An enlarged heart muscle

e. A heart rate of less than 60 beats per minute

f. A localized dilation in a blood vessel wall

g. Nitroglycerine

h. Narrowing of aorta

i. Cerebrovascular accident

j. Abnormal heart sound

k. Coumadin

l. Dysrhythmia

Skill Drills

1. List the eight questions recommended for obtaining a cardiovascular patient's history.

a. _____

b. _____

c. _____

d. _____

e. _____

f. _____

g. _____

h. _____

2. List six symptoms associated with a transient ischemic attack.

a. _____

b. _____

c. _____

d. _____

e. _____

f. _____

Multiple Choice

1. What statements about the cardiovascular system are accurate?
   a. Disorders of the cardiovascular system may adversely affect other body systems.
   b. Lack of oxygen and nutrients has no effect on symptoms.
   c. Symptoms may include nausea and vomiting, ulcers that do not heal, and pain that increases with ambulation.
   d. *a* and *c*

2. Pericarditis is an inflammation of the sac that covers the heart. Which statements are accurate?
   a. It usually results from a localized infection.
   b. Signs and symptoms include sharp pain in the same locations expected with a myocardial infarction.
   c. Pain increases on inspiration and in lying down.
   d. *b* and *c*

3. Causes of congestive heart failure (CHF) may include
   a. coronary artery disease.
   b. valvular heart disease.
   c. hypotension.
   d. *a* and *b*

4. Cardiac arrhythmia will NOT occur as a
   a. primary disorder.
   b. secondary response to a systemic problem.
   c. result of gradual weight loss.
   d. reaction to drug toxicity or electrolyte imbalance.

5. Which statement is NOT accurate about the sinoatrial (SA) node?
   a. It is the normal pacemaker of the heart.
   b. The SA node is located in the left ventricle.
   c. The rhythm is called sinus rhythm.
   d. An electrical impulse in an adult at rest occurs 60–100 times a minute.

6. An arrhythmia of the SA node may occur
   a. if the SA node is damaged.
   b. if a blockage occurs in the conduction pathway.
   c. with bradycardia or tachycardia.
   d. *a, b,* and *c*

7. Which of the following statements is not accurate about ventricular tachycardia?
   a. Ventricular tachycardia is a serious medical disorder.
   b. It occurs when some of the electrical impulses originate in the ventricles, rather than the SA node.
   c. When the ventricles beat at a very rapid rate, too much blood is pumped out of the heart.
   d. Less blood is pumped into circulation, which means less oxygen to the tissues, causing dizziness, unconsciousness, or cardiac arrest.

8. Which of the following statements about valvular heart disease are accurate?
   a. It is characterized by stenosis and obstructed blood flow or backflow.
   b. Disease of the valves occurs only due to congenital abnormality.

   c. Rheumatic heart disease may occur 10–21 days after an upper respiratory incident caused by group A β-hemolytic streptococci.
   d. *a* and *c*

9. Symptoms of coronary artery disease (CAD) include all but one of the following. Identify the one that is incorrect.
   a. Edema, especially of the extremities
   b. Excessive fatigue or fainting
   c. Unexplained cough without general respiratory symptoms
   d. Angina pectoris

10. Angina pectoris pain will not include
    a. pain radiating to the jaw or neck.
    b. pain radiating to the shoulder, arm, or back.
    c. pain relieved by rest.
    d. migrainelike headache lasting several hours.

11. Which of the following statements is NOT accurate about diagnostic and therapeutic procedures for cardiovascular disorders?
    a. The procedures are only noninvasive.
    b. Some tests may be done during a routine general physical by auscultation.
    c. Chest radiography and ECG are often part of an annual physical examination.
    d. Weight, temperature, pulse, respiratory rate, and blood pressure are an important part of a patient's cardiac history.

12. An electrocardiogram (EKG or ECG) is a graphic record of the electrical current as it progresses through the heart. Which of the following statements is NOT accurate about an ECG?
    a. It cannot be performed on a patient who is experiencing chest pain.
    b. The medical assistant may be responsible for applying the electrodes and running the ECG machine.
    c. ECGs help with diagnosing ischemia, delays in conduction, hypertrophy of cardiac chambers, and arrhythmia.
    d. It can be used to detect heart murmurs.

Critical Thinking Practice

1. Your cousin has been diagnosed with atherosclerosis. Because you work in the health care field, he comes to you to find out what you know about the disease. What can you tell him about ways he may be able to change or reverse the risks associated with the disease?

_____

_____

_____

_____

2. A 57-year-old man phones the medical clinic where you work. He is having what he states is "a little chest pain." How can you differentiate whether he may be having angina or myocardial infarction?

_____

_____

_____

_____

Patient Education

1. Hypertension is a common medical diagnosis and contributes to other circulatory problems. You have been asked to do a presentation to a small group of senior citizens on the topic of essential and malignant hypertension. What are some of the points you would make?

_____

_____

_____

_____

34

Gastroenterology

CHAPTER COMPETENCIES

Review the information in your text that supports the following course objectives.

Learning Objectives

Upon successfully completing this chapter, you will be able to:

1. Spell and define the key terms.

2. Describe common disorders of the alimentary canal and accessory organs.

3. Explain the purpose of various diagnostic procedures associated with the GI system.

4. Discuss the role of the medical assistant in diagnosing and treating disorders of the GI system.

Performance Objectives

Upon successfully completing this chapter, you will be able to:

1. Assist with colon procedures (Procedure 34-1).

2. Instruct a patient on collecting a stool specimen (Procedure 34-2).

3. Test a stool specimen for occult blood (Procedure 34-3).

CHAPTER OUTLINE

	NOTES
Common Gastrointestinal Disorders	
Mouth Disorders	
Esophageal Disorders	
Stomach Disorders	
Intestinal Disorders	
Liver Disorders	
Gallbladder Disorders	
Pancreatic Disorders	
Common Diagnostic and Therapeutic Procedures	
History and Physical Examination of the Gastrointestinal System	
Blood Tests	
Radiologic Studies	
Nuclear Imaging	
Ultrasonography	
Endoscopic Studies	
Fecal Tests	

LEARNING SELF-ASSESSMENT EXERCISES

Key Terms

Define the following key terms:

anorexia _____

ascites _____

dysphagia _____

guaiac _____

hematemesis _____

hepatomegaly _____

hepatotoxin _____

insufflator _____

leukoplakia _____

malocclusion _____

melena _____

metabolism _____

obturator _____

peristalsis _____

sclerotherapy _____

stomatitis _____

turgor _____

Matching

Match the term in Part 1 with the correct definition in Part 2.

PART 1

_____ 1. Anorexia

_____ 2. Ascites

_____ 3. Dysphagia

_____ 4. Guaiac

_____ 5. Hematemesis

_____ 6. Hepatotoxin

_____ 7. Hepatomegaly

PART 2

a. Substance used in laboratory tests for occult blood in the stool

b. Accumulation of serous fluid in the peritoneal cavity

c. Difficulty swallowing

d. Loss of appetite

e. An enlarged liver

f. Vomiting blood or bloody vomitus

g. Substance that can be damaging to the liver.

Skill Drills

1. List five types of hepatitis and tell how each is transmitted.

a. _____

b. _____

c. _____

d. _____

e. _____

2. List five diagnostic tests for liver disorders.

a. _____

b. _____

c. _____

d. _____

e. _____

Multiple Choice

1. Which of the following functions is not part of the gastrointestinal (GI) system?
   a. Ingestion
   b. Digestion
   c. Transportation
   d. Turgor

2. Which of the following is not related to disorders within the GI system?
   a. Alimentary canal (the GI tract)
   b. Liver, gallbladder
   c. Spleen
   d. Gallbladder, pancreas

3. Which of the following statements best explains why dentists and other health care professionals should examine the mouth for disorders?
   a. Insurance forms require the examination and documentation.
   b. Mouth disorders reflect nutrition, digestion, and health status of the patient.
   c. Dental caries will cause further damage if not treated.
   d. Early prevention will decrease loss of teeth.

4. What is malocclusion?
   a. Abnormal contact between the teeth in the upper and lower jaw
   b. An inflammation of the mucous membranes of the mouth
   c. An opportunistic yeast that is always present in the oral cavity
   d. White spots or patches caused by the irritation of cigarette smoke

5. What is a common defect in the esophageal diaphragm?
   a. Bronchospasm
   b. Laryngeal paralysis
   c. Hiatal hernia
   d. Umbilical hernia

6. What are the predisposing factors of esophageal cancer?
   a. Varicose veins, atherosclerosis, hypertension
   b. Chronic gastroesophageal reflux, smoking, drinking alcohol
   c. Spicy diet, alcohol consumption, refined sugar consumption
   d. Dysphagia, overuse of antacids, high fat diet

7. Which organism is thought to cause gastritis by residing in the mucous lining of the stomach and secreting enzymes that attack the mucous membrane?
   a. *Escherichia coli*
   b. Herpes simplex
   c. Tubercle bacillus
   d. *Helicobacter pylori*

8. What is the caustic chemical secreted by the lining of the stomach that may cause erosion if too much is secreted?
   a. Pepsin
   b. Insulin
   c. Hydrochloric acid
   d. Retsina

9. What is usually the first study ordered to aid in diagnosis of a disorder of the GI tract?
   a. Barium enema
   b. CT scan
   c. Flexible sigmoidoscopy
   d. Upper GI series

10. How does the duodenum differ significantly from the stomach?
    a. The pH is alkaline and the mucosa not as well protected.
    b. The pH is acid and the mucosa is more protected than the stomach mucosa.
    c. There is no significant difference.
    d. Ulcerative lesions are more likely to perforate the lining of the small intestine.

Critical Thinking Practice

1. What is celiac sprue? How does this disorder affect an individual on a daily basis? Look in your pantry and read a few food product labels. List some you found that contain wheat or wheat by-products.

_____

_____

_____

_____

2. A common functional disorder of the GI tract is constipation. Working in a clinical setting, you will frequently be counseling people about treatment. What will you tell these patients?

_____

_____

_____

_____

Patient Education

1. A patient needs to have a flexible sigmoidoscopy to determine the cause of abdominal pain accompanied by bloody diarrhea. After you explain the preparation, the patient has concerns about the procedure. Explain both the preparation and the procedure.

_____

_____

_____

_____

35

Neurology

CHAPTER COMPETENCIES

Review the information in your text that supports the following course objectives.

Learning Objectives

Upon successfully completing this chapter, you will be able to:

1. Spell and define the key terms.

2. Identify common diseases of the nervous system.

3. Describe the physical and emotional effects of degenerative nervous system disorders.

4. Explain the medical assistant's role in caring for a patient having a seizure.

5. List potential complications of a spinal cord injury.

6. Name and describe the common procedures for diagnosing nervous system disorders.

Performance Objectives

Upon successfully completing this chapter, you will be able to:

1. Assist with a lumbar puncture (Procedure 35-1).

CHAPTER OUTLINE

	NOTES
Common Nervous System Disorders	
Infectious Disorders	
Degenerative Disorders	
Seizure Disorders	
Developmental Disorders	
Trauma	
Brain Tumors	
Headaches	
Common Diagnostic Tests for Disorders of the Nervous System	
Physical Examination	
Radiological Tests	
Electrical Tests	
Lumbar Puncture	

LEARNING SELF-ASSESSMENT EXERCISES

Key Terms

Define the following key terms:

cephalagia _____

concussion _____

contusion _____

convulsion _____

dysphagia _____

dysphasia _____

electroencephalogram (EEG) _____

herpes zoster _____

meningocele _____

migraine _____

myelogram _____

myelomeningocele _____

Queckenstedt test _____

Romberg test _____

seizure _____

spina bifida occulta _____

Matching

Match the term in Part 1 with the correct definition in Part 2.

PART 1

_____ 1. Cephalagia

_____ 2. Concussion

_____ 3. Dysphagia

_____ 4. Meningocele

_____ 5. Dysphasia

_____ 6. Migraine

_____ 7. Myelogram

PART 2

a. Difficulty swallowing

b. Difficulty speaking

c. Brain injury due to trauma

d. Meninges protruding though the spinal column

e. A headache

f. A type of severe headache, usually unilateral, may appear in cluster

g. Invasive radiological test in which dye is injected into the spinal fluid

Skill Drills

1. List three types of paralysis with cause and results:

Type	Cause	Result

2. List the 12 cranial nerves with their type and function(s).

Nerve (number)	Type	Function(s)

Multiple Choice

1. What are the two divisions of the nervous system?
   a. Autonomic nervous system and central nervous system
   b. Arterial nervous system and vascular nervous system
   c. Central nervous system and peripheral nervous system
   d. Peripheral nervous system and lateral nervous system

2. Disorders of the nervous system include which of the following?
   a. Infectious, degenerative, developmental, traumatic
   b. Irritable, spastic, chronic
   c. Expanding, interfering, blocking
   d. Suppressed, incited, nonreactive

3. Which statement about viral meningitis is not correct?
   a. It usually is precipitated by an upper respiratory infection.
   b. It is characterized by inflammation of the meninges.
   c. It is life threatening.
   d. It most often occurs in children.

4. Which statement about encephalitis is not accurate?
   a. It frequently follows a viral infection of varicella, measles, or mumps.
   b. There is a strain that is transmitted by mosquitos.
   c. Diagnosis is made through a lumbar puncture and analysis of the CSF.
   d. Symptoms may include insomnia, headache, and fever.

5. What is shingles?
   a. A painful outbreak of papules on the skin
   b. Papules caused by herpes zoster, the chickenpox virus
   c. A virus that follows the nerve pathway and has an anesthetic effect
   d. *a* and *b*

6. What new dimension of poliomyelitis has been identified in the past few years?
   a. PPMA syndrome in documented cases of patients who had polio as children.
   b. Acute phase requires palliative and supportive treatment.
   c. The virus can live outside the body for several months.
   d. The incidence has been greatly reduced in the United States.

7. What is lockjaw?
   a. An infection of nervous tissue caused by *Clostridium tetani*
   b. A postanesthesia syndrome caused by reaction to the medication
   c. A clamp used for neurological testing
   d. A spontaneous nervous behavior demonstrated by autistic patients

8. Rabies is caused by a virus that is commonly transmitted by animal saliva through a bite wound. Who is at highest risk?
   a. Farmers
   b. Forest rangers
   c. Children
   d. Patients with suppressed immune systems

9. Reye syndrome is a devastating nervous system illness. What is the cause?
    a. Varicella virus in an acute phase
    b. Combination of a child with viral illness and the use of aspirin
    c. The early phase of multiple sclerosis
    d. Severe reaction to immunizations, such as MMR

10. What is a grand mal seizure?
    a. A four-phase seizure: aura, loss of consciousness, incontinence, recovery
    b. A three-phase seizure: aura, loss of consciousness, postictal
    c. A two-phase seizure: ictal, recovery
    d. A two-phase seizure followed by increased fatigue and drowsiness

Critical Thinking Practice

1. Working in a medical clinic, you will have phone calls regarding children or infants who have hit their heads during some type of accident. Why are children a high-risk group for head injuries? What signs or symptoms result? How are traumatic head injuries diagnosed?

_____

_____

_____

_____

_____

2. What are three types of headaches? How do they differ? How are they treated?

_____

_____

_____

_____

_____

Patient Education

1. Joan Davies phones the clinic to report that her 6 year old has measles, but her main concern is the axillary temperature of 102°. She is worried the child may have a febrile seizure. What will you tell her about management of fever?

_____

_____

_____

_____

_____

36

Allergy and Immunology

CHAPTER COMPETENCIES

Review the information in your text that supports the following course objectives.

Learning Objectives

Upon successfully completing this chapter, you will be able to:

1. Spell and define the key terms.

2. Describe disorders of the lymphatic and immune systems.

3. Identify laboratory tests and clinical procedures related to the lymphatic and immune systems.

4. Describe what is meant by immunity.

5. Explain what a vaccine is and identify some of the common vaccines in use today.

6. Discuss HIV, ARC, and AIDS.

CHAPTER OUTLINE	NOTES
The Lymphatic and Immune Systems	
The Lymphatic System	
The Immune System	
Antigens and Antibodies	
Types of Immunity	
Common Lymphatic Disorders	
Lymphadenitis	
Mononucleosis	
Hodgkin's Disease	
Common Immune Disorders	
Allergies	
Autoimmunity	
Immunodeficiency Diseases	
Common Diagnostic and Therapeutic Procedures	
Allergy Testing	
Laboratory Testing for HIV	

LEARNING SELF-ASSESSMENT EXERCISES

Key Terms

Define the following key terms:

acquired immunodeficiency syndrome (AIDS) _____

allergen _____

allergy _____

antibodies _____

antigen _____

antihistamine _____

attenuated _____

complement _____

ELISA _____

histamine _____

immune globulins _____

immunity _____

interferon _____

Kaposi sarcoma _____

opportunistic infection _____

retrovirus _____

titer _____

toxoid _____

vaccine _____

Western blot _____

Matching

Match the term in Part 1 with the correct definition in Part 2.

PART 1

_____ 1. Antihistamine

_____ 2. Titer

_____ 3. Western blot

_____ 4. immunity

_____ 5. ELISA—enzyme-linked immunosorbent assay.

_____ 6. antibodies

_____ 7. attenuated

PART 2

a. A measure of the amount of an antibody in serum

b. Complex glycoproteins produced by B lymphocytes in response to the presence of an antigen

c. A test used to screen blood for antibody to the AIDS virus

d. A medication that opposes the action of a histamine

e. Diluted or weakened; pertaining to reduced virulence of a pathogenic microorganism

f. A specific, confirmatory antibody test for the presence of HIV in blood

g. The process of becoming insusceptible to a disease

Skill Drills

1. List four types of gamma globulins and their function.

Globulin	Function

2. List 10 signs and symptoms frequently associated with HIV and AIDS.

a. _____

b. _____

c. _____

d. _____

e. _____

f. _____

g. _____

h. _____

i. _____

j. _____

Multiple Choice

1. What are the organs of the lymphatic system?
   a. Tonsils, kidneys, thymus
   b. Tonsils, spleen, thymus
   c. Tonsils, pancreas, thymus
   d. Tonsils, pancreas, spleen

2. How do the organs of the lymphatic system perform their role?
   a. Functioning as filters, removing microorganisms
   b. Stimulating the natural defense mechanisms
   c. Changing the pH of the urinary and respiratory tract
   d. Stimulating increased urine output, increasing body temperature, increasing perspiration

3. Which of the following is not one of the barrier defenses?
   a. Intact skin, digestive enzymes, tears
   b. Interferon, produced by cells that are infected with viruses
   c. Acidity of the genitourinary tract
   d. Protective reflexes (coughing, sneezing, vomiting, diarrhea)

4. What type of immunity is acquired through the injection of gamma globulins, or antibodies, after presumed exposure to an infectious disease?
   a. Passive acquired natural immunity
   b. Active acquired artificial immunity
   c. Active acquired natural immunity
   d. Passive acquired artificial immunity

5. A vaccine made with live virus, treated with heat to weaken them, is what type of vaccine?
   a. Titer
   b. Booster
   c. Attenuated
   d. Toxoid

6. What are infections that result from a defective immune system that cannot defend against pathogens normally found in the environment?
   a. Opportunistic
   b. Debilitating
   c. Secondary
   d. Low grade

7. The Epstein-Barr virus causes which of the following disorders?
   a. Lymphadenitis
   b. Mononucleosis
   c. Hodgkin's disease
   d. HIV

8. What is an individual's hypersensitivity reaction to particular antigens called?
   a. Autoimmunity
   b. Acquired immunity
   c. Allergy
   d. Barrier defense

9. Which of the following statements about Hodgkin's disease is not accurate?
   a. There is a high probability of cure with available treatments.
   b. It is diagnosed by identifying the Reed-Sternberg cell in the lymph nodes.
   c. Symptoms are fever, weakness, anorexia, and weight loss.
   d. It most commonly affects young women.

10. For what specific reason should emergency equipment be in date and available in an allergist's office?
    a. Because of potential anaphylactic reactions to testing and immunizations
    b. Patients often faint because of the high number of scratch tests.
    c. Many patients who have allergies also have asthma.
    d. Allergy staff members are not as well trained in CPR as those in other settings.

Critical Thinking Practice

1. A patient comes to the allergy clinic for testing. *Why should the patient not take antihistamines prior to allergy testing?* The patient will be given 24 scratch tests for various environmental proteins: dust mites, molds, animal dander, plant antigens, etc. *How can you tell if the test result is positive? Why should the patient remain in the office at least 30 minutes after the testing is complete?*

_____

_____

_____

_____

2. What are the nonspecific defenses? What role does interferon play in the defense system? Why is it not necessary to treat a low-grade fever with antipyretics?

_____

_____

_____

_____

Patient Education

1. The doctor is referring one of the patients to an allergist for testing. The patient is very apprehensive. Explain scratch tests, intradermal injections, and patch tests to the patient to help reduce anxiety.

_____

_____

_____

_____

37

Urology

CHAPTER COMPETENCIES

Review the information in your text that supports the following course objectives.

Learning Objectives

Upon successfully completing this chapter, you will be able to:

1. Spell and define the key terms.

2. Identify and explain the primary organs of the urinary system.

3. List and describe the disorders of the urinary system and the male reproductive system.

4. Describe and explain the purpose of various diagnostic procedures associated with the urinary system.

5. Discuss the role of the medical assistant in diagnosing and treating disorders of the urinary system and the male reproductive system.

Performance Objectives

Upon successfully completing this chapter, you will be able to:

1. Perform a female urinary catheterization (Procedure 37-1).

2. Perform a male urinary catheterization (Procedure 37-2).

3. Instruct a male patient on the self-testicular examination (Procedure 37-3).

CHAPTER OUTLINE	NOTES
Common Urinary Disorders	
Renal Failure	
Calculi	
Tumors	
Hydronephrosis	
Urinary System Infections	
Common Disorders of the Male Reproductive System	
Benign Prostatic Hyperplasia	
Prostate Cancer	
Testicular Cancer	
Hydrocele	
Cryptorchidism	
Inguinal Hernia	
Infections	
Impotence	

CHAPTER OUTLINE   *continued*

Common Diagnostic and Therapeutic Procedures	NOTES
Urinalysis	
Blood Tests	
Cystoscopy, or Cystourethroscopy	
Intravenous Pyelogram and Retrograde Pyelogram	
Ultrasound	
Rectal and Scrotal Examinations	
Vasectomy	

LEARNING SELF-ASSESSMENT EXERCISES

Key Terms

Define the following key terms:

anuria _____

blood urea nitrogen _____

catheterization _____

cystoscopy _____

dialysis _____

dysuria _____

enuresis _____

hematuria _____

impotence _____

incontinence _____

intravenous pyelogram (IVP) _____

lithotripsy _____

nephrostomy _____

nocturia _____

oliguria _____

prostate-specific antigen _____

proteinuria _____

psychogenic _____

pyuria _____

retrograde pyelogram _____

specific gravity _____

ureterostomy _____

urinalysis _____

urinary frequency _____

Matching

Match the term in Part 1 with the correct definition in Part 2.

PART I

_____ 1. Anuria

_____ 2. Specific gravity

_____ 3. Pyuria

_____ 4. Psychogenic

_____ 5. Proteinuria

_____ 6. Lithotripsy

_____ 7. Oliguria

PART 2

a. Crushing of a stone by use of sound waves

b. Of psychological origin

c. The relative density of a liquid such as urine

d. The presence of protein in the urine

e. The presence of pus in the urine

f. Scanty urine production

g. Failure of the kidneys to produce urine

Skill Drills

1. List four causes for acute renal failure.
   a. _____
   b. _____
   c. _____
   d. _____

2. List four causes for chronic renal failure.
   a. _____
   b. _____
   c. _____
   d. _____

Multiple Choice

1. What is the name of the surgical creation of an opening to the outside of the body from the ureter to facilitate the drainage of urine from an obstructed kidney?
   a. Ureterostomy
   b. Ileostomy
   c. Nephrostomy
   d. Cystoscopy

2. What is dysuria?
   a. Small amount of urine
   b. Inability to urinate
   c. Pain or difficulty when urinating
   d. Pus in the urine

3. What is an intravenous pyelogram (IVP)?
   a. Direct visualization of the urinary bladder through a special instrument
   b. Radiography using contrast medium to evaluate kidney function
   c. Radiography of the urinary tract using contrast medium injected into the bladder and ureters

d. Procedure for introducing a flexible tube into the bladder to drain urine

4. Which of the following statements is not accurate about the lithotripsy procedure?
   a. Treatment is required for both small and large renal calculi.
   b. The stones are crushed using ultrasound.
   c. The chemical makeup of the stones is analyzed.
   d. The procedure is done at a surgery center.

5. Why is peritoneal dialysis not appropriate for patients who have had invasive abdominal surgery?
   a. It will cause the patient more discomfort.
   b. The risk of puncturing internal organs is greater.
   c. Surgery leaves scar tissue that disrupts the continuity of the peritoneal membrane.
   d. There is no reason why these patients cannot have peritoneal dialysis.

6. How is a rectoscope used during a TURP?
   a. Inserted through the male urethra to drain the bladder

b. Inserted through the male urethra, rotated into the prostate

c. Suprapubic insertion into the bladder

d. Inserted rectally and rotated into the prostate

7. Which of the following is not a probable symptom of renal calculi?
   a. Severe low abdominal pain
   b. Severe flank (midback) pain
   c. Pale, clammy, with nausea and vomiting
   d. Hematuria

8. What are the symptoms of hydronephrosis?
   a. Flank pain, hematuria, pyuria, fever, and chills
   b. Abdominal pain, pyuria, fever, and chills
   c. Flank pain, hematuria, fever, and chills
   d. Hematuria, frequency

9. Which of the following disorders may occur in children 1 to 4 weeks after a streptococcal infection?
   a. Renal calculi
   b. Kidney failure
   c. Glomerulonephritis
   d. Pyelonephritis

10. Why are women more likely than men to experience cystitis?
    a. The mucous membrane of the urethra has a more receptive pH.
    b. The urethra is shorter so it is easier for microorganisms to spread to the bladder.
    c. Some women have never been taught to wipe from front to back after voiding.
    d. It is not known why women tend to have cystitis more than men.

Critical Thinking Practice

1. Many couples choose vasectomy as a birth control option. Though it is a choice, some men are still very anxious about having such personal surgery. Explain the procedure and follow-up in lay terms for a patient.

_____

_____

_____

_____

2. Some men worry about sexual function following a vasectomy. What can you say to reassure a patient and why is follow-up with the doctor important?

_____

_____

_____

_____

Patient Education

1. Jeff Sands, a college student, has come in for a sports physical. He tells you he has been lifting increasingly heavy weights. His coach told him to ask to be checked for inguinal hernia, and he is curious about this. Explain to him what the hernia is and why it occurs in men.

_____

_____

_____

_____

38

Obstetrics and Gynecology

CHAPTER COMPETENCIES

Review the information in your text that supports the following course objectives.

Learning Objectives

Upon successfully completing this chapter, you will be able to:

1. Spell and define the key terms.

2. List and describe common gynecological and obstetric disorders.

3. Identify your role in the care of gynecological or obstetric patients.

4. Describe the components of prenatal and postpartum patient care.

5. Explain the diagnostic and therapeutic procedures associated with the female reproductive system.

6. Identify the various methods of contraception.

7. Describe menopause.

Performance Objectives

Upon successfully completing this chapter, you will be able to:

1. Instruct the patient on the breast self-examination (Procedure 38-1).

2. Assist with the pelvic examination and Pap smear (Procedure 38-2).

3. Assist with colposcopy and cervical biopsy (Procedure 38-3).

CHAPTER OUTLINE	NOTES
Gynecological Disorders	
Dysfunctional Uterine Bleeding	
Premenstrual Syndrome	
Endometriosis	
Uterine Prolapse and Displacement	
Leiomyomas	
Ovarian Cysts	
Gynecological Cancers	
Infertility	
Sexually Transmitted Diseases	
Common Diagnostic and Therapeutic Procedures	
The Gynecological Examination	
Colposcopy	
Hysterosalpingography	
Dilation and Curettage	

CHAPTER OUTLINE *continued*	NOTES
Obstetric Care	
Diagnosis of Pregnancy	
First Prenatal Visit	
Subsequent Prenatal Visits	
Onset of Labor	
Postpartum Care	
Obstetric Disorders	
Ectopic Pregnancy	
Hyperemesis Gravidarum	
Abortion	
Preeclampsia and Eclampsia	
Placenta Previa and Abruptio Placentae	
Common Obstetric Tests and Procedures	
Pregnancy Test	
Alpha Fetoprotein	
Fetal Ultrasonography	
Contraction Stress Test and Nonstress Test	
Contraception	
Menopause	

LEARNING SELF-ASSESSMENT EXERCISES

Key Terms

Define the following key terms:

abortion _____

amenorrhea _____

amniocentesis _____

Braxton-Hicks contractions _____

Chadwick's sign _____

colpocleisis _____

colporrhaphy _____

colposcopy _____

culdocentesis _____

curettage _____

cystocele _____

dysmenorrhea _____

dyspareunia _____

Goodell's sign _____

gravid _____

gravida _____

gravidity _____

hirsutism _____

human chorionic gonadotropin (HCG) _____

hysterosalpingogram _____

labor _____

laparoscopy _____

lightening _____

lochia _____

menorrhagia _____

menarche _____

menses _____

metrorrhagia _____

multipara _____

nulligravida _____

nullipara _____

parity _____

pessary _____

polymenorrhea _____

primigravida _____

primipara _____

proteinuria _____

puerperium _____

rectocele _____

salpingo-oophorectomy _____

Matching

Match the term in Part 1 with the correct definition in Part 2.

PART I

_____ 1. Parity

_____ 2. Metrorrhagia

_____ 3. Menorrhagia

_____ 4. Hirsutism

_____ 5. Gravida

_____ 6. Dysmenorrheal

_____ 7. Cystocele

_____ 8. Dyspareunia

_____ 9. Colpocleisis

_____ 10. Lightening

PART 2

a. Surgery to occlude the vagina

b. Pregnancies that resulted in a viable birth

c. Painful menstruation

d. Irregular uterine bleeding

e. Painful coitus or sexual intercourse

f. Abnormal or excessive growth of hair in women

g. The descent of the fetus farther into the pelvis

h. Herniation of the urinary bladder into the vagina

i. A pregnant woman

j. Excessive bleeding during menstruation

Skill Drills

1. List seven warning signs of breast cancer.
   a. _____
   b. _____
   c. _____
   d. _____
   e. _____
   f. _____
   g. _____
   h. _____

2. List four warning signs of ovarian cancer.
   a. _____
   b. _____
   c. _____
   d. _____

Multiple Choice

1. What is amenorrhea?
   a. Before menarche or onset of menses
   b. A condition of not menstruating
   c. Painful menstrual cycle
   d. Exceptionally short menstrual cycle

2. What is the period of time (about 6 weeks) from childbirth until reproductive structures return to normal?
   a. Puerperium
   b. Menarche
   c. Metrorrhagia
   d. Dyspareunia

3. What is the gestational status of a woman who has given birth to more than one viable fetus?
   a. Gravida
   b. Multipara
   c. Multigravida
   d. Polipara

4. What is the process of viewing the internal abdominal cavity and its contents?
   a. Cystoscopy
   b. Colposcopy
   c. Endoscopy
   d. Laparoscopy

5. What is the condition of having abnormally frequent menstrual periods?
   a. Parity
   b. Polymenorrhea
   c. Dysmenorrhea
   d. Multigravida

6. What is the softening of the cervix that occurs in early pregnancy called?
   a. Braxton's sign
   b. Hick's sign

   c. Goodell's sign
   d. Ortolani's sign

7. What is the procedure of scraping a body cavity such as the female uterus?
   a. Pap smear
   b. Curettage
   c. Cystocele
   d. Culdocentesis

8. What is a salpingo-oophorectomy?
   a. Suturing of the vagina
   b. Surgical puncture of, and aspiration of fluid from, the vaginal cul-de-sac for diagnostic/therapeutic purposes
   c. Surgical procedure for tying the fallopian tubes to prevent pregnancy
   d. Surgical excision of both the fallopian tube and the ovary

9. What is a radiograph called that is taken of the uterus and fallopian tubes after injection with contrast medium?
   a. Uterosalpingogram
   b. Hysterosalpingogram
   c. Salpingogram
   d. Hysterogram

10. What is an amniocentesis?
    a. Herniation of the rectum into the vaginal area
    b. Surgery to occlude the vagina
    c. A device that supports the uterus when inserted into the vagina
    d. Puncture of the amniotic sac to remove fluid for testing

Critical Thinking Practice

1. Make two columns and parallel the signs and symptoms of preeclampsia and eclampsia. Also, explain treatment for each.

_____

_____

_____

_____

2. Karen Jung, a 24-year-old primipara patient in her 14th gestational week, phones the office to report persistent nausea and vomiting. She has not been able to keep food or liquid down for 48 hours. She thought it was a bad case of morning sickness but now feels dehydrated and weak. What do you think the treatment will include? Is it something that may be accomplished in the medical clinic?

_____

_____

_____

_____

Patient Education

1. A 44-year-old woman comes in for her annual physical. As you complete the form for her Pap smear, you ask when the first day of her last menstrual cycle occurred. She states it has been 3–4 months ago and voices some dread about "going through the change." What can you tell her about menopause that may help her think about the process in a less anxious manner?

_____

_____

_____

_____

39

Pediatrics

CHAPTER COMPETENCIES

Review the information in your text that supports the following course objectives.

Learning Objectives

Upon successfully completing this chapter, you will be able to:

1. Spell and define the key terms.

2. List safety precautions for the pediatric office.

3. Explain the difference between a well-child and a sick-child visit.

4. List types and schedule of immunizations.

5. Describe the types of feelings a child might have during an office visit.

6. List and explain how to record the anthropometric measurements obtained in a pediatric visit.

7. Identify two injection sites to use on an infant and two used on a child.

8. Describe the role of the parent during the office visit.

9. List the names, symptoms, and treatment for common pediatric illnesses.

Performance Objectives

Upon successfully completing this chapter, you will be able to:

1. Measure infant weight and length (Procedure 39-1).

2. Measure head and chest circumference (Procedure 39-2).

3. Apply a pediatric urine collection device (Procedure 39-3).

CHAPTER OUTLINE	NOTES
The Pediatric Practice	
Safety	
Types of Pediatric Office Visits	
Child Development	
Psychological Aspects of Care	
Physiological Aspects of Care	
The Pediatric Physical Examination	
The Pediatric History	
Obtaining and Recording Measurements and Vital Signs	
Using Restraints	
Administering Medications	
Oral Medications	
Injections	

CHAPTER OUTLINE *continued*

CHAPTER OUTLINE *continued*	NOTES
Collecting a Urine Specimen	
Understanding Child Abuse	
Pediatric Illnesses and Disorders	
Impetigo	
Meningitis	
Encephalitis	
Tetanus	
Cerebral Palsy	
Croup	
Epiglottitis	
Cystic Fibrosis	
Asthma	
Otitis Media	
Tonsillitis	
Obesity	
Attention Deficit Hyperactivity Disorder	

LEARNING SELF-ASSESSMENT EXERCISES

Key Terms

Define the following key terms:

aspiration _____

autonomous _____

congenital anomaly _____

immunization _____

neonatologist _____

pediatrician _____

pediatrics _____

psychosocial _____

restrain _____

sick-child visit _____

varicella zoster _____

well-child visit _____

Matching

Match the age range in Part 1 with the correct development stage in Part 2.

PART 1

_____ 1. Infancy (0–1 year)

_____ 2. Toddler (1–3 years)

PART 2

a. Self-control—initiative

b. Sits and stands—trust

_____ 3. Preschool (3–6 years)

_____ 4. School age (6–12 years)

_____ 5. Adolescent (12–18 years)

c. Identity and place in the world—identity

d. Growth rate slows—autonomy

e. Self-concept—industry

Skill Drills

1. List five types of feelings children may have about being in a doctor's office.

_____

_____

_____

_____

2. List five warning signs of child abuse.

_____

_____

_____

_____

Multiple Choice

1. Which of the following may be a hidden, or nonobvious, sign of abuse?
   a. Dislocations
   b. Bruises
   c. Burns
   d. Poor hygiene

2. If a child has a febrile seizure during an illness, what are the long-term implications?
   a. The child will probably be subject to grand mal seizures as an adult.
   b. This increases the likelihood that child will be epileptic.
   c. This will lead to epilepsy, but only a mild form.
   d. This does not mean that the child will be prone to seizures.

3. Why should parents be advised never to give aspirin to young children with viral fevers?
   a. Tylenol has proven to be a better antipyretic in most cases.
   b. Aspirin has been associated with a condition known as Reye syndrome.
   c. Viral fevers do not respond to aspirin.
   d. Studies are inconclusive about the use of aspirin in pediatric patients.

4. Which of the following statements about laryngotracheobronchitis is not accurate?
   a. Whooping cough is the lay term.
   b. Treatment may include hospitalization, cool mist vaporizers, and medications to decrease the swelling.
   c. It is caused by a viral infection of the larynx resulting in swelling and narrowing of the airway.
   d. Symptoms include a high-pitched crowing wheeze (stridor) on inspiration and a sharp barking cough.

5. Cystic fibrosis is an inherited disease that affects the exocrine glands of the body. Which statement is correct?
   a. The most serious complications are usually respiratory.
   b. The most serious complications are of the circulatory system.
   c. Current treatment of cystic fibrosis includes antihypertensives.
   d. There is little hope for a cure.

6. What is the primary reason for restraining a child during a medical examination?
   a. So the parents will not have to hold the child.
   b. Some children will not cooperate but will kick and hit the examiner.
   c. To protect the child from injury.
   d. To help get the examination over with as quickly as possible.

7. What is the least important reason to weigh a child at each visit?
   a. So the parents may keep an accurate medical history in the baby book.
   b. Many medication doses are based on weight.

c. Growth charts are kept on file to check for normal growth factors.

d. It helps to identify nutritional or metabolic problems.

8. When is poliomyelitis (IPV) 0.5 mL given subcutaneously (SC)?

a. At 4 months, 8 months, 12 months, and 4–6 years

b. At 6 months, 12 months, and 2 years

c. At 2 months, 4 months, 6–12 months, and 4–6 years.

d. At 5 years, 10 years, and prior to high school

9. Varicella zoster (VZV) is also known as what?

a. Chickenpox

b. Smallpox

c. Measles

d. Mumps

10. What is the least important reason for the medical assistant to have a broad knowledge of child growth and developmental patterns?

a. To know when to administer childhood immunizations

b. To anticipate age-appropriate behavior

c. To provide proper psychological support and physical care

d. So expectations of actions are within the child's developmental age

Critical Thinking Practice

1. What is pharyngitis? How is it diagnosed and what might be the role for a medical assistant? What treatment will be prescribed?

_____

_____

_____

_____

2. What safety precautions are important to address in a pediatric office?

_____

_____

_____

_____

Patient Education

1. The mother of a 7 year old phones to talk to the medical assistant. She is concerned that her child may have ADHD, and she wonders how it is diagnosed. What can you tell her?

_____

_____

_____

_____

40

Geriatrics

CHAPTER COMPETENCIES

Review the information in your text that supports the following course objectives.

Learning Objectives

Upon successfully completing this chapter, you will be able to:

1. Spell and define the key terms.

2. Explain how aging affects thought processes.

3. Describe methods to increase compliance with health maintenance programs among the elderly.

4. Discuss communication problems that may occur with the elderly and list steps to maintain open communication.

5. Recognize and describe the coping mechanisms used by the elderly to deal with multiple losses.

6. Name the risk factors and signs of elder abuse.

7. Explain the types of long-term care facilities available.

8. Describe the effects of aging on the way the body processes medication.

9. Discuss the responsibility of medical assistants with regard to teaching elderly patients.

10. List and describe physical changes and diseases common to the aging process.

CHAPTER OUTLINE	NOTES
Concepts of Aging	
Reinforcing Medical Compliance in the Elderly	
Reinforcing Mental Health in the Elderly	
Coping with Aging	
Alcoholism	
Suicide	
Long-term Care	
Elder Abuse	
Medications and the Elderly	
Systemic Changes in the Elderly	
Diseases of the Elderly	
Parkinson's Disease	
Alzheimer's Disease	

CHAPTER OUTLINE *continued*	NOTES
Maintaining Optimum Health	
Exercise	
Diet	
Safety	

LEARNING SELF-ASSESSMENT EXERCISES

Key Terms

Define the following key terms:

activities of daily living (ADL) _____

biotransform _____

bradykinesia _____

cataracts _____

cerebrovascular accident (CVA) _____

compliance _____

degenerative joint disease (DJD) _____

dementia _____

dysphagia _____

gerontologist _____

glaucoma _____

Kegel exercises _____

keratosis (senile) _____

kyphosis (dowager's hump) _____

lentigines _____

osteoporosis _____

potentiation _____

presbycusis _____

presbyopia _____

senility _____

syncope _____

transient ischemic attack (TIA) _____

vertigo _____

Matching

Match the term in Part 1 with the correct definition in Part 2.

PART 1

_____ 1. Dysphagia

_____ 2. Presbycusis

_____ 3. Presbyopia

_____ 4. Senility

PART 2

a. Vision change (farsightedness) associated with aging

b. Sensation of whirling of oneself or the environment

c. Inability or difficulty in swallowing

d. A generalized mental deterioration associated with the elderly

_____ 5. Vertigo

_____ 6. Compliance

_____ 7. Gerontologists

e. Loss of hearing associated with aging

f. Specialists who study the processes of aging

g. The willingness of a patient to follow a prescribed course of treatment

Skill Drills

1. List four systems that benefit from exercise and describe how it is beneficial.

_____

_____

_____

_____

2. List five challenges the elderly face in trying to maintain good nutritional status.

a. _____

b. _____

c. _____

d. _____

e. _____

Multiple Choice

1. What is keratosis (senile)?
   a. Premalignant overgrowth or thickening of epithelium or horny layer of the skin
   b. Tan or brown macules on skin after prolonged sun exposure; also known as liver spots
   c. Abnormal porosity of the bone found in the elderly, predisposing the affected bony tissue to fracture
   d. Abnormally slow voluntary movements

2. Which of the following is not one of seven stages of Alzheimer's disease?
   a. Presenile dementia
   b. Inability to remember facts, faces, and names
   c. Late dementia
   d. Acceptance of the disease process

3. What type of care will the patient in stage VII, late dementia, require?
   a. Assisted living facility with minimal supervision
   b. Full-time care and is rarely seen in the office setting
   c. Assistance with meals, but still eating all textures with little difficulty
   d. Assistance with bathing and meals, but otherwise independent

4. Which of the following is not appropriate when dealing with a patient who does not remember you?
   a. Respond with the utmost patience and compassion.
   b. Speak calmly and without condescension.

   c. Remind the patient how many times he or she has seen you in the past.
   d. Be nonthreatening and remind the patient who you are and what you must do.

5. Why may Parkinson patients become depressed and embarrassed?
   a. They have an increased problem with swallowing and choking.
   b. They must use public restrooms designed for the handicapped.
   c. There is increased media information available to the public.
   d. They are aware of the outward signs of the disease.

6. Which of the following are most likely reasons why a patient is not compliant with a prescribed treatment plan?
   a. Poor hearing, lack of understanding, forgetfulness
   b. Fixed income and unable to pay for recommended medications or treatments
   c. Lack of interest or depressed about aging and losing independence
   d. All of the above

7. Why do Americans stereotype the elderly in a subtle and usually unconscious way?
   a. To dissociate ourselves from the prospect of growing old
   b. Mass marketing is geared toward antiaging products.

c. Fitness is encouraged by burgeoning athletic clubs.

d. Antiaging drugs are big business.

8. Why is adjusting to pain or disability often easier than adjusting to loss of social interaction or dependency?

a. Adapting to a role of dependency is very difficult (loss of mobility to outside world).

b. After a lifetime of social interaction may come loss of peers and family members

c. Mental pain is more intense than physical pain.

d. *a* and *b*

9. Many elderly patients feel overwhelmed with stress and grief. How can you best help these patients to cope with stress?

a. Listen to their fears and concerns, respecting their right to have these feelings.

b. Encourage them to think about more positive things.

c. Suggest they speak to the doctor about an antidepressant.

d. Give them some hobby ideas or a list of places to volunteer.

10. What coping behavior will some elderly patients adopt that may be mistaken for dementia, TIAs, or other CNS impairments?

a. Smoking marijuana

b. Drinking alcohol

c. Buying street drugs such as heroine or angel dust

d. Mixing Rx pain medications with additional OTC pain medications

Critical Thinking Practice

1. What are some examples of passive and active neglect that may constitute elder abuse? How might you become of aware of these examples while working as a medical assistant?

_____

_____

_____

_____

2. If you become of aware that an elderly patient may be the victim of elder abuse, what should you do? Who is responsible for reporting possible elder abuse? Who are the authorities?

_____

_____

_____

_____

Patient Education

1. What home safety tips can you give the adult children of an aging parent?

_____

_____

_____

_____

41

Introduction to the Clinical Laboratory

CHAPTER COMPETENCIES

Review the information in your text that supports the following course objectives.

Learning Objectives

Upon successfully completing this chapter, you will be able to:

1. Spell and define the key terms.

2. List reasons for laboratory testing.

3. Outline the medical assistant's responsibility in the clinical laboratory.

4. Name the kinds of laboratories where medical assistants work and the functions of each.

5. List the types of personnel in laboratories and describe their jobs.

6. Name the types of departments found in most large laboratories and give their purposes.

7. Explain how to use a package insert to determine the procedure for a laboratory test.

8. List the equipment found in most small laboratories and give the purpose of each.

9. List and describe the parts of a microscope.

10. Explain the significance of the Clinical Laboratory Improvement Amendments and how to follow their regulations to ensure quality control.

11. Define OSHA and state its purpose.

12. List the laboratory safety guidelines.

Performance Objective

Upon successfully completing this chapter, you will be able to:

1. Care for the microscope (Procedure 41-1).

CHAPTER OUTLINE	NOTES
Types of Laboratories	
Reference Laboratory	
Hospital Laboratory	
Physician's Office Laboratory	
Laboratory Departments	
Hematology	
Coagulation	
Clinical Chemistry	
Toxicology	
Urinalysis	
Immunohematology	

CHAPTER OUTLINE *continued*	NOTES
Immunology	
Microbiology	
Anatomical and Surgical Pathology	
Laboratory Personnel	
Physician Office Laboratory Testing	
Laboratory Equipment	
Cell Counter	
Microscope	
Chemistry Analyzers	
Centrifuges	
Incubator	
Refrigerators and Freezers	
Glassware	
Laboratory Safety	
Occupational Safety and Health Administration (OSHA)	
Safety Guidelines	
Incident Reports	
Clinical Laboratory Improvement Amendments	
Levels of Testing	
Laboratory Standards	

LEARNING SELF-ASSESSMENT EXERCISES

Key Terms

Define the following key terms:

aerosol _____

anticoagulant _____

calibration _____

capillary action _____

centrifugal force _____

Clinical Laboratory Improvement Amendments (CLIA) _____

material safety data sheet (MSDS) _____

National Committee for Clinical Laboratory Standards (NCCLS) _____

normal values _____

quality assurance (QA) _____

quality control (QC) _____

reagents _____

reportable range _____

specimens _____

Matching

Match the term in Part 1 with the correct definition in Part 2.

PART 1

_____ 1. Toxicology

_____ 2. Partial prothrombin time

_____ 3. Hematology department

_____ 4. POL

_____ 5. QC procedures

_____ 6. Coagulation

PART 2

a. PTT

b. Laboratory in a doctor's office that performs only a few types of tests on a limited number of patients

c. Testing measuring blood levels of both therapeutic drugs and drugs of abuse

d. Testing evaluating reaction to injury of blood vessels and affect of medications like Coumadin

e. Checking instruments, performing daily maintenance, and running control specimens

f. Common tests done include CBC, WBC, RBC, Hgb, Hct, differential, ESR, etc.

Skill Drills

1. List seven types of glassware used in a medical laboratory.

a. _____

b. _____

c. _____

d. _____

e. _____

f. _____

g. _____

2. List the seven important sections of a Material Safety Data Sheet.

a. _____

b. _____

c. _____

d. _____

e. _____

f. _____

g. _____

Multiple Choice

1. What does the simplest cell counter count?
   a. Only red and white blood cells and performs hemoglobin and hematocrit testing
   b. Only white cells
   c. Only red cells
   d. Only hemoglobin and hematocrit determinations

2. What type of microscope is commonly used in the medical office?
   a. 7× to 45× trinocular stereo zoom boom microscope
   b. 3.75× to 35× stereo zoom boom microscope
   c. Articulating arm stereo zoom boom microscope
   d. Compound microscope—a two-lens system in which ocular and objective lenses together provide the total magnification.

3. Which of the following statements is a very important guideline for use of the centrifuge?
   a. Only spin two tubes at a time.
   b. It is permissible to open the lid before the spinning stops.
   c. Tubes must always be counterbalanced.
   d. Centrifuges require no routine cleaning.

4. Which statement is not correct?
   a. Refrigerators in laboratories are used to store reagents, kits, and patient specimens.
   b. The temperature is critical and must be measured and recorded daily.
   c. Food may be stored in these refrigerators if food containers are covered.
   d. They vary in size and can be purchased according to office needs and space.

5. Why is laboratory testing most commonly ordered?
   a. Detecting and diagnosing disease
   b. As part of pharmaceutical research project
   c. Meeting legal requirements (e.g., drug testing, a marriage license)
   d. In response to patient request

6. Which of the following is not accurate information about a reference laboratory?
   a. It is a large facility in which thousands of tests are performed each day.
   b. Direct patient contact is limited to its satellite specimen procurement stations.
   c. It receives specimens from hospitals and clinics from the region it serves.
   d. The specimens are mailed as low-priority shipments.

7. What are the most common tests done in a clinic laboratory?
   a. Blood glucose, Lyme disease, medication toxicity, mononucleosis and streptococcus tests
   b. Urinalysis, blood cell counts, blood glucose, rapid streptococcus and pregnancy tests
   c. Blood typing, Rh immune globulin (RhIg), and HIV testing
   d. Mononucleosis, streptococcus, diabetic testing, and kidney function

8. What are the three types of hazards found in a laboratory?
   a. Liquid, gas (flame), ergonomic
   b. Splash or spray, inhalation, skin contact
   c. Physical, chemical, and biological hazards
   d. Noise pollution, eyestrain, neck pain

9. What does BLUE represent in the National Fire Protection Association (NFPA) classification system section?
   a. Health hazard
   b. Fire hazard
   c. Reactive hazard
   d. Blank to list specific hazard

10. According to OSHA requirements, what are employers required to provide free to their employees?
    a. Hepatitis C vaccine series
    b. Testing for sexually transmitted diseases (STDs)
    c. Hepatitis B virus vaccine series
    d. Hepatitis laboratory screen to establish baseline of status

11. If there is a biological spill, what is the best order for safe cleanup?
    a. Cover spill, flood with disinfectant, put on gloves, wipe up, dispose of waste
    b. Put on gloves, cover spill, flood with disinfectant, wipe up, dispose of waste
    c. Flood with disinfectant, cover the area, put on gloves, wipe up, dispose of waste
    d. Put on gloves, cover the area with disposable towels, wipe up, dispose of waste

Critical Thinking Practice

1. Briefly explain who or what OSHA is and how the standards are meant to provide a safe work environment.

_____

_____

_____

_____

2. OSHA Bloodborne Pathogens Standard has set some specific training and safety provisions for the employer to make available for the employees. What are these provisions?

_____

_____

_____

_____

Patient Education

1. A patient has been sent to your medical clinic for a urine drug screen. She knows her employment may hinge on the results of the test, and she asks if there is any chance that someone else's laboratory results will be reported as hers. Explain the Chain of Custody procedure in lay terms. The purpose of having each person who has a role in processing the specimen rechecks the name on the sample and on the accompanying document before signing the Chain of Custody form. This extra precaution is to ensure the lab results will be hers.

_____

_____

_____

_____

2. A patient phones your medical clinic and states that the surgeon he was referred to is going to be doing abdominal surgery in 2 weeks. The patient wants to come in to the clinic to have blood taken and held on reserve in case he has to have a blood transfusion. Explain to the patient why blood for transfusion is not taken in the clinic setting.

_____

_____

_____

_____

42 Microbiology

CHAPTER COMPETENCIES

Review the information in your text that supports the following course objectives.

Learning Objectives

Upon successfully completing this chapter, you will be able to:

1. Spell and define the key terms.

2. List and describe primary microorganisms.

3. Identify various bacterial illustrations.

4. Describe how bacteria are named.

5. Describe the classifications of fungi, rickettsiae, chlamydiae, protozoa, and metazoa.

6. State the factors necessary for microbial growth.

7. Describe the medical assistant's responsibilities in microbiological testing.

8. List the most common types of microbiological specimens collected in the physician's office laboratory.

9. State the differences between mixed cultures, secondary cultures, and pure cultures.

10. Describe the different types of medium used for microbial testing.

11. List the steps used in caring for media plates.

12. List each step in Gram staining and state the purpose of each step.

13. State the purpose of sensitivity testing and give the meaning of sensitive, resistant, and intermediate results.

Performance Objectives

Upon successfully completing this chapter, you will be able to:

1. Label and identify specimens for transportation and handling (Procedure 42-1).

2. Prepare a wet-mount slide.

3. Prepare a dry specimen smear (Procedure 42-2).

4. Prepare a specimen with Gram stain (Procedure 42-3).

5. Inoculate a tube of broth medium.

6. Inoculate a culture and conduct sensitivity testing (Procedure 42-4).

CHAPTER OUTLINE	NOTES
Microbiological Life Forms	
Bacteria	
Rickettsias and Chlamydiae	
Fungi	
Viruses	
Protozoa	
Metazoa	
Microbiological Testing: The Medical Assistant's Role	

CHAPTER OUTLINE   *continued*

	NOTES
Specimen Collection and Handling	
Types of Specimens	
Types of Culture Media	
Caring for the Media	
Transporting the Specimen	
Microscopic Examination of Microorganisms	
Smears and Slides	
Identification by Staining	
Microbiological Inoculation	
Sensitivity Testing	
Streptococcal Testing	

LEARNING SELF-ASSESSMENT EXERCISES

Key Terms

Define the following key terms:

aerobic _____

agar _____

anaerobic _____

bacilli (sing. bacillus) _____

bacteriology _____

centesis _____

Chlamydiae _____

cocci _____

diplococci _____

flagella (sing. flagellum) _____

media _____

morphology _____

mycology _____

nosocomial infections _____

obligate _____

opportunistic _____

pathogens _____

parasitology _____

Petri plate _____

primary cultures _____

rickettsia _____

secondary culture _____

spirochetes _____

staphylococci _____

streptococci _____

virology _____

Matching

Match the term in Part 1 with the correct definition in Part 2

PART 1

_____ 1. Helminths

_____ 2. Arthropods

_____ 3. Toxoplasma

_____ 4. Aerobic

_____ 5. Entamoeba

_____ 6. Anaerobic

_____ 7. Pathogen

_____ 8. Mycology

_____ 9. Flagella

_____ 10. Giardia

PART 2

a. Diarrhea, dysentery, and liver and lung disorders

b. Living without oxygen

c. Science and study of fungi

d. Giardiasis, diarrhea, and malabsorption of nutrients

e. Mites, lice, ticks, and fleas, bees, spiders, wasps, mosquitoes, and scorpions

f. Requiring oxygen to live

g. Round worms, flat worms, and flukes

h. Toxoplasmosis and fetal abnormalities

i. Microorganisms that can produce disease

j. Hairlike, motile process on the extremity of a bacterium or protozoan

Skill Drills

1. What eight administrative and clinical skills may a medical assistant be expected to perform in microbiological testing?

_____
_____
_____
_____
_____
_____
_____

2. List the five elements that bacteria require for survival.

a. _____

b. _____

c. _____

d. _____

e. _____

Multiple Choice

1. How are laboratory specimens drawn from the body?
   a. Centesis (surgical puncture)
   b. Sputum, stool, or urine
   c. Venipuncture
   d. *a* and *c*

2. What microorganisms are likely to present problems in the health care field?
   a. Those that thrive between 96°F and 101°F in a basically neutral environment
   b. Those that do not require oxygen to thrive

c. Those that do require oxygen to thrive

d. Those that thrive between 100°F and 104°F in an acidic environment

3. When a microorganism is recognized by its morphology, this means what?

a. It is recognized by its size.

b. It is recognized by its shape.

c. It is recognized by the color of stain it retains.

d. It is recognized by the number of nuclei it has.

4. Which of the following statements best states the purpose of a Gram stain?

a. Staining is just a standard procedure for many smear samples.

b. Most bacteria are colorless and hard to see or to identify.

c. Bacteria that retain the purple color are said to be Gram-positive.

d. Bacteria that do not retain crystal violet will stain red and are Gram-negative

5. Which statement about bacilli is not accurate?

a. Bacilli are bacteria with a rodlike shape.

b. Bacilli are usually anaerobic.

c. Bacilli may be Gram-positive or Gram-negative.

d. Bacilli include tetanus, botulism, gas gangrene, tuberculosis, etc.

6. Which statement about spirochetes is not accurate?

a. They are long, spiral, flexible organisms.

b. They are classified as spirilla if they are rigid rather than flexible.

c. Spirochetes are responsible for syphilis and Lyme disease.

d. They are responsible for salmonellosis, certain pneumonias, and otitis media.

7. What is the morphology of vibrios?

a. They are curved, comma-shaped bacteria and are very motile.

b. They are clusters of cocci that appear to vibrate under microscopic examination.

c. They are strings (5–6) of rods.

d. They are single cocci with a flagellum.

8. What microorganisms in our environment often produce spores to protect themselves under adverse conditions?

a. Spirochetes form an elongated capsule and become dormant.

b. Bacilli form a capsule around themselves and enter a resting state.

c. Tubercle bacilli are the only microorganisms that form a protective capsule.

d. Herpes viruses can form a protective barrier.

9. Which of the following are specialized forms of bacteria that are referred to as *obligate*?

a. *Pseudomonas* and fungus

b. *Neisseria gonorrhoeae* and *Klebsiella*

c. Protozoa and metazoa

d. *Rickettsia* and chlamydia

10. Fungi are small organisms like bacteria and are often opportunistic. What does this mean?

a. When another pathogen is present, they mutate and spread rapidly.

b. They become pathogenic when the host's normal flora cannot counterbalance.

c. Primary fungal infections give secondary infections the opportunity to thrive.

d. They multiply rapidly in the presence of glucose

Critical Thinking Practice

1. Amy Rogers, a 29-year-old patient, has a severely compromised immune system due to recent chemotherapy. What opportunistic mold infections should you be aware of in her case? How might they affect her?

_____

_____

_____

_____

2. Commercially prepared culture media contained in disposable plastic Petri plates are available for use in medical offices. How should these plates be cared for? What quality control measures need to be followed?

_____

_____

_____

_____

Patient Education

1. Virginia Gerber, a 40-year-old patient, spent a few weeks visiting rural Appalachia. She has not felt well since her return home. Symptoms she reports are generalized aches and pains with fatigue. She is concerned about the possibility of having contracted Lyme disease, but she is not familiar with how it is spread or what additional symptoms might be. How would you respond to Ms. Gerber's questions?

_____

_____

_____

_____

2. In our fast-service society, many people feel that they do not have time to be sick. Some people have concerns about lost wages if they cannot work. You will often receive phone calls from patients who report symptoms of mild upper respiratory symptoms and who want antibiotic treatment. First, what screening questions will you ask (refer to Chapter 2, Medical History and Patient Assessment)? Is an appointment advisable (refer to Chapter 13, Ophthalmology and Otolaryngology)? How can you respond to the request for antibiotics?

_____

_____

_____

_____

43

Urinalysis

CHAPTER COMPETENCIES

Review the information in your text that supports the following course objectives.

Learning Objectives

Upon successfully completing this chapter, you will be able to:

1. Spell and define the key terms.

2. Describe the methods of urine collection.

3. List and explain the physical and chemical properties of urine.

4. State the conditions that can be detected by abnormal urinalysis findings.

5. List and describe the components that can be found in urine sediment and describe their relationships to chemical findings.

Performance Objectives

Upon successfully completing this chapter, you will be able to:

1. Explain to and/or assist a patient in obtaining a clean-catch midstream urine specimen (Procedure 43-1).

2. Explain the method of obtaining a 24-hour urine collection (Procedure 43-2).

3. Determine color and clarity of urine (Procedure 43-3).

4. Accurately interpret chemical reagent strip reactions (Procedure 43-4).

5. Perform copper reduction test (Procedure 43-5).

6. Perform a nitroprusside reaction (Acetest) for ketones (Procedure 43-6).

7. Perform acid precipitation test (Procedure 43-7).

8. Perform diazo tablet test (Ictotest) for bilirubin (Procedure 43-8).

9. Prepare urine sediment (Procedure 43-9).

10. Prepare urine sediment for microscopic examination.

CHAPTER OUTLINE	NOTES
Specimen Collection Methods	
Clean-Catch Midstream Urine Specimen	
Bladder Catheterization	
Suprapubic Aspiration	
24-Hour Urine Collection	
Physical Properties of Urine	
Color	
Clarity	
Specific Gravity	

CHAPTER OUTLINE *continued*	NOTES
Chemical Properties of Urine	
pH	
Glucose	
Ketones	
Proteins	
Blood	
Bilirubin	
Urobilinogen	
Nitrite	
Leukocyte Esterase	
Urine Sediment	
Structures Found in Urine Sediment	
Urine Pregnancy Testing	
Urine Drug Testing	

LEARNING SELF-ASSESSMENT EXERCISES

Key Terms

Define the following key terms:

ammonia _____

bilirubinuria _____

creatinine _____

culture _____

diurnal variation _____

Ehrlich units _____

electrolytes _____

esterase _____

galactosuria _____

glycosuria _____

hemoglobinuria _____

lyse _____

nitroprusside _____

particulate matter _____

phosphates _____

precipitation _____

quantitative _____

sulfosalicylic acid _____

threshold _____

urates _____

Matching

Match the term in Part 1 with the correct definition in Part 2.

PART 1

_____ 1. Glycosuria

_____ 2. Phosphates

_____ 3. Galactosuria

_____ 4. Creatinine

_____ 5. Esterase

_____ 6. Electrolytes

_____ 7. Ammonia

_____ 8. Bilirubinuria

PART 2

a. An enzyme that helps fight urinary tract infections

b. Elements dissolved in the blood that carry an electrical charge

c. Bilirubin in the urine

d. A substance produced by decomposition of nitrogen

e. Important in the balance of acid–base balance

f. A substance formed from creatine metabolism

g. Sugar in the urine

h. Increased levels of galactose in the blood and urine

Skill Drills

1. List the nine tests included on a urine test strip with the expected range. Can you give one example of a cause for an abnormal reading for each of the nine tests?

Test	Expected Range	Abnormal Reading Cause
a.		
b.		
c.		
d.		
e.		
f.		
g.		
h.		
i.		

2. List four things that can change the color of urine. What color would you expect in the urine for each of the causes?

_____

_____

_____

_____

Multiple Choice

1. What is urinalysis (UA)?
   a. A breakdown of base elements in a urine sample
   b. Determination of physical components in a urine sample
   c. A physical and chemical examination of urine to assess renal function
   d. Analysis of reactions to multitest reagent strips

2. Unless otherwise specified by a physician, what type of urine sample is collected?
   a. A 24-hour urine collection
   b. A random urine sample, freshly voided, clean catch, midstream
   c. Sample collected at the first voiding of the morning
   d. Straight catheter sample obtained by aseptic technique

3. What is one guideline that all culture samples have in common?
   a. They are all collected with a sterile swab.
   b. All must be collected and placed in a sterile tube with a preservative.
   c. All are collected early in the day.
   d. All cultures require that the specimen not be contaminated during collection.

4. Why is it important to give the patient proper instructions about how to obtain a clean-catch sample?
   a. Microorganisms from the perineal area may produce misleading results.
   b. It reduces any embarrassment the patient may feel about obtaining the sample.
   c. To charge for a clean-catch urine, it must be a clean-catch urine sample.
   d. It is the only way to guarantee that the sample is fresh.

5. What are two tests that require a first-morning urine sample?
   a. Urine sugar and ketones to check diabetes
   b. Bilirubin and pH
   c. 2-hour postprandial specimens and pregnancy test
   d. Nitrates and leukocyte esterase

6. Which of the following statements about urine collection by catheterization is not accurate?
   a. A thin sterile tube (catheter) is placed into the bladder through the urethra.
   b. A medical assistant may be trained by a physician to perform catheterizations.
   c. Catheterization is performed when a patient cannot provide a clean-catch sample.
   d. Only physicians and licensed nurses may perform this procedure.

7. Urine odors can indicate specific patient conditions. Which statement is not true?
   a. A diabetic patient's urine may smell sweet.
   b. A sour urine smell may be due to high blood pressure.
   c. Ingestion of asparagus may give urine a faint odor of the vegetable.
   d. Presence of bacteria may give urine a foul odor.

8. What may be the cause of hazy urine?
   a. Normal, freshly voided urine
   b. Presence of particulate matter
   c. Low concentration of phosphates
   d. Absence of blood cells

9. Which statement about specific gravity is not accurate?
   a. The specific gravity reflects the concentration of a urine specimen.
   b. The weight of the urine is compared with the weight of blood.
   c. Normal urine is heavier than water by a small amount.
   d. Specific gravity for a normal urine specimen is 1.003 to 1.035.

10. What may increased numbers of epithelial cells in urine indicate?
    a. An irritation, such as inflammation, somewhere in the urinary system
    b. A normal part of the aging and thinning process of skin
    c. The patient is overly dehydrated.
    d. The urine sample has sat too long before examination.

Critical Thinking Practice

1. Dark-yellow urine may indicate an elevated bilirubin level. One of your patients has just given a clean-catch sample that is quite dark. What care or precautions need to be taken with this sample? If you suspect the presence of bilirubin, what clue might that give you about the patient's health?

_____

_____

_____

_____

2. Why would a bowel obstruction cause a rise in serum levels of bilirubin and urobilinogen? What test is used to determine the presence of urobilinogen?

_____

_____

_____

_____

Patient Education

1. Mark Green phones the clinic with concerns about the sudden onset of red urine. He denies fever, burning, urgency, or flank pain. What dietary information might be helpful? Should a urinalysis be ordered?

_____

_____

_____

_____

2. One of your patients is curious. To him, normal urine looks clear, as if there is nothing present. He wonders why he needs to pay for a urinalysis when he has his annual physical. What can you tell him?

_____

_____

_____

_____

44

Phlebotomy

CHAPTER COMPETENCIES

Review the information in your text that supports the following course objectives.

Learning Objectives

Upon successfully completing this chapter, you will be able to:

1. Define and spell the key terms.

2. Identify equipment and supplies used to obtain a routine venous specimen and a routine capillary skin puncture.

3. List the major anticoagulants, their color codes, and the suggested order in which they are filled from a venipuncture.

4. Describe the location and selection of the blood collection sites for capillaries and veins.

5. Explain the importance of correct patient identification and complete specimen and requisition labeling.

6. Describe the steps in preparation of the puncture site for venipuncture and skin puncture.

7. Describe care for a puncture site after blood has been drawn.

8. List precautions to be observed when drawing blood.

Performance Objectives

Upon successfully completing this chapter, you will be able to:

1. Obtain a blood specimen from a patient by venipuncture (Procedure 44-1).

2. Obtain a blood specimen from a patient by skin puncture (Procedure 44-2).

3. Use a butterfly collection system.

CHAPTER OUTLINE	NOTES
General Blood Drawing Equipment	
Blood Drawing Station	
Gloves	
Antiseptics	
Spill Kit Supplies and Instructions	
Gauze Pads	
Bandages	
Needle and Sharps Disposal Containers	
Venipuncture Equipment	
Tourniquets	
Needles	
Blood Collection Systems	
Evacuated Tube System	

CHAPTER OUTLINE   *continued*

CHAPTER OUTLINE *continued*	NOTES
Tube Additives	
Syringe System	
Winged Infusion Set	
Order of Draw	
Skin Puncture (Microcollection) Equipment	
Lancets	
Microhematocrit Tubes	
Microcollection Containers	
Filter Paper Test Requisitions	
Warming Devices	
Patient Preparation	
Performing a Venipuncture	
Selection of the Venipuncture Site	
Complications of Venipuncture	
Performing a Skin Puncture	
Complications of Skin Puncture	

LEARNING SELF-ASSESSMENT EXERCISES

Key Terms

Define the following key terms:

antecubital space _____

anticoagulant _____

antiseptic _____

bevel _____

evacuated tube _____

gauge _____

gel separator _____

hematoma _____

hemoconcentration _____

hemolysis _____

Luer adapter _____

multisample needle _____

order of draw _____

palpate _____

prophylaxis _____

sharps container _____

syncope _____

Matching

Match the term in Part 1 with the correct definition in Part 2.

PART I

_____ 1. Syncope

_____ 2. Hemolysis

_____ 3. Gauge

_____ 4. Palpate

_____ 5. Antiseptic

_____ 6. Hematoma

PART 2

a. The rupture of erythrocytes with the release of hemoglobin.

b. Helps locate veins and determine their size, depth, and direction

c. Fainting

d. Formation caused by blood leaking into the tissues during or after venipuncture

e. Indicates size based on the lumen (bore size or opening)

f. Inhibits the growth of bacteria

Skill Drills

1. List five steps you should follow if you ever experience potential exposure to blood-borne pathogens.

a. _____
b. _____
c. _____
d. _____
e. _____

2. List six situations that may trigger hematoma formation.

a. _____
b. _____
c. _____
d. _____
e. _____
f. _____

Multiple Choice

1. Which of the following would be found in a biohazardous spill kit?
   a. Nitrile disposable gloves, absorbant material or product, PPE
   b. A mop and garbage can with a 3-mil plastic liner
   c. Sterile towels, latex gloves, and floor cleaner with water 50:50 dilution
   d. Laboratory coat, vinyl gloves, state reporting form to complete and mail

2. What are the first two steps in the chain of response for a biohazard spill?
   a. Apply disinfectant to the area, pour adsorbent material over the spill
   b. Secure spill area, locate a spill cleanup kit
   c. Wear gloves during cleanup, secure spill area
   d. Wear gloves and wipe up blood with an absorbent towel

3. What methods are used to collect blood specimens?
   a. Arterial puncture, venipuncture
   b. Arterial puncture, skin puncture, and venipuncture
   c. Skin puncture and venipuncture
   d. Venipuncture only

4. What is the purpose of collecting an arterial specimen?
   a. To evaluate cardiac function
   b. To evaluate the filtration system of the kidneys
   c. To evaluate respiratory function
   d. To determine the percentage of mitral valve regurgitation

5. What features need to be considered when preparing a phlebotomy station?
   a. Bed or reclining chair available for patients with a history of fainting
   b. Wall color—research shows that blue or lavender relaxes patients
   c. Aquariums, which provide essential distraction and help reduce anxiety
   d. Easy-listening music, which helps keep a pleasant atmosphere

6. Which of the following statements about use of gloves is not correct?
   a. A new pair of gloves must be used for each patient.
   b. Latex, nitrile, vinyl, and polyethylene nonsterile, disposable gloves are acceptable.
   c. Glove fit is not important for drawing blood. They are just for protection.
   d. Gloves dusted with powder can contaminate some tests.

7. What is the purpose of a bevel?
   a. They are silicon-coated, which enables them to penetrate the skin.
   b. The bevel decreases the amount of discomfort involved in a venipuncture.
   c. The degree of bevel helps to identify the gauge of the needle.
   d. A bevel allows the needle to penetrate the vein easily and prevents *coring.*

8. Which of the following needles has the largest bore size or opening?
   a. 30 gauge
   b. 18 gauge
   c. 22 gauge
   d. 25 gauge

9. Why would you not want to draw blood using a small-gauge needle?
   a. There is greater likelihood of it breaking off in the vein.
   b. Blood cells will rupture, causing hemolysis of the specimen.
   c. The luer adaptor will not fit venipuncture cuffs.
   d. The small needles are awkward to hold and manipulate.

10. What example explains the best advantage of using the evacuated tube system?
    a. Multiple tubes may be filled from a single venipuncture.
    b. The tubes are color coded according to the tests to be done.
    c. The vacuum draws the blood into the tubes.
    d. It is a universal system, used in all phlebotomy laboratories around the country

11. What safety features are available for the holder used with the evacuated tube system?
    a. Shields that cover the needle, or devices that retract the needle into the holder
    b. A self-locking cover for recapping the needle
    c. A gripper to clamp the holder to the Vacutainer tube, preventing slippage
    d. Orange color as a reminder to discard in biohazard container

12. Which of the following is not an additive found in Vacutainer tubes?
    a. Anticoagulants to prevent the blood from coagulating or clotting
    b. Clot activators to enhance coagulation
    c. Thixotropic gel separator
    d. Ethyl alcohol 2%

Critical Thinking Practice

1. Needlestick injuries are contributing to the overall burden of health care worker injuries. Estimates indicate that 600,000 to 800,000 such injuries occur annually, about half of which go unreported. What are some reasons you think there is such a high percentage of unreported exposures? What risks are the unreported individuals placing on themselves, their family, and their patients?

_____

_____

_____

_____

2. What are some techniques for drawing blood with a syringe successfully?

_____

_____

_____

_____

Patient Education

1. The physician has ordered a chemistry panel, a lipid panel, a CBC, a TSH, and a PSA for one of the patients. The patient's next appointment is a month from today. The patient will need to have the lab work done at least 5 days before the appointment, so the physician can review results with the patient. Your role is to complete the patient information on the laboratory order and to give the patient instructions for fasting. What will you tell the patient? Why encourage hydration?

_____

_____

_____

_____

45

Hematology

CHAPTER COMPETENCIES

Review the information in your text that supports the following course

Learning Objectives

Upon successfully completing this chapter, you will be able to:

1. Spell and define the key terms.

2. List the parameters measured in the complete blood count and their normal ranges.

3. State the conditions associated with selected abnormal complete blood count findings.

4. Explain the functions of the three types of blood cells.

5. Describe the purpose of testing for the erythrocyte sedimentation rate.

6. List the leukocytes seen normally in the blood and their functions.

7. Explain the hemostatic mechanism of the body.

8. List and describe the tests that measure the body's ability to form a fibrin clot.

9. Explain how to determine the prothrombin time and partial thromboplastin time.

Performance Objectives

Upon successfully completing this chapter, you will be able to:

1. Use a Unopette system for diluting blood specimens (Procedure 45-1).

2. Perform a manual white blood cell count (Procedure 45-2).

3. Make a peripheral blood smear (Procedure 45-3).

4. Stain a peripheral blood smear (Procedure 45-4).

5. Determine a white blood cell differential (Procedure 45-5).

6. Perform a red blood cell count (Procedure 45-6)

7. Perform a hemoglobin determination (Procedure 45-7).

8. Perform a microhematocrit determination (Procedure 45-8).

9. Determine a Wintrobe erythrocyte sedimentation rate (Procedure 45-9).

10. Determine a bleeding time (Procedure 45-10).

CHAPTER OUTLINE	NOTES
Formation of Blood Cells	
Hematological Testing	
Complete Blood Count	
White Blood Cell Count and Differential	
Red Blood Cell Count	
Hemoglobin	
Hematocrit	
Mean Cell Volume	

CHAPTER OUTLINE   *continued*

	NOTES
Mean Cell Hemoglobin and Mean Cell Hemoglobin Concentration	
Platelet Count	
Erythrocyte Sedimentation Rate	
Coagulation Tests	
Prothrombin Time	
Partial Thromboplastin Time	
Bleeding Time	

LEARNING SELF-ASSESSMENT EXERCISES

Key Terms

Define the following key terms:

anisocytosis _____

enzyme _____

erythrocyte _____

erythropoietin _____

femtoliter _____

folate _____

granulocytes _____

hematocytometer (hemocytometer) _____

hematopoiesis _____

hemolytic anemia _____

hemostasis _____

leukocytes _____

morphology _____

poikilocytosis _____

sickle cell anemia _____

thrombocytes _____

thromboplastin _____

Matching

Match the term in Part 1 with the correct definition in Part 2.

PART 1

_____ 1. Hematology

_____ 2. Erythropoietin

_____ 3. Vasoconstriction

_____ 4. Granulocytes

PART 2

a. Neutrophils, eosinophils, and basophils

b. The primary monitor of Coumadin anticoagulant therapy

c. Constriction of the vein to reduce blood loss

d. Study of hemostasis, or the ability of the patient to maintain blood in a fluid state within the vessels

_____ 5. Iron

_____ 6. PT

_____ 7. Morphology

e. A hormone that is released from the kidneys

f. Substance that gives RBCs their distinctive red color

g. Description of the physical characteristics of blood cells

Skill Drills

1. List four factors that contribute to conditions with diminished numbers of leukocytes (leukopenia).

   a. _____

   b. _____

   c. _____

   d. _____

2. List five sources that can cause leukocytosis (increased numbers of WBCs).

   a. _____

   b. _____

   c. _____

   d. _____

   e. _____

Multiple Choice

1. Why is a WBC differential performed?
   a. To check for anemia
   b. To determine amounts of various WBC types present in the peripheral blood
   c. To determine clotting time
   d. To determine blood type and Rh factor

2. When checking a slide for neutrophils, lymphocytes, monocytes, eosinophils, and basophils, why is the slide stained?
   a. Because it helps differentiate the blue nuclei from the red nuclei
   b. Because the shape of each nucleus is more defined
   c. Because small cells do not show up as well as large cells
   d. Because all of these types of leukocytes are colorless

3. Which of the following statements about basophils is not accurate?
   a. Basophils are least numerous, representing less than 1% of circulating WBCs.
   b. The nucleus is four-lobed, resembling a clover.
   c. Basophils appear to be involved in allergic asthma and contact allergies.
   d. They are present in hypothyroidism and chronic myeloid leukemia.

4. Which statement about the hematocrit is not accurate?
   a. To measure a hematocrit, blood is centrifuged to pack the RBCs.
   b. The normal range is 37–48% in men and 45–52% in women.
   c. Automated instruments calculate the hematocrit from the RBC count and mean cell volume (MCV).
   d. The purpose of measuring the hematocrit is to detect anemia.

5. Which statement about thrombocytopenia (decreased platelets) is not accurate?
   a. It may be associated with increased bleeding.
   b. Treatment requires a specific diagnosis of the cause of the thrombocytopenia.
   c. The risk of bleeding decreases as the platelet count decreases.
   d. Causes may include anemia, infectious disease, drugs, and acute leukemia.

6. Which of the following is not a method for determining ESR?
   a. Warner method
   b. Wintrobe method
   c. Westergren method
   d. *a* and *b*

7. What is platelet plug formation?
   a. Platelets adhere to a wound and form a plug, temporarily slowing or stopping the blood flow.
   b. Platelets group with monocytes to enhance phagocytosis of foreign material
   c. It is a desired ratio that is out of balance in patients with hemophilia.
   d. It is a common test for determining how well a fibrin clot can form.

8. Monocytes are the third most abundant leukocytes. What statement is also true?
   a. Monocytes stay in the bloodstream for about 3 days and then move into tissues.
   b. The monocyte nucleus tends to be egg shaped.
   c. It is much smaller than the lymphocyte and closer in size to the neutrophil.
   d. The normal percentage of monocytes is 1–5%.

9. Blood cells are formed in several areas of the body. Identify the exception.
   a. Blood cells are formed in the bone marrow.
   b. The long bones, skull, pelvis, and sternum usually manufacture these cells.
   c. Alternative sites include the liver and spleen.
   d. The placenta of the developing fetus also produces blood cells.

10. What is a feature of sickle cell anemia?
   a. Each hemoglobin molecule contains four protein chains called globins.
   b. Defects in the globin chains result in abnormal hemoglobins such as S.
   c. Alpha and beta globins are the most common, with some gamma.
   d. It can only be identified by the HemoCue system.

Critical Thinking Practice

1. The complete blood count (CBC) or hemogram is one of the most frequently ordered tests in the laboratory.
   a. List eight common parameters.

   b. Give a reason why leukopenia may be present.

   c. Why would the normal percentage of neutrophils increase?

2. Maria Young, a 49-year-old patient, is receiving chemotherapy for acute leukemia and is experiencing some unsteadiness. She has thrombocytopenia and just completed a transfusion of platelets. She asks you to assist her to the restroom, and you say you will help her as soon as you complete another task. When you return, Maria is exiting from the restroom rubbing her hip. She tells you she could not wait, and while in the restroom, she lost her balance and fell backward onto the toilet. What will you do? What are some symptoms of thrombocytopenia? Do you think this fall may alter the benefit of the platelet infusion she just received?

Patient Education

1. One of the clinic patients is scheduled for hip replacement surgery in 2 weeks. The doctor asks you to perform a bleeding time determination. Explain to the patient why you are doing this test. What medications do you need to advise the patient to avoid prior to surgery?

_____

_____

_____

_____

46

Serology and Immunohematology

CHAPTER COMPETENCIES

Review the information in your text that supports the following course objectives.

Learning Objectives

Upon successfully completing this chapter, you will be able to:

1. Spell and define the key terms.

2. List the indications for serological testing.

3. Describe the antigen-antibody reaction.

4. Name and describe the two most common methods of enhancing the antigen-antibody reaction for testing purposes.

5. List areas to address to ensure quality assurance and quality control in serological testing.

6. Explain the storage and handling of serological test kits.

7. List and describe serological tests most commonly encountered through the medical office.

Performance Objectives

Upon successfully completing this chapter, you will be able to:

1. Perform an agglutination test.

2. Perform an enzyme immunoassay test.

3. Perform a mononucleosis test (Procedure 46-1).

4. Perform an HCG pregnancy test (Procedure 46-2).

5. Perform a group A rapid strep test (Procedure 46-3).

CHAPTER OUTLINE	NOTES
Antigens and Antibodies	
Serology Test Methods and Principles	
Agglutination Test	
Enzyme Linked Immunosorbent Assays	
Reagent and Kit Storage and Handling	
Following Test Procedures	
Quality Assurance and Quality Control	
External Controls	
Internal Controls	
Serology Tests	
Rheumatoid Factor and Rheumatoid Arthritis	
Infectious Mononucleosis	
Rapid Plasma Reagin Test for Syphilis	
Pregnancy Test	
Group A Streptococcus	

CHAPTER OUTLINE *continued*	NOTES
Other Serological Tests	
Immunohematology	
Blood Group Antigens	
Blood Group Testing	
Blood Supply	

LEARNING SELF-ASSESSMENT EXERCISES

Key Terms

Define the following key terms:

agglutination _____

donor _____

immunohematology _____

sensitivity _____

serology _____

specificity _____

false positive _____

false negative _____

external control _____

internal control _____

Matching

Match the term in Part 1 with the correct definition in Part 2.

PART 1

_____ 1. Serology

_____ 2. Donor

_____ 3. Mononucleosis

_____ 4. Specificity

_____ 5. Sensitivity

PART 2

a. Epstein-Barr

b. Refers to the source of most samples, the liquid part of blood called serum

c. An antibody has a particularly strong attraction for its antigen, requiring trace amounts to trigger response

d. One who contributes blood

e. Each antibody produced by the body combines with and destroys only one antigen

Skill Drills

List six or seven helpful guidelines for ensuring that reagents will be accurate.

_____

_____

_____

_____

_____

_____

_____

Multiple Choice

1. What biohazard precautions are used during testing described in this chapter?
   a. Respiratory precautions
   b. Standard precautions
   c. Wound precautions
   d. Isolation precautions

2. Which statement about antigens or antibodies is not accurate?
   a. Antigens are substances recognized as foreign to the body.
   b. Antibodies are proteins produced in response to a specific antigen.
   c. Antibodies remain in the liver and kidneys to help filter out antigens.
   d. Antigens cause the body to initiate a defense response.

3. Which statement about tests using antigen–antibody is true?
   a. Tests using antigen–antibody reactions as their bases are specific and sensitive.
   b. These tests require large amounts of a substance to pick it out of a solution.
   c. These tests results are rarely dependable.
   d. These tests are costly to perform, so are rarely ordered.

4. In serology, when substances are tested, what are the expected outcomes?
   a. Sensitivity to treatment is determined.
   b. Resistance to treatment is determined.
   c. A substance is identified or the amount present (quantity) is measured.
   d. A ratio is calculated or projected.

5. For agglutination testing, what two things are necessary?
   a. The patient's sample and a urine reagent strip
   b. A reagent containing the antibody and the patient's sample
   c. A reagent containing the antigen and the patient's sample
   d. A blood sugar glucometer and a patient sample

6. What happens if agglutination does not occur?
   a. The test solution remains clear and transparent.
   b. The test solution appears smooth and milky.
   c. The test solution appears granular.
   d. The test solution becomes pale blue.

7. What method is used to test for infectious mononucleosis, rheumatoid arthritis, syphilis, and rubella?
   a. Specific antibody in reagent and patient's serum
   b. Nonspecific antibody in reagent and patient's serum
   c. Specific antigen in reagent and the patient's serum
   d. Nonspecific antigen in reagent and the patient's serum

8. What is an external control?
   a. A solution similar to a patient sample that has a known outcome
   b. A solution similar to a suspected diagnosis, tested against a patient sample
   c. A control solution that will always produce a positive result
   d. A control solution that will always produce a negative result

9. What test method is used to identify rheumatoid arthritis?
   a. Reagent test
   b. Enzyme-linked immunosorbent assays
   c. Agglutination test
   d. Rapid plasma reagin

10. If the controls do not give the expected results, what should you do with the patient results?
    a. Report them with a notation that results are inconclusive.
    b. Report them with a notation that results are 50% accurate.
    c. Do not report them and repeat the test with accurate controls.
    d. Do not report them until the controls give the result you want

Critical Thinking Practice

1. A false-positive RPR result can be seen in patients with lupus erythematosus, infectious mononucleosis, hepatitis, and rheumatoid arthritis, and in pregnancy and the elderly. Improper rotation of specimen can also cause a false-negative result. What is the RPR test? Look at each diagnosis mentioned in which a false positive might result. Imagine a patient for each diagnosis. How do you think each patient might react if told he or she has a positive RPR result?

_____

_____

_____

_____

_____

_____

2. False-negative and false-positive results can occur because of biological conditions of patients. They can also be due to technical difficulty with samples or performance of the test. Testing personnel cannot control the biological conditions, but they can sometimes control the technical conditions. What are some ways in which testing personnel can ensure the accuracy of test results?

_____

_____

_____

_____

Patient Education

1. The test for pregnancy is based on the detection of the hormone human chorionic gonadotropin (HCG). Modern pregnancy tests can detect pregnancy before the first missed menses. Considering what you have learned about the possibility of false-positive and false-negative results, what would you advise if a patient asks you if a home pregnancy test is as accurate as one done in a laboratory? For additional information, check www.WebMD.com or call a local laboratory and ask about the accuracy of home test kits.

_____

_____

_____

_____

47

Clinical Chemistry

CHAPTER COMPETENCIES

Review the information in your text that supports the following course objectives.

Learning Objectives

Upon successfully completing this chapter, you will be able to:

1. Spell and define the key terms.

2. List the common electrolytes and explain the relationship of electrolytes to acid-base balance.

3. Describe the nonprotein nitrogenous compounds and name conditions with abnormal values.

4. List and describe the substances commonly tested in liver function assessment.

5. Explain thyroid function and the hormone that regulates the thyroid gland.

6. Describe how an assessment for a myocardial infarction is made with laboratory tests.

7. Describe how pancreatitis is diagnosed with laboratory tests.

8. Describe glucose use and regulation and the purpose of the various glucose tests.

9. Describe the function of cholesterol and other lipids and their correlation to heart disease.

Performance Objectives

Upon successfully completing this chapter, you will be able to:

1. Determine blood glucose (Procedure 47-1).

2. Perform a glucose tolerance test (Procedure 47-2).

CHAPTER OUTLINE

CHAPTER OUTLINE	NOTES
Instruments and Methodology	
Renal Function	
Electrolytes	
Nonprotein Nitrogenous Compounds	
Liver Function	
Bilirubin	
Enzymes	
Thyroid Function	
Thyroid-Stimulating Hormone	
Cardiac Function	
Creatine Kinase-MB	
Troponin	
Pancreatic Function	
Pancreatic Enzymes	
Pancreatic Hormones and Carbohydrate Metabolism	

CHAPTER OUTLINE *continued*	NOTES
Lipids and Lipoproteins	
Cholesterol	
Low-Density Lipoprotein	
High-Density Lipoprotein	
Triglycerides	

LEARNING SELF-ASSESSMENT EXERCISES

Key Terms

Define the following key terms:

amylase _____

bicarbonate _____

bile _____

body fluids _____

creatine _____

extracellular _____

gestational diabetes _____

intracellular _____

ions _____

lipase _____

lipids _____

lipoproteins _____

nitrogenous _____

Matching

Match the term in Part 1 with the correct definition in Part 2.

PART 1

_____ 1. Body fluids

_____ 2. Electrolytes

_____ 3. Sodium (chemical symbol, Na)

_____ 4. Potassium (chemical symbol, K)

_____ 5. Hypophosphatemia

_____ 6. Alkaline phosphatase

_____ 7. Creatine kinase (CK)

PART 2

a. The major cation of the extracellular fluid

b. Phosphorus level below 2.5 mg/dL

c. Fluids that accumulate in the body's compartments

d. The major cation of the intracellular fluid

e. Ions (chemicals that carry a charge)

f. Found almost exclusively in skeletal muscle and myocardium

g. Present in the bones, liver, intestines, kidneys, and placenta

Skill Drills

1. Hypoglycemia is a syndrome characterized by fasting blood sugar levels below 45 mg/dL. List seven symptoms of hypoglycemia.

   a. _____
   b. _____
   c. _____
   d. _____
   e. _____
   f. _____
   g. _____

2. List four substances commonly tested in liver function assessment.

   a. _____
   b. _____
   c. _____
   d. _____

Multiple Choice

1. In which of the following systems does the pancreas function?
   a. The endocrine and exocrine systems
   b. The renal and endocrine systems
   c. The vascular and exocrine systems
   d. The pulmonary and endocrine systems

2. What is produced by the salivary glands?
   a. Phosphates
   b. Creatinine
   c. Lipase
   d. Amylase

3. Troponin is a protein specific to heart muscle. Which statement is true?
   a. Levels can be measured to monitor the effectiveness of thrombolytic therapy.
   b. It is a predictor of future myocardial infarction.
   c. The level is reduced for several hours after a myocardial infarction.
   d. The level increases for several hours after a stroke.

4. Where is creatine kinase (CK) found?
   a. It is only found in the large skeletal muscles.
   b. It is found in smooth muscle and the liver.
   c. Almost exclusively in skeletal muscle and myocardium
   d. It is only found in the myocardium.

5. In the absence of disease, when additional thyroid hormones are needed, what is secreted to stimulate the thyroid gland?
   a. T_4
   b. TSH
   c. T_3
   d. Thyroxine

6. Which of the following statements about the liver is not accurate?

   a. The liver is the largest gland of the body and one of the most complex.
   b. One of its major functions is the metabolism of bile.
   c. It aids metabolism of many compounds used by the body.
   d. It detoxifies substances found in the blood that could prove dangerous.

7. What is the body's normal pH range?
   a. 6.9 to 7.35
   b. 7.00 to 7.50
   c. 7.45 to 8.25
   d. 7.35 to 7.45

8. What factors may result in hypophosphatemia (phosphorus level below 2.5 mg/dL)?
   a. Inadequate absorption, gastrointestinal losses, electrolyte shifts
   b. Fluid overload, endocrine disorders.
   c. Sodium retention
   d. Additional loss of calcium

9. What may cause hypercalcemia?
   a. Inadequate intake of fish and poultry
   b. Osteoporosis or excessive exercise
   c. Hypoparathyroidism or excessive calcium absorption
   d. Hyperparathyroidism or excessive calcium absorption

10. What factors may lead to hypokalemia (potassium level below 3.5 mEq/L)?
    a. Insulin therapy, gastrointestinal losses, and renal disease
    b. Cell injuries and renal failure
    c. Red blood cell lysis, as may occur with a traumatic venipuncture
    d. Excessive intake of sport drinks

Critical Thinking Practice

1. Why is it important for medical assistant students to spend time learning about laboratory testing when very few tests are actually done in a physician's medical practice?

_____

_____

_____

_____

2. The kidneys rid the body of waste products and help maintain fluid balance and acid–base balance. What happens when kidneys begin to fail? What tests will the doctor order to evaluate renal function?

_____

_____

_____

_____

Patient Education

1. The disease gout is characterized by a high uric acid accumulation in the joints; the joints become inflamed and painful. Jim Ray is 45 and weighs 60 lb over his ideal weight. He takes hydrochlorothiazide for hypertension. His lipid levels usually run high, and he has told you in the past that he is a "meat and potatoes man." Now he is being seen for an acute episode of pain (the doctor told him it is gout) in his right foot. This is an educational opportunity. What information might you share with Mr. Ray?

_____

_____

_____

_____

48

Making the Transition: Student to Employee

CHAPTER COMPETENCIES

Review the information in your text that supports the following course objectives.

Learning Objectives

1. Spell and define the key terms

2. Explain the purpose of the externship experience

3. List your professional responsibilities during externship

4. Understand the evaluation process for the extern student

5. List personal and professional attributes necessary to ensure a successful externship

6. Determine your best career direction based on your skills and strengths

7. Identify the steps necessary to apply for the right position and be able to accomplish those steps

8. Draft an appropriate cover letter

9. List guidelines for an effective interview that will lead to employment

10. Identify the steps that you need to take to ensure proper career advancement

Performance Objectives

1. Write a résumé to properly communicate skills and strengths

2. Complete an employment application

CHAPTER OUTLINE	NOTES
Externships	
Types of Facilities	
Extern Sites	
Benefits of Externship	
Benefits to the Student	
Benefits to the Medical Assisting Program	
Benefits to the Externship Site	
Responsibilities of Externship	
Responsibilities of the Student	
Responsibilities of the Medical Assisting Program	
Responsibilities of the Externship Site	
Guidelines for a Successful Externship	
Procedural Performance	
Preparedness	

CHAPTER OUTLINE *continued*

CHAPTER OUTLINE *continued*	NOTES
Attendance	
Appearance	
Attitude	
Externship Documentation	
Time Records	
Site Evaluation	
Self-Evaluation	
Establish the Job for You	
Setting Employment Goals	
Self-Analysis	
Finding the Right Job	
Applying for the Job	
Answering Newspaper Advertisements	
Preparing Your Résumé	
Preparing Your Cover Letter	
Completing an Employment Application	
Interviewing	
Preparing for the Interview	
Crucial Interview Questions	
Follow-up	
Why Some Applicants Fail to Get the Job	
Keep the Job or Move On?	
Employment Laws	

LEARNING SELF-ASSESSMENT EXERCISES

Key Terms

Define the following key terms:

externship _____

networking _____

portfolio _____

preceptor _____

résumé _____

Matching

Match the definition in part 1 with the correct term in part 2.

PART 1

_____ 1. Works with the student the same as the instructor did in the classroom

_____ 2. Part of the training of medical assistants that
gives them hands-on experience

_____ 3. It is imperative for the medical assistant to
stay

_____ 4. To know your strengths as well as your weakness comes from being able to conduct a

_____ 5. Using friends, colleagues, and family members to advance in the job market is known as

PART 2

a. Self-analysis

b. Externship

c. Flexible

d. Preceptor

e. Networking

Skill Drills

1. State the personal attributes of a good medical assistant.

_____

_____

_____

_____

2. Define what a résumé is for, how it is to appear, and what is and is not to be included.

_____

_____

_____

_____

3. State the purpose of a cover letter.

_____

_____

_____

_____

4. What is the correct procedure for leaving a position?

_____

_____

_____

_____

Multiple Choice

1. Which of the following is considered *not* to be professional in appearance?
a. Long, brightly colored fingernails
b. Strong perfume
c. Untidy uniforms
d. All of the above

2. Which of the following is *not* a responsibility of
the student in the clinical facility?
a. Dependability
b. Professionalism
c. Well-groomed appearance
d. Scheduling of tasks

3. Studies show that the majority of available positions are never advertised in the media.
   a. True
   b. False

4. Which of the following is *not* a resource to identify potential job opportunities?
   a. Government employment offices
   b. School placement offices
   c. Medical facilities
   d. Calling various medical offices

5. Which document allows you to state the position you desire, stress your skills, and request an interview?
   a. Cover letter
   b. Résumé
   c. Vita
   d. All of the above

6. The best way to set a goal and eventually get what you want in a job is to
   a. Study your strengths and weaknesses
   b. Ask your family or instructors
   c. Seek the highest pay
   d. Never apply for a job that is challenging

7. A thank-you letter should be sent to the prospective employer within
   a. 2 days
   b. 2 weeks
   c. Immediately after the interview
   d. 1 week

8. When applying for a job, which question would you not ask at an interview?
   a. What are the job responsibilities of the position?
   b. Why is the current employee leaving?
   c. What does the benefit package include?
   d. How many vacations days and sick days?

9. Employment laws are enforced by
   a. EEOC
   b. EEC
   c. EOC
   d. State legislation

10. Which of these questions is it illegal for the interviewer to ask?
    a. How old are you?
    b. How many children do you have?
    c. What does your spouse do for a living?
    d. All of the above

Critical Thinking Practice

1. What are the three questions most interviewers ask, and why will a negative answer to any of these most likely mean you will not get the job?

2. What is meant by "attitude determines altitude"?

3. In an interview it is clear to you that the interviewer is concerned with confidentiality. How do you let this potential employer know that you can keep patient information confidential?

This section of your study guide contains lecture notes that will closely follow the PowerPoint slide presentation of your instructor's lecture. The pages are perforated, and can be taken out and brought to class. Key points in the lectures are intentionally blank. To promote active listening skills and to reinforce your understanding of the lectures, you will need to fill in the key points as they are covered in class.

These notes can be used with or without the PowerPoint presentation. Either way, they will be an important study tool when reviewing for your quizzes and exams.

Chapter 1

Medicine and Medical Assisting

MEDICINE AND MEDICAL ASSISTING

Medical assisting

- Fascinating, challenging career
- One of fastest-growing specialties in medicine
- _____ health professional

HISTORY OF MEDICINE

Greatest medical advances occurred in 20th century

Most advances in past 100 to 150 years

- Antibiotics
- X-ray machines
- Anesthesia

ANCIENT MEDICAL HISTORY

Egypt, 4000 B.C.

- Records of tuberculosis, pneumonia, arteriosclerosis

- Brain surgery
- Fractures with splints

Early medicines

- Digitalis
- Opium
- Supplemental iron

ANCIENT MEDICAL HISTORY
(continued)

Moses

- First public health officer
- Rules for sanitation
  - Eat only freshly slaughtered animals
  - Wash dishes and utensils

ANCIENT MEDICAL HISTORY
(continued)

Aesculapius

- Greek god of healing
  - Massage
  - Exercise
- Often pictured holding staff with serpent

Mercury

- Roman god
- Caduceus

ANCIENT MEDICAL HISTORY
(continued)

_____ , *called the Father of Medicine, turned medicine into a science and erased the element of mysticism that it once held.*

Hippocratic oath

- Still part of medical school graduation ceremony

ANCIENT MEDICAL HISTORY
(continued)

_____

- Greek physician
- Father of Experimental Physiology
- Dissected apes and swine
- Anatomic findings mostly incorrect

ANCIENT MEDICAL HISTORY
(continued)

Roman Empire

- Strides in public health
  - Clean drinking water
  - Sewer system
  - Encouraged personal cleanliness

Dark Ages

- Few medical advances
- Bubonic plague killed 20 million people in two epidemics

CHECKPOINT QUESTION 1

Why were Galen's anatomic findings considered incorrect?

Answer

_____

_____

_____

_____

MODERN MEDICAL HISTORY

Renaissance

- Andreas Vesalius
  - Father of Modern Anatomy
- Anton von Leeuwenhoek
  - Invented microscope
  - Observed bacteria under a lens
- John Hunter
  - Father of Scientific Surgery

MODERN MEDICAL HISTORY
(continued)

_____

- Discovered smallpox vaccine

Jenner's discovery of the smallpox vaccine led to more emphasis on _____ of diseases rather than on cures.

_____

- Founder of modern nursing

MODERN MEDICAL HISTORY
(continued)

Benjamin Rush

- Advocate for mentally ill
- Began modern psychiatry

Louis Pasteur

- Father of Bacteriology
- _____, eliminating bacteria in liquids through heat

MODERN MEDICAL HISTORY
(continued)

Ignaz Semmelweiss

- Advocated handwashing, especially in delivering babies

Joseph Lister

- Applied antiseptics to wounds to prevent infection

Crawford Williamson Long

- Founded modern anesthesia
- Nitrous oxide

MODERN MEDICAL HISTORY
(continued)

Elizabeth Blackwell

- First woman in United States to complete medical school

In 1869, Blackwell established her own medical school in Europe for women only, opening the door for a rapidly expanding role for women in the medical field.

Clara Barton

- Founded American Red Cross

MODERN MEDICAL HISTORY
(continued)

X-rays were discovered in 1895 by Wilhelm Konrad Roentgen when he discovered that a previously unknown ray generated by a cathode tube could pass through soft tissue and outline underlying structures.

Marie Curie and Pierre Curie

- Discovered polonium and radium

MODERN MEDICAL HISTORY
(continued)

Sir Alexander Fleming

- Discovered penicillin (accidentally)

Jonas Salk and Albert Sabin

- Discovered polio vaccine

 CHECKPOINT QUESTION 2

What did Louis Pasteur discover about bacteria found in liquids?

Answer

_____

_____

RECENT MEDICAL HISTORY

1980s

- Radiology advances
  - Computed tomography (CT)
  - Magnetic resonance imaging (MRI)

2000s

- Cloning
- Human gene mapping

RECENT MEDICAL HISTORY
(continued)

Role of medical assistant will expand as medicine advances

THE AMERICAN HEALTH CARE SYSTEM

Changed greatly over past 2 decades

Insurance evolved into managed care to control health care costs

Medical facilities required to adhere to government regulations

THE MEDICAL OFFICE

Different environment from past years

- Often owned by larger company
- Paperless
- Computers
- Legal aspects very important

THE MEDICAL OFFICE *(continued)*

Typical office

- One or more physicians
- Physician assistant/nurse practitioner
- Administrative staff
  - Financial management
- Clinical staff
  - Patient care

CHECKPOINT QUESTION 3

Which members of the health care team are considered providers?

Answer

_____

_____

_____

_____

MEDICAL SPECIALTIES

Physicians choose area of specialty

- Family or internal medicine
- Cosmetic surgery
- Vascular surgery

CHECKPOINT QUESTION 4

What is the specialty that treats newborn babies?

Answer

_____

_____

_____

THE MEDICAL ASSISTING PROFESSION

What is a medical assistant?

Duties of a medical assistant

- _____ duties
- _____ duties
- _____ duties

WHAT IS A MEDICAL ASSISTANT?

A medical assistant is a multiskilled allied health professional, a member of the health care delivery team who performs administrative and clinical procedures.

Employed in physician offices and ambulatory care settings

Working conditions vary greatly

DUTIES OF A MEDICAL ASSISTANT

Administrative tasks

Clinical tasks, including laboratory duties

ADMINISTRATIVE DUTIES

Make office more efficient and productive

Tasks such as:

- _____
- _____
- _____
- _____
- _____
- _____
- _____

CLINICAL DUTIES

Tasks vary among employers and state laws

Tasks such as:

- _____
- _____
- _____
- _____
- _____
- _____

LABORATORY DUTIES

- _____
- _____

CHECKPOINT QUESTION 5

What are five administrative duties and five clinical or laboratory duties performed by a medical assistant?

Answer

Examples of administrative duties:

- ▪ _____
- ▪ _____
- ▪ _____
- ▪ _____
- ▪ _____

Answer (continued)

Examples of clinical duties:

- ▪ _____
- ▪ _____
- ▪ _____
- ▪ _____
- ▪ _____

CHARACTERISTICS OF A PROFESSIONAL MEDICAL ASSISTANT

Medical assistants play a key role in creating and maintaining a professional image for their employers.
- ▪ Appear neat and well groomed
- ▪ Wear minimal makeup and jewelry
- ▪ Be dependable and reliable
- ▪ Be flexible and adaptable

CHARACTERISTICS OF A PROFESSIONAL MEDICAL ASSISTANT *(continued)*

Additional important characteristics:

- ▪ Excellent communicator
- ▪ Maturity
- ▪ Accuracy

Careless errors can cause harm to the patient and result in legal action against the physician.
- ▪ Respect for confidentiality
- ▪ Empathy
- ▪ Courtesy
- ▪ Initiative and responsibility

 CHECKPOINT QUESTION 6

What are eight characteristics that a professional medical assistant should have?

Answer

_____
_____
_____
_____

MEMBERS OF THE HEALTH CARE TEAM

A multidisciplinary team is a group of specialized professionals who are brought together to _____ _____.

PHYSICIANS

Lead the team

Diagnose and treat patients

Have undergraduate, medical school, and residency training

Must pass state licensure

PHYSICIAN ASSISTANTS

Perform many physician tasks

- ▪ Physical examinations
- ▪ Basic diagnoses and treatments

Minimum of 2 years training

NURSES

Implement various patient care needs

Inpatient or hospital setting

Various levels of nursing education

NURSE PRACTITIONERS

May practice medicine independently or work closely with a physician

- ▪ Write prescriptions
- ▪ Operate offices
- ▪ Admit patients to hospitals

All NPs are experienced RNs, usually with master's degrees and special training

ALLIED HEALTH PROFESSIONALS

Large section of health care team

Education requirements vary

Responsibilities vary greatly

All are supported by professional organizations

THE HISTORY OF MEDICAL ASSISTING

1934–first medical assisting school opened by Dr. Mandl

The need for a highly trained professional with a background in administrative and clinical skills led to the formation of an alternative field of allied health care.

1955–American Association of Medical Assistants (AAMA) founded in Kansas City

1959–National office founded in Chicago

1963–Certification examination developed

THE HISTORY OF MEDICAL ASSISTING *(continued)*

1991–Board of Trustees of AAMA approved the current definition of medical assisting:

"Medical assisting is an allied health profession whose practitioners function as members of the health care delivery team and perform administrative and clinical duties."

 CHECKPOINT QUESTION 7

What prompted the establishment of a school for medical assistants?

Answer

_____

_____

_____

_____

MEDICAL ASSISTING EDUCATION

Prepares students to enter the profession

Programs found in:

- Postsecondary schools
- Two-year colleges
- Community colleges

Six months to two years long

Accredited programs include externship

Continue education after graduation

 CHECKPOINT QUESTION 8

What is an externship?

Answer

_____

_____

_____

_____

MEDICAL ASSISTING PROGRAM ACCREDITATION

As of 1998: CMA examination open only to graduates of accredited medical assisting programs

Accreditation = professional peer review to evaluate programs according to standards

Medical assisting accreditation based on AAMA Role Delineation Chart: Occupational Analysis of the Medical Assisting Profession

MEDICAL ASSISTING PROGRAM ACCREDITATION

Accrediting bodies:

- The Commission on Accreditation of Allied Health Education Programs (CAAHEP)
- The Accrediting Bureau of Health Education Schools (ABHES)

MEDICAL ASSISTING CERTIFICATION

Certification examinations:

- _____ (CMA)
- _____ (RMA)

CERTIFIED MEDICAL ASSISTANT

CMA examination immediately open to CAAHEP- and ABHES-accredited program graduates

Certified Medical Assistant (CMA) designation upon passing

Must recertify every 5 years

- Retest
- Continuing education

REGISTERED MEDICAL ASSISTANT

Open to ABHES-accredited program graduates

Open to medical assistants employed for 5-year minimum

Recertification not necessary but available through STEP program

 WHAT IF?

You plan to work in a state that does not require certification to work as a medical assistant in a physician's office. Why become certified?

 CHECKPOINT QUESTION 9

What is required to maintain current status as a CMA?

Answer

_____

_____

_____

MEDICAL ASSISTING AND RELATED ALLIED HEALTH ASSOCIATIONS

Association Membership

- American Association of Medical Assistants
- American Medical Technologists
- Professional Coder Associations
- American Health Information Management Association
- American Association of Medical Transcription

ASSOCIATION MEMBERSHIP

Many benefits for members

- _____
- _____
- _____
- _____
- _____
- _____

AMERICAN ASSOCIATION OF MEDICAL ASSISTANTS

AAMA purpose

- Promote professional identity and stature of members
- Educate and grant credentials

CMA Today **journal**

- Informative articles
- CEU opportunities

Reduced dues for students

AMERICAN MEDICAL TECHNOLOGISTS

Similar organization to AAMA

Members also include medical technologists, laboratory technicians, phlebotomy technicians, dental assistants, and allied health instructors

PROFESSIONAL CODER ASSOCIATIONS

American Academy of Professional Coders (AAPC)

Offers certified professional coder (CPC) credential

AMERICAN HEALTH INFORMATION MANAGEMENT ASSOCIATION

Dedication to medical records/health information specialists

Offers certified coding specialist (CCS) and certified coding specialist—physician-based (CCS-P)

AMERICAN ASSOCIATION OF MEDICAL TRANSCRIPTION

Represents medical transcription practitioners

Two-part examination for certified medical transcriptionist (CMT) credential

CHECKPOINT QUESTION 10

What are the two organizations that accredit medical assisting programs?

Answer

_____

_____

_____

EMPLOYMENT OPPORTUNITIES

The outlook for medical assisting employment is

_____.

Can work in variety of settings:

- ▪ _____
- ▪ _____
- ▪ _____
- ▪ _____
- ▪ _____
- ▪ _____

CHECKPOINT QUESTION 11

List the settings that may employ a medical assistant.

Answer

_____

_____

_____

Chapter 2
Law and Ethics

LAW AND ETHICS

Ethics deals with concepts of _____ and _____

Laws written to carry out ethics

THE AMERICAN LEGAL SYSTEM

Ensures rights of all citizens

Protection from wrongdoings of others

Basic understanding of legal system necessary for medical assistants

- ▪ _____
- ▪ _____
- ▪ _____

Know roles and responsibilities as physician's agent

SOURCES OF LAW

_____ = enforced rules of conduct

Three sources of law in United States:

- Stare decisis = legal decisions based on previous legal decisions (precedents)
- Statutes = laws made by legislative bodies
- Administrative = laws made by government agencies

BRANCHES OF LAW

Two main branches:

- _____ law
- _____ or civil law

PUBLIC LAW

Focuses on issues between government and citizens

- Criminal law = issues of citizen welfare
- Constitutional law = laws of legislature
- Administrative law = laws made by government agencies
- International law = treaties between countries

PRIVATE OR CIVIL LAW

Focuses on issues between private citizens

Main concern in medical law

- _____ = concerns those involved in contracts
- _____ = righting wrongs caused by wrongdoing

CHECKPOINT QUESTION 1

Which branch of law covers a medical assistant charged with practicing medicine without a license?

Answer

_____
_____
_____

THE RISE IN MEDICAL LEGAL CASES

_____ = action by health care worker that harms a patient

Rise in cases increases cost of malpractice insurance

Four primary reasons for malpractice claims:

- _____
- _____
- _____
- _____

PHYSICIAN–PATIENT RELATIONSHIP

Rights and responsibilities of the patient and physician

Contracts

Consent

RIGHTS AND RESPONSIBILITIES OF THE PATIENT AND PHYSICIAN

Patients' rights:

- _____
- _____
- _____
- Know in advance:
  - What treatment consists of
  - Effects
  - Dangers

RIGHTS AND RESPONSIBILITIES OF THE PATIENT AND PHYSICIAN
(continued)

Physicians' rights:

- _____
- _____
- _____

CONTRACTS

Contract = _____

Three components:

- _____
- _____
- _____

Invalid without all three components

CONTRACTS *(continued)*

Contract offer made when _____ _____

Offer accepted when _____

Two types of contracts between physicians and patients:

- Implied contracts
- Expressed contracts

IMPLIED CONTRACTS

Most common type

_____

Example: patient calls for appointment

- Patient requested appointment on his own (offer)
- Physician accepts patient for care (acceptance)
- Patient pays for services (consideration)

EXPRESSED CONTRACTS

Consist of specific details

Mutual sharing of responsibilities

Less common in medical setting than implied contracts

CHECKPOINT QUESTION 2

An orthopedic surgeon decides to make a change in his services. He wants to limit his practice to nonsurgical patients. What action should the physician take?

Answer

_____

_____

_____

TERMINATION OR WITHDRAWAL OF THE CONTRACT

Patient may end contract at any point

Physician must follow legal protocol to end relationship with patient

PATIENT-INITIATED TERMINATION

Patient should notify physician through written correspondence with reasons for termination

Place in medical record

Physician letter to patient:

- _____
- _____
- _____

PHYSICIAN-INITIATED TERMINATION

Physician may terminate if patient is _____ **or** _____

Physician's letter to patient should include:

- _____
- _____
- _____
- _____
- _____

Sent _____

Copy and return receipt to medical record

ABANDONMENT

If a contract is not properly terminated, the physician can be sued for _____.

Patient care must be supplied by substitute if physician unavailable

CHECKPOINT QUESTION 3

What five elements must be in a physician's termination intent letter?

Answer

_____

_____

_____

_____

_____

CONSENT

Patients must consent to be touched, examined, treated

Given _____,

_____, _____

Durable power of attorney gives patient's representative ability to make health care decisions

IMPLIED CONSENT

Patients' actions usually imply consent

- Rolling up sleeve prior to injection
- Emergency situation

INFORMED OR EXPRESSED CONSENT

Physician must obtain permission for invasive treatments

- Surgery
- Experimental drugs

Informed consent is based on the patient's right to know every possible benefit, risk, or alternative to the suggested treatment and the possible outcome if no treatment is initiated.

INFORMED OR EXPRESSED CONSENT *(continued)*

Patient must give permission and understand implications

Consent form includes:

- _____
- _____
- _____
- _____
- _____
- _____
- _____

INFORMED OR EXPRESSED CONSENT *(continued)*

Never coerce (force or compel against his or her wishes) a patient into signing a consent form.

Mentally competent adults may sign consent form

Minors under certain conditions:

- Armed services
- Communicable diseases
- Pregnancy, abortion, birth control
- Drug or alcohol abuse
- Emancipated minors

 CHECKPOINT QUESTION 4

Under what circumstances should a patient never be asked to sign a consent form?

Answer

_____

_____

_____

REFUSAL OF CONSENT

Patients must sign form if refusing treatment

Document refusal to protect physician

RELEASING MEDICAL INFORMATION

Medical record is a legal document

- Information belongs to _____
- Document belongs to _____

Patient rights:

- Right to medical information
- Deny sharing information

Requests for records are common

 WHAT IF?

A well-meaning family member asks for information about her mother's condition. What should you say?

LEGALLY REQUIRED DISCLOSURES

Legally required disclosures = patient information that health care facilities must report to government agencies

- _____
- _____
- _____
- _____
- _____
- _____

VITAL STATISTICS

Birth certificates

Stillborn reports

Death certificates

MEDICAL EXAMINER'S REPORTS

Death:

- From an unknown cause
- From a suspected criminal or violent act
- Not attended by a physician
- Within 24 hours of hospital admission

INFECTIOUS OR COMMUNICABLE DISEASES

Reported to local health department

Information used for statistics or disease tracking

- Telephone reports (diphtheria, meningitis, plague)
- Written reports (hepatitis, leprosy, polio, TB)
- Trend reports (high incidence of flu)

NATIONAL CHILDHOOD VACCINE INJURY ACT OF 1986

Requires providers to report side effects of vaccines

Must also report:

- Date administered
- Lot number and manufacturer
- Adverse reactions
- Name, title, address of person administering

ABUSE, NEGLECT, OR MALTREATMENT

Must report abuse, neglect, or maltreatment for any patient incapable of self-protection

Federal Child Abuse Prevention and Treatment Act

- Threats to a child's well-being must be reported
- Workers who report abuse are not identified to parents
- Reporting workers are protected against liability

Relay abuse concerns to physician

Spousal abuse

Elder abuse

VIOLENT INJURIES

Providers obligated to report suspected criminal acts

- Weapons
- Assault

- Attempted suicide
- Rape

OTHER REPORTS

Cancer diagnoses

Epilepsy

Positive PKU results in newborns

Infantile hypothyroidism

 CHECKPOINT QUESTION 5

What are six situations and conditions you are legally required to report?

Answer

_____

_____

_____

_____

_____

_____

SPECIFIC LAWS AND STATUTES THAT APPLY TO HEALTH PROFESSIONALS

Medical practice acts

Licensure, certification, and registration

Controlled Substances Acts

- Good Samaritan Act

MEDICAL PRACTICE ACTS

Unique to each state

Similar elements:

- _____
- _____
- _____
- _____
- _____
- _____

MEDICAL PRACTICE ACTS *(continued)*

A physician may have his or her license revoked or suspended by the board of medical examiners in most states for a variety of reasons, including certain criminal offenses, unprofessional conduct, fraud, or professional or personal incompetence.

MEDICAL PRACTICE ACTS *(continued)*

Medical assistant must report:

- Illegal acts
- Unethical behavior
- Signs of incompetence

LICENSURE, CERTIFICATION, AND REGISTRATION

_____ practitioners must maintain license to practice; regulated by laws

_____ practitioners must meet basic requirements, pass standard test, gain approval from governing body

_____ = voluntary process regulated by professional organization

LICENSURE, CERTIFICATION, AND REGISTRATION *(continued)*

CMA/RMA credentials recognized nationally

Medical assistants:

- Not licensed
- Not limited to certain duties
- Physician or employer sets limits on responsibilities

CONTROLLED SUBSTANCES ACT

Federal law enforced by Drug Enforcement Administration (DEA)

Regulates

_____

Designed to prevent substance abuse by medical professionals

CONTROLLED SUBSTANCES ACT
(continued)

Offices with stock for dispensing must use triplicate order form issued by DEA

Transaction records must be kept for _____ years

Must be available for inspection by DEA at any time

All substances must be in _____ _____

Prescription pads must be kept secure

Theft must be immediately reported to local police and DEA

GOOD SAMARITAN ACT

Good Samaritan acts ensure that caregivers are immune from liability suits as long as they give care in good faith and in a manner that a reasonable and prudent person would in a similar situation.

Covers acts outside of formal medical practice

BASICS OF MEDICAL LAW

Tort law

Negligence and malpractice (unintentional torts)

TORT LAW

Tort = _____

- **_____ = harm was intended**
- **_____ = the defendant did not intend harm**

90% of suits against physicians fall into the latter category

NEGLIGENCE AND MALPRACTICE (UNINTENTIONAL TORTS)

Negligence is performing an act that a reasonable health care worker or provider would not have done

or the omission of an act that a reasonable professional or provider would have done.

Called malpractice if physician involved

NEGLIGENCE AND MALPRACTICE (UNINTENTIONAL TORTS) *(continued)*

Three types of malpractice:

- **_____ = incorrect treatment**
- **_____ = treatment performed incorrectly**
- **_____ = treatment delayed or not given**

NEGLIGENCE AND MALPRACTICE (UNINTENTIONAL TORTS) *(continued)*

Standard of care determines reasonable actions

Standards of care are written by various professional agencies to clarify what the reasonable and prudent physician or health care worker would do in a given situation.

NEGLIGENCE AND MALPRACTICE (UNINTENTIONAL TORTS) *(continued)*

For negligence to be proved, the plaintiff's attorney must prove four elements were present:

_____, _____, _____, and _____.

DUTY

Present when patient and physician have formed contract

Easiest of four elements to prove

DERELICTION OF DUTY

Plaintiff must prove physician did not meet guidelines of standards of care

DIRECT CAUSE

Plaintiff must prove derelict act directly caused harm to patient

Difficult to prove in patients with extensive medical history

DAMAGE

Plaintiff must prove damages (injury) occurred

Must have documentation of diagnosis

JURY AWARDS

Three types of awards for damages:

- _____ = small compensation for minimal injury
- _____ = money awarded for injury; moderate to significant amount
- _____ = money is awarded to punish practitioner; costly

CHECKPOINT QUESTION 6

What four elements must be proved in a negligence suit?

Answer

_____

_____

_____

_____

INTENTIONAL TORTS

Act takes place with malice and intent to harm

- _____
- _____
- _____
- _____
- _____
- _____
- _____

ASSAULT AND BATTERY

Assault = _____

Battery = _____

DURESS

_____

Example:

- Staff persuades pregnant mother of four to have an abortion
- Patient signs form, and procedure is performed
- Later, patient sues, saying she was coerced into signing the form (duress) and that abortion was performed against her wishes (assault, battery)

INVASION OF PRIVACY

Patients have right to privacy

Must sign authorization to release information to insurance company

Written permission from patient needed to:

- Release records or personal data
- Publish case histories in medical journals
- Make photographs of patients
- Allow observers

INVASION OF PRIVACY (continued)

Example:

- Patient seen for skin biopsy
- Insurer asks for information regarding bill and requests biopsy report
- Information is given
- Patient had not signed release form

DEFAMATION OF CHARACTER

_____

_____

- Libel = written statements
- Slander = verbal statements

Example:

- Patient asks for referral to specific surgeon
- Medical assistant claims that surgeon has a history of alcoholism

FRAUD

_____

_____

- Raising false expectations
- Improper instruction on possible side effects of a procedure
- Filing false insurance claims

TORT OF OUTRAGE

_____

_____

Plaintiff's attorney must prove:

- Intent to inflict emotional distress
- Physician acted in amoral or unethical manner
- Caused severe distress

UNDUE INFLUENCE

_____

_____

Example:

- Deceiving an elderly or mentally incompetent patient to undergo expensive or unnecessary procedure

 CHECKPOINT QUESTION 7

What is the difference between assault and battery?

Answer

_____

_____

_____

_____

THE LITIGATION PROCESS

Patient consults attorney

Attorney obtains medical record

Attorney files complaint

Defendant answers complaint

Discovery phase–interrogations; depositions

THE LITIGATION PROCESS _(continued)_

Trial phase

- Jury selection
- Opening statements
- Plaintiff presents case
  - Expert witnesses, evidence, witnesses examined
- Defense presents opposing arguments
- Closing arguments
- Verdict
- Awards or dismissal of charges

DEFENSES TO PROFESSIONAL LIABILITY SUITS

Defenses include:

- _____
- _____
- _____
- _____
- _____
- _____

MEDICAL RECORDS

The best and most solid defense the caregiver has is

_____.

"If it's not in the chart, it did not happen."

All documentation should be:

- _____
- _____
- _____

STATUTE OF LIMITATIONS

Length of time a patient has to sue a caregiver

Typically 1 to 3 years

Often exceptions for minors or wrongful death

ASSUMPTION OF RISK

Defendant claims patient was informed and accepted potential for injury

Example:

- Patient informed of adverse effects of chemotherapy
- Patient understands risks and receives therapy
- Decides to sue for hair loss (alopecia)
- Signed consent form proves patient accepted risk

RES JUDICATA

"The thing has been decided"

Losing party may not countersue once settlement reached

Example:

- Physician loses malpractice suit
- Cannot sue patient for defamation

CONTRIBUTORY NEGLIGENCE

Physician admits negligence but claims patient made injury worse

Example:

- Patient laceration stitched with fewer sutures than required
- Physician instructs patient to limit movement
- Patient plays baseball, laceration opens, becomes infected with scarring
- Both physician and patient contributed to injury

Awards not usually given for contributory negligence

COMPARATIVE NEGLIGENCE

Award of damages based on percentage of contribution to negligence

Example:

- Court decides negligence is equally shared
- Award is $20,000
- Physician responsible for $10,000

IMMUNITY

Federal Tort Claim Act of 1946 = no suit against U. S. government facility

- Veterans hospitals
- Military bases

Immunity for ordinary negligence, not intentional torts

DEFENSE FOR THE MEDICAL ASSISTANT

Respondeat superior = literally "let the master answer"

Also called _____

The physician is responsible for your actions as a medical assistant as long as your actions are within your scope of practice.

DEFENSE FOR THE MEDICAL ASSISTANT (continued)

Example:

- Patient calls, but physician has left for the day
- Medical assistant tells patient to take medication and call back tomorrow
- Patient dies during the night
- Physician claims medical assistant not instructed to give advice over the phone
- Medical assistant not covered by respondeat superior

DEFENSE FOR THE MEDICAL ASSISTANT (continued)

Refer to job description

Practice within guidelines

Never hesitate to seek clarification from a physician.

Malpractice insurance

CHECKPOINT QUESTION 8

What is the law of agency, and how does it apply to the medical assistant?

Answer

_____

_____

_____

_____

_____

EMPLOYMENT AND SAFETY LAWS

Civil Rights Act of 1964, Title VII

Occupational Safety and Health Act

Other legal considerations

CIVIL RIGHTS ACT OF 1964, TITLE VII

Protects employees from discrimination

Enforced by Equal Employment Opportunity Commission (EEOC)

Governs:

- Hiring practices
- Workplace conduct
- Accessibility

SEXUAL HARASSMENT

Defined as

_____

When conduct:

- Is a condition of hiring
- Is a condition of advancement
- Interferes with work performance

AMERICANS WITH DISABILITIES ACT

Prohibits discrimination against disabled

Applies to all employment practices

Applies to employers with 15 or more employees

Employers must make reasonable accommodations for disabled employees

ADA designed to protect employees, not require unreasonable accommodations

AMERICANS WITH DISABILITIES ACT *(continued)*

Require public buildings to be accessible

- Entrance ramps
- Widened rest rooms
- Braille signs
- Special phone service

OCCUPATIONAL SAFETY AND HEALTH ACT

Occupational Safety and Health Administration (OSHA) monitors _____

_____

OSHA rules protect health care workers from _____ **pathogen exposure and all body fluids**

OTHER LEGAL CONSIDERATIONS

Clinical Laboratory Improvement Amendments (CLIA)

- Specific rules for laboratory safety

Joint Commission on Accreditation of Healthcare Organizations (JCAHO)

- Standards for health care administration

 CHECKPOINT QUESTION 9

What are blood-borne pathogens? Which government agency governs their control in the medical office?

Answer

_____

_____

_____

_____

MEDICAL ETHICS

Medical ethics = principles of ethical and moral conduct governing behavior and conduct of health care professionals

Ethics are guidelines specifying _____ and are enforced by peer review and professional organizations.

_____ = issues and problems affecting a patient's life

AMERICAN MEDICAL ASSOCIATION (AMA) CODE OF ETHICS

States AMA's expectations of its members' behavior

Guidelines for disciplinary actions

- Censure = verbal or written reprimand
- Suspension = temporary removal of privileges and association with organization
- Expulsion = formal discharge from organization

MEDICAL ASSISTANT'S ROLE IN ETHICS

Medical assistants must:

- Protect patient confidentiality
- Follow state and federal laws
- Be honest in all actions

Medical assistants must apply ethical standards to all duties

Provide objective care for all patients

 WHAT IF?

A patient is hearing impaired, and you cannot communicate with him. What should you do?

PATIENT ADVOCACY

Your primary responsibility as a medical assistant is to be a patient advocate at all times.

Consider _____ above all else

PATIENT CONFIDENTIALITY

Information obtained during care of patient may not be revealed without patient's authorization

HONESTY

Report _____ to supervisor and physician

The mark of a true professional is the ability to admit mistakes and take full responsibility for all actions.

Speak honestly to patients

 CHECKPOINT QUESTION 10

What are the three ethical standards a CMA, as an agent of the physician, should follow?

Answer

_____

_____

_____

BIOETHICS

Moral issues and problems affecting human life

Examples: abortion, genetic engineering

What may be right for one patient may be wrong for another; that is the foundation of bioethics.

AMA COUNCIL ON ETHICAL AND JUDICIAL AFFAIRS

AMA subcommittee reviews principles and interprets them in clinical situations

Four categories:

- Social policy
- Relations with colleagues and hospitals
- Administrative office procedures
- Professional rights and responsibilities

Outside medical assistant's scope, but you will face their consequences during career

SOCIAL POLICY ISSUES

Guidelines for physician decision making related to:

- Allocation of resources
- Clinical investigation and research
- Obstetric dilemmas
- Organ transplantation
- Withholding or withdrawing treatment

ALLOCATION OF RESOURCES

Organs for transplantation

Funds for research

Funds for health care

Hospital beds and professional care

CLINICAL INVESTIGATIONS AND RESEARCH

Research must be part of systematic program with controls

Goal must be to obtain scientifically valid data

Utmost care and respect to patients

Obtain patient's permission

Patient's decision must be voluntary

Advise patients of experiment

Check and balance system

OBSTETRIC DILEMMAS

Technologic advances create new legal and ethical situations in obstetrics practice

- Abortion
- Genetic testing
- Artificial insemination

ORGAN TRANSPLANTATION

Need far exceeds availability of organs

Council's views:

- Treat rights of donor and recipient equally
- Donors must be given every opportunity to live
- Donor's death must be confirmed by physician not involved with transplant team
- Receive consent from donor and recipient

WITHHOLDING OR WITHDRAWING TREATMENT

Physicians must promote quality of life by sustaining life and relieving suffering

Patients may refuse treatment or request that life support be withheld

Advance directive = statement of wishes for medical decisions prior to a critical event

Must be written; copy given to next of kin

 CHECKPOINT QUESTION 11

What is an advance directive? How can a patient be sure his or her wishes will be followed?

Answer

_____

_____

_____

_____

PROFESSIONAL CONDUCT AND BEHAVIOR

All health care professionals are required to report unethical practices

No professional should engage in an ethically or morally inappropriate act

ETHICAL ISSUES IN OFFICE MANAGEMENT

Medical assistant involved in council's administrative guidelines:

- Financial interests should not come above patient care

- Physicians must warn patients of fees for canceling appointments
- Medical record should not be held against nonpayment
- Fees cannot be excessive
- Interest on past due accounts may be charged with prior notification

ETHICAL ISSUES IN OFFICE MANAGEMENT *(continued)*

No fees may be charged for referrals or hospital admission

No fees for completing or filing simple insurance forms

Use caution with computers to maintain confidentiality

Advertise honestly

Notify all patients if practice closes or physician dies

 CHECKPOINT QUESTION 12

What steps should be taken when a physician closes his or her practice?

Answer

_____

_____

_____

_____

Chapter 3

Fundamental Communication Skills

FUNDAMENTAL COMMUNICATION SKILLS .

Communication = _____

Verbal or otherwise

FUNDAMENTAL COMMUNICATION SKILLS *(continued)*

Medical assistant's role:

- Accurate and appropriate information sharing
- First point of contact for patients
- Be positive, pleasant
- Use good communication skills at all times

BASIC COMMUNICATION FLOW

Three elements:

- _____
- _____
- _____

Two or more people alternate as sender and receiver

BASIC COMMUNICATION FLOW *(continued)*

Medical assistant communicates in therapeutic manner

- Office procedures
- Policies
- Patient care

BASIC COMMUNICATION FLOW *(continued)*

Other communication responsibilities:

- Clarifying messages
- Validating patient perceptions

- Adapting messages to patient's understanding
- Verifying message as received

CHECKPOINT QUESTION 1

What three elements must be present for communication to occur?

Answer

_____

_____

_____

FORMS OF COMMUNICATION

Verbal communication

Nonverbal communication

VERBAL COMMUNICATION

Verbal communication involves an exchange of messages using _____; it is the most commonly used form and is usually the initial form of communication.

Oral communication = sending and receiving messages using spoken language

Be pleasant, polite

Use proper English and grammar

VERBAL COMMUNICATION
(*continued*)

Gear your conversation to the patient's educational level.

Consider:

- "Heart attack" vs. "myocardial infarction"

Do not talk down to patients

VERBAL COMMUNICATION
(*continued*)

Paralanguage = _____

Nonlanguage = _____

_____

"It's not what you say, it's how you say it."

VERBAL COMMUNICATION
(*continued*)

Written communication =

_____

Must be clear, concise, and accurate

Unclear messages may hinder treatment

Example:

- "Return to the office if you don't feel better."
  OR
- "If your temperature is not back to normal in 24 hours, call to schedule a revisit."

CHECKPOINT QUESTION 2

List five examples of paralanguage.

Answer

_____

_____

_____

_____

_____

NONVERBAL COMMUNICATION

Nonverbal communication—exchanging messages without using words—is sometimes called

_____.

- Kinesics
- Proxemics
- Touch

NONVERBAL COMMUNICATION
(*continued*)

Kinesics = _____

_____

- Facial expressions
- Gestures
- Eye movements

Can reveal patient's true feelings more accurately than verbal communication

Learn to read patients' actions and nonverbal clues for information

NONVERBAL COMMUNICATION
(continued)

Proxemics =

_____

3-foot area around patient considered personal space

Must enter personal space to deliver care

Because some individuals become uncomfortable when their space is invaded, it is essential to approach the patient in a professional manner and explain what you plan to do.

NONVERBAL COMMUNICATION
(continued)

Touch

Can be therapeutic

- Indicates support, concern

Some patients threatened by touch

Assess patient's demeanor for clues before applying touch

ACTIVE LISTENING

Ensures messages are correctly received

- _____
- _____
- _____

Develop active listening skills with practice

INTERVIEW TECHNIQUES

Medical assistant's responsibility to gather patient information

- Patient interviewing
  - Ask questions
  - Interpret responses

Goal is to gather accurate and pertinent information

INTERVIEW TECHNIQUES *(continued)*

New patients

- Medical and family history
- Review of body systems
- Social history

Established patients

- Review chart
- Make a list of questions
- Reconfirm medications and treatments

INTERVIEW TECHNIQUES *(continued)*

Conducting an interview

- Listen actively
- Ask appropriate questions
- Record answers

Introduce yourself

Know what questions to ask and in which order

Eliminate distractions

INTERVIEW TECHNIQUES *(continued)*

Six interviewing techniques:

- _____
- _____
- _____
- _____
- _____
- _____

REFLECTING

_____

Allow patients to complete sentences

Reflection encourages the patient to _____.

Example:

- "Mrs. Rivera, you were saying that your back hurts you. . .."

Do not overuse

PARAPHRASING OR RESTATEMENT

_____

Paraphrasing can help verify that you have accurately understood what was said.

Allows patients to clarify

Example:

- "You are saying that. . .."

ASKING FOR EXAMPLES OR CLARIFICATION

_____

Such as:

- "Can you describe one of those dizzy spells?"

ASKING OPEN-ENDED QUESTIONS

_____

- Be careful about asking "why" questions, because they can often sound judgmental or accusing.

Example:

- "How did you get that large bruise on your arm?"

ASKING OPEN-ENDED QUESTIONS (continued)

Avoid closed-ended questions

Example:

- "Are you taking your medications?"

SUMMARIZING

_____

Gives patient chance to clarify or correct misinformation

Also helps you organize your information

Example:

- "You told me that you have been feeling dizzy for the past 3 days and that you frequently stumble when walking."

ALLOWING SILENCES

Silences can be beneficial

Silences are natural parts of conversations and can give patients time to formulate their thoughts, reconstruct events, evaluate their feelings, or assess what has already been said.

CHECKPOINT QUESTION 3

What are six interviewing techniques?

Answer

_____

_____

_____

_____

_____

_____

FACTORS AFFECTING COMMUNICATION

Messages may not be received despite best efforts

Common causes:

- _____
- _____
- _____
- _____

FACTORS AFFECTING COMMUNICATION (continued)

Clichés

Example:

- "Don't worry. Rome wasn't built in a day."

Patient may interpret message to mean she is slow or old

Better statement:

- "I can see you're making progress."

FACTORS AFFECTING COMMUNICATION *(continued)*

Unclear or inappropriate message

Example:

- "I have scheduled you for a PET scan in radiology tomorrow at 8:00 a.m."

Patients may not understand technical language

Better statement:

- "The doctor wants you to have a test called a PET scan; here is a brochure that explains it."

FACTORS AFFECTING COMMUNICATION *(continued)*

Patients may be anxious or distracted

- Pain
- Positive or negative news

FACTORS AFFECTING COMMUNICATION *(continued)*

Environmental distractions

- Noises
- Interruptions

CULTURAL DIFFERENCES

Patients' perceptions and values are influenced by cultural, social, and religious beliefs

Patients have a variety of ethnic and cultural backgrounds

Medical assistants must understand differences for effective communication

CULTURAL DIFFERENCES

Consider:

- Personal questions during a medical history
- Eye contact
- Shyness

STEREOTYPING AND BIASED OPINIONS

All patients must be treated fairly, respectfully, and with dignity, regardless of their cultural, social, or personal values

_____ = judging all members of an ethnic or cultural group based on oversimplified negative characterizations

Stereotyping and bias prohibit therapeutic relationships

STEREOTYPING AND BIASED OPINIONS *(continued)*

Treat patients impartially

Guard against discrimination

Remain nonjudgmental

Avoid stereotypes

Maintain professional demeanor

LANGUAGE BARRIERS

Because it is crucial for you to give and receive accurate information, you will need to use an _____ to help bridge any language barriers.

- Staff member
- Family member
- Phrase book

LANGUAGE BARRIERS *(continued)*

Additional suggestions:

- Do not shout
- Demonstrate or pantomime
- Speak to patient with interpreter in line of vision

- Speak slowly, simply
- Avoid slang
- Avoid distractions
- Learn basic phrases of other languages in your area

Answer

_____

_____

_____

SPECIAL COMMUNICATION CHALLENGES

Assess situation and patient's ability to comprehend

Include patients in exchange

Examples:

- Hearing- or sight-impaired patients
- Speech impairments
- Mental health illness
- Distressed patients
- Children
- Grieving patients

HEARING-IMPAIRED PATIENTS

Many forms of impairment

- Anacusis = complete hearing loss
- Presbycusis = partial hearing loss, common in older patients

Tact, diplomacy, and patience are needed for effective communication

HEARING-IMPAIRED PATIENTS
(continued)

Other suggestions for effective communication:

- Touch gently to gain attention
- Talk directly, face-to-face
- Illuminate face
- Lower voice pitch
- Notepads, demonstrations, pictograms
- Short sentences
- Eliminate distractions

 CHECKPOINT QUESTION 4

What is the term for complete hearing loss?

WHAT IF?

You need to call a hearing-impaired patient. What should you do?

SIGHT-IMPAIRED PATIENTS

Range from complete blindness to blurred vision

Lose valuable nonverbal communication

SIGHT-IMPAIRED PATIENTS
(continued)

Suggestions for improving communication:

- Identify yourself by name
- Maintain normal speaking voice
- Keep patient informed; notify before touching
- Allow patient to touch table, chair, counter, etc.
- Offer to escort patient in office
- Tell patient when entering or leaving room
- Explain machine sounds

SPEECH IMPAIRMENTS

Variety of types

- Dysphasia = difficulty with speech; usually a neurological problem
- Dysphonia = voice impairment; usually a physical condition
- Stuttering

SPEECH IMPAIRMENTS *(continued)*

Suggestions for communicating effectively:

- Allow patient time to gather thoughts
- Allow time for communicating
- Do not rush conversation
- Offer a notepad
- Consider speech therapist

CHECKPOINT QUESTION 5

What is the medical term for difficulty with speech? What does dysphonia mean?

Answer

_____

_____

_____

MENTAL ILLNESS

Mental illness can affect communication:

- Outbursts
- Muteness
- Patients may hear voices

In-depth training required with moderate to severe mentally ill patients

Keep communication professional, nonjudgmental, and encouraging

MENTAL ILLNESS *(continued)*

Suggestions for improving communication:

- Tell patient what to expect and when
- Focused and professional conversation
- Do not force patient to answer
- Alert supervisor if you feel unsafe
- Do not confirm hearing voices
- If necessary, orient patient to reality

ANGRY OR DISTRESSED PATIENTS

With upset patients, prevent escalation of problem

Keep patients informed:

- Wait times
- Billing or insurance charges
- Office policies

ANGRY OR DISTRESSED PATIENTS *(continued)*

Most patients take sad news calmly

- Offer assistance
- Provide written information

- Be supportive
- Be honest
- Avoid false reassurances
- Do not belittle patient's problem
- Ensure safety with angry patients

CHILDREN

Tailor communication to child's comprehension level

Other suggestions:

- Maintain eye contact
- Use low-pitched, gentle voice
- Slow, visible movements
- Rephrase questions as needed

CHILDREN *(continued)*

- Child may return to lower development level for comfort
- Use play to gain cooperation
- Allow expression (fear, crying)
- With adolescents:
  - Assess situation before including parent
  - Remain objective

COMMUNICATING WITH A GRIEVING PATIENT OR FAMILY MEMBER

Grief = great sadness caused by a loss

Also called mourning

Five stages:

- _____
- _____
- _____
- _____
- _____

COMMUNICATING WITH A GRIEVING PATIENT OR FAMILY MEMBER *(continued)*

Patients may want to discuss:

- Feelings
- Fears
- Concerns for loved ones

Allow time for expression

Listen actively

Offer appropriate education

Shows respect

Sets professional tone

Avoid pet names

COMMUNICATING WITH A GRIEVING PATIENT OR FAMILY MEMBER (continued)

Focus on _____, not
_____

_____ can help you recognize a patient's fear and discomfort so you can do everything possible to provide support and reassurance.

Sympathy can compromise professional relationship with patient.

 CHECKPOINT QUESTION 6

What are the five stages of grieving?

Answer

_____

_____

_____

_____

_____

ESTABLISHING POSITIVE PATIENT RELATIONSHIPS

To establish and maintain positive relationships with patients, speak respectfully and exhibit an appropriate demeanor during all interactions.

PROPER FORM OF ADDRESS

Use proper form of address when greeting patients

Example:

- "Good morning, Mr. Jones."

PROPER FORM OF ADDRESS (continued)

Referring to the patient as a medical condition sends the message that the staff values the patient as nothing more than an illness, which can lead to increased anxiety.

PROFESSIONAL DISTANCE

Establish level of communication to deliver patient care

Personal involvement may jeopardize ability to make objective decisions

Maintain professional distance

Avoid revealing intimate personal details

TEACHING PATIENTS

One of fundamental communication skills necessary for medical assistants

May be simple or complex

TEACHING PATIENTS (continued)

Guidelines for effective patient education:

- Be knowledgeable
- Know special services in area
- Have printed information available
- Allow enough teaching time
- Minimize disruptions
- Be clear, concise, organized
- Give patient time to assimilate
- Ask questions to determine patient understanding
- Invite follow-up call

PROFESSIONAL COMMUNICATION

Communicating with peers

Communicating with physicians

Communicating with other facilities

COMMUNICATING WITH PEERS

Professional and appropriate at all times

Avoid non–work-related topics

Be honest, accurate

Become involved in local and national professional organizations

COMMUNICATING WITH PHYSICIANS

Be professional

Address physician as _____ _____ unless otherwise specified

Use correct medical terminology

Be honest

- If unsure, explain condition rather than guessing at a term

COMMUNICATING WITH OTHER FACILITIES

Maintain patient confidentiality

Observe legal requirements

Use caution with fax, e-mail

Provide only the facts

Be objective

Confirm receipt

Chapter 4
Patient Education

- _____
- _____

PATIENT EDUCATION

Patients require extensive and exhaustive education

One of the most challenging and rewarding roles in medical assisting

Education performed under physician's direction

PATIENT EDUCATION PROCESS

To educate patients effectively, you need to help them accept their illness, involve them in the process of gaining knowledge, and provide positive reinforcement.

Five steps:

- _____
- _____
- _____

ASSESSMENT

Assess your feelings and attitudes

Set aside personal feelings and experiences

Gather information on patient's needs and abilities

Sources of information:

- Medical record
- Physician
- Family members
- Spouse or significant other

CHECKPOINT QUESTION 1

What is the purpose of the assessment step during patient education?

Answer

_____

_____

_____

_____

_____

_____

_____

PLANNING

Planning involves using the information you have gathered during the assessment phase to determine how you will approach the patient's learning needs.

Learning goal: _____

Learning objectives: _____

- Specific
- Measurable

IMPLEMENTATION

Implementation is the process used to

_____

Carried out over several steps

EVALUATION

Evaluation is the process that indicates how well patients are adapting or applying new information to their lives.

_____ *is the patient's inability or refusal to follow a prescribed order.*

- Determine reason for noncompliance
- Notify the physician

Evaluation is an _____ *process, so you should expect to update and modify your plan periodically.*

CHECKPOINT QUESTION 2

What is the purpose of evaluation during patient education?

Answer

_____

_____

DOCUMENTATION

Includes recording of all teaching

Consists of:

- _____
- _____
- _____
- _____
- _____

Requires your _____

Document all telephone conversations too

DOCUMENTATION *(continued)*

Documentation is essential because from a legal viewpoint, procedures are considered to have been done only if they are recorded.

CONDITIONS NEEDED FOR PATIENT EDUCATION

Learning cannot occur without motivation or a perceived need to learn.

MASLOW'S HIERARCHY OF NEEDS

Abraham Maslow: people are motivated by needs, and certain basic needs must be met before a person can progress to higher-level needs

Applies to patients too

MASLOW'S HIERARCHY OF NEEDS *(continued)*

Physiologic needs: _____

Safety and security needs: _____

_____

Affection needs: _____

Esteem needs: _____

Self-actualization: _____

CHECKPOINT QUESTION 3

What are the basic physiologic needs outlined in Maslow's pyramid?

Answer

_____

_____

_____

_____

ENVIRONMENT

Must be conducive to learning

Quiet

Well lit

Limited distractions

Patients must feel relaxed and comfortable

EQUIPMENT

A psychomotor skill requires the participant to

_____.

Equipment should be available and functional

Teaching a psychomotor skill:

- Demonstrate entire skill
- Demonstrate step-by-step
- Have patient demonstrate skill with your help
- Have patient demonstrate skill without your help

KNOWLEDGE

Person teaching a skill must know the material

Research subject

RESOURCES

Use multiple resources or techniques

- Hearing
- Seeing
- Touch

Family or significant others should be present

Patients should wear necessary sensory devices

Use an interpreter if necessary

FACTORS THAT CAN HINDER EDUCATION

Recognize factors and intervene

If necessary:

- Delay teaching plan
- Revise teaching plan as necessary

EXISTING ILLNESSES

Patients' illnesses affect ability to learn

- Moderate to severe pain
- Poor prognosis or limited rehabilitation potential
- Weakness or general malaise
- Impaired mental health or cognitive abilities
- More than one chronic illness
- Respiratory distress

CHECKPOINT QUESTION 4

What types of conditions or illnesses may hinder your patient's ability to learn effectively? List six.

Answer

_____

_____

_____

_____

_____

_____

COMMUNICATION BARRIERS

Age

Educational background

Physical impairments

Other barriers

AGE

Educate at age-appropriate level

Safety education is a primary teaching focus for
_____ *and*
_____.

CHECKPOINT QUESTION 5

What is the primary teaching focus for small children and their parents?

Answer

_____

_____

_____

_____

_____

EDUCATIONAL BACKGROUND

Consider patient's:

- Educational background
- Ability to read
- Interest in preventive care

PHYSICAL IMPAIRMENTS

Impairments may hinder learning

Consult an occupational therapist

Consult physician for referrals

OTHER FACTORS

Patient's culture

Financial troubles

Assess patient's readiness to learn

Remove obstacles

TEACHING SPECIFIC HEALTH CARE TOPICS

Topics depend on:

- Patient
- Type of medical office
- Physician's preferences

PREVENTIVE MEDICINE

Preventive health care tips:

- Regular physical examinations
- Regular flu and pneumonia vaccinations
- Adult immunizations
- Childhood immunizations
- Regular dental examinations
- Breast self-examinations
- Mammograms
- Papanicolaou tests
- Prostate-specific antigen tests

PREVENTIVE MEDICINE *(continued)*

Preventable injury is the leading cause of death in persons aged 1 to 21.

Fall prevention tips should be taught to all older patients or any patient who has a problem with maintaining balance or uses an ambulation device (cane, walker).

CHECKPOINT QUESTION 6

Which patients should you teach fall prevention tips?

Answer

_____

_____

_____

_____

_____

MEDICATIONS

Pharmaceutical companies offer in-depth medication information for health care providers and patients concerning the chemical makeup of the drug, physiologic reactions in the body, prescribed dosage and route, and possible side effects.

_____

_____

_____

_____

MEDICATIONS *(continued)*

When preparing a medication therapy teaching tool, you must consider such factors as the patient's financial abilities, social or cultural demands, physical disabilities, and age.

Include over-the-counter medications

Include scheduling

Before developing a medication schedule, evaluate the patient's daily routine to see how adhering to the schedule may affect the patient's lifestyle.

MEDICATIONS *(continued)*

Pillboxes assist in scheduling

Consider route of medication administration

NUTRITION

Nutrition is focused not only on what people consume but also on how the body uses the food it ingests to maintain and repair itself.

Basic facts:

- No quick methods for weight loss
- Moderation is key
- Limit salt and sodium
- Eat three balanced meals daily
- Drink plenty of water

THE FOOD GUIDE PYRAMID

The pyramid consists of five main food group categories and one "other" category:

_____

_____

BREAD, CEREAL, GRAINS, AND PASTA

Darker breads

Best cereals = oat, bran, whole grain cereal

Avoid cheese or butter crackers

Avoid pasta sauces

VEGETABLES AND FRUITS

Fresh or frozen

Avoid butter or cream sauces

Limit boiling time

MILK, YOGURT, AND CHEESE

Skim milk or 1% milk fat

Low-fat or nonfat yogurt

1% or 2% milk fat cottage cheese

MEAT, POULTRY, AND FISH

USDA Select grade beef

Limit bacon

Fresh fish

FATS, OILS, AND SWEETS

Use oil sparingly

Avoid mayonnaise and salad dressing

Low-fat snacks

OTHER FOOD PYRAMIDS

Children 2 to 6 years

Adults over 70 years

Ethnic food pyramids

 CHECKPOINT QUESTION 7

What are the five main food groups listed in the USDA pyramids?

Answer

_____

_____

_____

_____

DIETARY GUIDELINES

USDA guidelines:

- Variety of foods
- Healthy weight
- Low-fat diet
- Vegetables, fruits, grains
- Limit sugar and salt
- Limit alcohol

DIETARY GUIDELINES *(continued)*

Encourage patients to read the labels on food containers; these labels provide important information on the nutritional values of the food, specific ingredients used, or any additives.

DIETARY GUIDELINES *(continued)*

Total fat

- Grams
- Percent of daily allowed fat in one serving

Carbohydrates

Carbohydrates are the _____
_____ *for our bodies.*
- Important factor for diabetic patients

Sodium, cholesterol, protein

DIETARY GUIDELINES *(continued)*

Healthy serving sizes

- A thumb = 1 ounce
- The palm = 3 ounces
- A handful = 2 ounces
- A fist = 1 cup

DIETARY GUIDELINES *(continued)*

Healthy food preparation

- Broil, boil, bake, roast or grill
- Trim fat
- Use a cooking rack
- Remove skin
- Use unsaturated oils

DIETARY GUIDELINES *(continued)*

The patient's age, culture, religion, geographic background, and social and financial circumstances may influence how well the patient complies with diet modification.

EXERCISE

If done in moderation, exercise can help relieve stress, maintain healthy body weight, and increase circulation and muscle tone.

Patients who are under age 35 and are in good health usually do not need a medical clearance before starting a routine exercise program.

EXERCISE *(continued)*

Patients with known medical disorders should check with the physician before exercising.

If patients are unable to perform exercises without assistance, it may be necessary to instruct them or their family members on range-of-motion (ROM) exercises.

EXERCISE *(continued)*

In most cases, ROM exercises are ordered by the physician to prevent further loss of motion or disfigurement after a musculoskeletal injury, surgery, or neurological damage.

If the patient is unable to perform the exercise on the affected area, passive ROM is performed.

 CHECKPOINT QUESTION 8

Why is teaching range-of-motion (ROM) exercises important?

Answer

_____

_____

_____

_____

_____

ALTERNATIVE MEDICINE

$300 billion/year industry

50% of Americans have used some form

Numerous types:

- Acupuncture
- Acupressure
- Hypnosis
- Yoga

ACUPUNCTURE

Acupuncture is one of the oldest forms of Chinese medicine.

Commonly used to treat:

- Addiction
- Fibromyalgia
- Asthma
- Chronic back pain

ACUPRESSURE

Similar to acupuncture

No needles

Commonly used for:

- Nausea and vomiting in chemotherapy patients
- Chronic pain
- Boosting the immune system

HYPNOSIS

Commonly used for:

- Weight reduction
- Obsessive-compulsive disorders
- Smoking cessation

YOGA

Yoga consists of a comprehensive discipline of physical exercise, posture, breathing exercises, and meditation.

HERBAL SUPPLEMENTS

Not regulated by the U. S. Food and Drug Administration (FDA)

Potentially dangerous side effects (ephedrine)

Advise patients to look for United States Pharmacopeia (USP) bar code

Placebo is the power of believing that something will make you better when there is no chemical reaction that warrants such improvement.

HERBAL SUPPLEMENTS (continued)

Assess patients' use of alternative therapies

- Length of use
- Side effects
- Notify physician

Recommend alternative therapies only when physician has approved

 CHECKPOINT QUESTION 9

What is a placebo?

Answer

_____

_____

_____

_____

STRESS MANAGEMENT

Stress comes from:

- Fear
- Anger
- Anxiety

Patients who are not capable of coping with stress on their own or with the help of instruction provided by the medical office staff may need professional counseling.

POSITIVE AND NEGATIVE STRESS

_____ *motivates individuals to work efficiently and perform to the best of their abilities.*

_____ *is the inability to relax after a stressful encounter.*

POSITIVE AND NEGATIVE STRESS
(continued)

Physical effects of unrelieved stress:

- Increased blood pressure
- Increased glucose levels
- Exhaustion

Coping mechanisms:

- Repression
- Denial
- Rationalization

POSITIVE AND NEGATIVE STRESS
(continued)

Coping strategies for patients:

- Reduce stressors
- Organize and limit activities
- Lessen fear of failure
- Talk about problems

RELAXATION TECHNIQUES

Breathing techniques

Visualization

Physical exercise

SMOKING CESSATION

Encourage patients to:

- Find local support groups
- Consult the Internet
  - American Heart Association
  - American Lung Association
- Patches, gums, other interventions

SUBSTANCE ABUSE

Substance abuse can be highly detrimental to your patients' health, so it is important that you give them information about substance abuse if they should ask.

Most common substance = _____

Other substances:

- Marijuana
- Cocaine, crack cocaine
- Stimulants, amphetamines
- Hallucinogens
- Narcotics

SUBSTANCE ABUSE (continued)

Detoxification is the process of clearing drugs out of the patient's body and treating the withdrawal symptoms.

CHECKPOINT QUESTION 10

What is the most commonly abused drug in our society? What does the term detoxification mean?

Answer

_____

_____

_____

_____

_____

PATIENT TEACHING PLANS

Developing a plan

Selecting and adapting teaching material

Developing your own material

DEVELOPING A PLAN

Because medical assistants are usually allotted only minimal time for patient teaching, you may often find yourself teaching without a written plan.

If you use preprinted teaching plans, be sure to adapt them to you particular patient's learning needs and abilities.

DEVELOPING A PLAN *(continued)*

Plans must contain:

- Learning goal
- Material to be covered
- Learning objectives
- Evaluations
- Comments

- Area for documenting:
  - When information presented
  - When objectives are completed

SELECTING AND ADAPTING TEACHING MATERIAL

When using preprinted material, consider the format, headings, illustrations, vocabulary, and writing style for overall clarity and readability.

Use commercially prepared materials to start a patient teaching library in the physician's office so you will have information at your fingertips when needed.

DEVELOPING YOUR OWN MATERIAL

Review available resources and teaching aids and adapt the information to benefit your patients.

- Identify the objective
- Personalize the information
- Use lists and outlines
- Avoid medical jargon
- Use simple diagrams

Chapter 5

The First Contact: Telephone and Reception

THE FIRST CONTACT: TELEPHONE AND RECEPTION

Your interaction with patient:

- Sets _____ for the visit
- Influences patient's perception

Project a caring, competent image

PROFESSIONAL IMAGE

Importance of a good attitude

The medical assistant as a role model

Courtesy and diplomacy in the medical office

First impressions

IMPORTANCE OF A GOOD ATTITUDE

Attitude = _____

- Positive or negative
- Shapes your behavior

Transmit a positive attitude to patients

By demonstrating empathy, interest, and concern, you can tell the patient that he or she is _____ and that _____.

WHICH INTERACTION IS POSITIVE?

"I know you feel terrible, Mr. Smith, but so does everyone else in the waiting room. It's flu season. Have a seat, and the doctor will see you shortly."

OR

"I'm sorry you don't feel well. Do you feel well enough to sit in the waiting room for about 10 minutes? The doctor will be ready to see you then."

_____

_____

_____

RECEPTION

Definition of a receptionist

Duties and responsibilities of the receptionist

Ergonomic concerns for the receptionist

THE MEDICAL ASSISTANT AS A ROLE MODEL

Good _____ and good _____ present a positive image to the patient.

Personal hygiene is important

DEFINITION OF A RECEPTIONIST

_____

_____

_____

COURTESY AND DIPLOMACY IN THE MEDICAL OFFICE

Positive attitude in all encounters

Courtesy and diplomacy are fundamental to successful human relations.

Diplomacy = _____

DUTIES AND RESPONSIBILITIES OF THE RECEPTIONIST

Prepare the office

Retrieve messages

Prepare the charts

Welcome patients and visitors

Register and orient patients

Manage waiting time

FIRST IMPRESSIONS

Are lasting

The patient's perception of the medical office is based in part on the impression you make.

 CHECKPOINT QUESTION 1

What are four ways that you can demonstrate a professional image to patients?

Answer

_____

_____

PREPARE THE OFFICE

Unlock doors

Disengage alarm system

Turn on lights, computers, printers, copiers

Check drop box

Systematic check of office

- Clean, tidy reception area
- Restock desk as necessary
- Check examination rooms if appropriate

RETRIEVE MESSAGES

Answering Service

Voice mail

Electronic mail

Facsimile machine

No matter how a message has been sent, all information must be treated _____.

CHECKPOINT QUESTION 2

From what four locations should you retrieve messages?

Answer

_____

_____

_____

_____

PREPARE THE CHARTS

Gather charts

Review charts

- Completeness
- Up-to-dateness
- Adequate clinical data available
- Test results

Charts for new patients with registration forms ready

WELCOME PATIENTS AND VISITORS

Greet patients personally

- Smile
- Cheerful greeting

Monitor waiting area for new arrivals

REGISTER AND ORIENT PATIENTS

Patient information sheet

- New patients
  - Personal information
  - Insurance information
  - Employment

- Marital status
- Social security number
- Referral

REGISTER AND ORIENT PATIENTS
(continued)

Orient new patients

- Brochures
- Policies and procedures
- Restroom and water fountain

MANAGE WAITING TIME

Tell patients if doctor is behind

Offer choices if wait will be longer than 30 minutes

ERGONOMIC CONCERNS FOR THE RECEPTIONIST

Having a good ergonomic workstation and good body mechanics:

- Prevents injuries
- Increases satisfaction
- Increases efficiency

ERGONOMIC CONCERNS FOR THE RECEPTIONIST *(continued)*

OSHA recommendations

Other recommendations:

- Carry small loads
- Frequently used items within reach
- Telephone headsets

CHECKPOINT QUESTION 3

What is the purpose of having an ergonomic workstation?

Answer

_____

_____

_____

_____

_____

THE WAITING ROOM

General Guidelines

- Designed for comfort, safety, and enjoyment
- Clean
- Uncluttered
- Ample walking room
- Low-key color scheme
- The reception area is a good place to set out patient education materials.

THE WAITING ROOM (continued)

Use television as an educational tool

- Lower volume
- Family-oriented programs
- Closed captioning

Check frequently

Monitor entrances, hallways, stairs

- Liability concerns

 CHECKPOINT QUESTION 4

What option should you offer hearing impaired patients if they wish to watch television?

Answer

_____

_____

_____

_____

_____

GUIDELINES FOR PEDIATRIC WAITING ROOMS

Most divided into two areas:

- _____ children
- _____ children

Monitor play area

Offer toys and books

AMERICANS WITH DISABILITIES ACT (ADA) REQUIREMENTS

The ADA Title III act requires that all public accommodations be _____ to everyone.

 WHAT IF?

A patient brings in his seeing eye dog and asks, "Can I keep the dog with me in the office?" What would you say?

 CHECKPOINT QUESTION 5

What act prohibits discrimination against patients with disabilities?

Answer

_____

_____

_____

_____

_____

INFECTION CONTROL ISSUES

_____ technique used in all aspects of work

- Standard precautions

_____ *is the most important practice for preventing the transmission of diseases.*

BIOHAZARD WASTE

All body fluids:

- Consider infectious
- Handle properly

Examples:

- Dressing supplies with bloodstains
- Tissues from patients with nosebleeds
- Vomit

COMMUNICABLE DISEASES

Exposure varies depending on office type

Communication among employees is essential

CHECKPOINT QUESTION 6

What is the most antiseptic technique for preventing the transmission of diseases?

Answer

_____

_____

_____

_____

_____

THE END OF THE PATIENT VISIT

Collect _____ or _____

Schedule follow-up appointment, if appropriate

Appointment reminder card

As patients leave the office, they should feel they have been well cared for by a competent and courteous staff.

TELEPHONE

Importance of the telephone in the medical office

Basic guidelines for telephone use

Routine incoming calls

Challenging incoming calls

Triaging incoming calls

Taking messages

Outgoing calls

Services and special features

IMPORTANCE OF THE TELEPHONE IN THE MEDICAL OFFICE

You must be able to use the tone and quality of your voice and speech to project a competent and caring attitude over the telephone.

BASIC GUIDELINES FOR TELEPHONE USE

Telephone communication is not effective if either party does not fully understand what is being said.

Effective conversation:

- Overcome obstacles
  - Noisy environment
  - Poor connection
  - Emotional distress
  - Patient's hearing

DICTION

How words are spoken and enunciated

Talk clearly

No gum or eating

Use a moderate pace of speech

PRONUNCIATION

Pronounce words correctly

Avoid:

- Unfamiliar terms
- Slang
- Medical terminology, where possible

WHICH QUESTION IS MORE APPROPRIATE?

"Are you dyspneic?"

OR

"Are you having trouble breathing?"

EXPRESSION

When talking,

- Sit up straight
- Smile
- Speak with a modulated pitch

LISTENING

Be attentive

Focus on conversation

Do not interrupt

Repeat message to verify

COURTESY

Speak politely

Never answer the telephone and immediately
_____.

Carefully monitor calls on hold

Balance between callers and patients in the office

CHECKPOINT QUESTION 7

What are the five basic guidelines for telephone use?

Answer

_____

_____

_____

_____

_____

ROUTINE INCOMING CALLS

An incoming call should be given the same courtesy and attention as an arriving visitor.

Typical calls:

- Appointments
- Billing inquiries
- Diagnostic test results
- Routine and satisfactory progress reports
- Test results
- Unsatisfactory progress reports and test results
- Prescription refills

APPOINTMENTS

New patients

- Appointments

Established patients

- Return visits

BILLING INQUIRIES

Inquiries concerning:

- Billing
- Fees
- Services
- Insurance

DIAGNOSTIC TEST RESULTS

Laboratory reports

Radiology reports

Record information

Report to physician

ROUTINE AND SATISFACTORY PROGRESS REPORTS

Patients

Hospitals

Home health agencies

Record information

Report to physician

TEST RESULTS

It is illegal to give information to anyone other than the patient without the patient's _____.

UNSATISFACTORY PROGRESS REPORTS AND TEST RESULTS

Never discuss unsatisfactory test results with a patient unless the doctor directs you to do so.

PRESCRIPTION REFILLS

Ensure that refills are _____

If in doubt, check with doctor

OTHER CALLS

Requests for referrals

Clarifying instructions for the patient

Routine administrative matters

CHALLENGING INCOMING CALLS

Unidentified callers

Irate patients

Medical emergencies

UNIDENTIFIED CALLERS

Do not interrupt physician

Take a message

IRATE PATIENTS

Calm the patient

Listen carefully

Take notes

Consult with physician if necessary

MEDICAL EMERGENCIES

As a medical assistant, you must be able to differentiate between _____ calls and _____ calls.

Call the caller

Ask specific questions

- Severe pain
- Profuse bleeding
- Chest pain
- High temperature

MEDICAL EMERGENCIES (continued)

Determine the patient's _____, _____, and _____ as quickly as possible in case you are disconnected or the patient is unable to continue the conversation.

Direct patients to nearest emergency room

Organize a list of the most common emergency calls and how to resolve them

TRIAGING INCOMING CALLS

Sorting calls into a _____

HOW WOULD YOU TRIAGE THESE CALLS?

Line 1: Wants to make appointment for her son, who has a 101.3° fever

Line 2: Wants to see the doctor this afternoon for chest pain

Line 3: Upset because she was disconnected 3 times and has a question about her bill

Line 4: Needs a prescription refill

TRIAGING INCOMING CALLS (continued)

Any patient with a potentially life-threatening problem needs to be taken first.

TAKING MESSAGES

Large part of daily responsibilities

Use phone message notepads

The minimum information needed for a telephone message includes the _____,

_____ *of the call,*
_____ *where the caller can*
be reached, a short _____ *of the*
caller's concern, and the _____
_____ *the message is*
routed.

CHECKPOINT QUESTION 8

What is the minimum information needed for taking messages?

Answer

_____

_____

_____

_____

_____

OUTGOING CALLS

General guidelines for outgoing calls

Calling emergency medical services

GENERAL GUIDELINES FOR OUTGOING CALLS

You should prepare for your calls carefully; have all information gathered and know what you want to say before you dial the number.

Verify time zones

Conference calls

- Notify all parties of time and date
- Provide access number and code in advance

CALLING EMERGENCY MEDICAL SERVICES

Patients needing immediate transport to hospital

Have the following information:

- _____
- _____
- _____
- _____

Speak slowly, calmly

CHECKPOINT QUESTION 9

What information about a patient should you know before calling emergency medical services for that patient?

Answer

_____

_____

_____

_____

_____

SPECIAL SERVICES AND FEATURES

Recall

Volume control

Intercom

Call forwarding

Caller identification

Cordless headset

TELECOMMUNICATIONS RELAY SYSTEM

ADA requirement

Used with hearing- or speech-impaired patients

Chapter 6

Managing Appointments

Review schedule carefully before making appointments

Along with notations in a patient's chart, the pages of the appointment book provide documentation of a patient's visit and any changes, such as cancellations and rescheduled appointments.

MANAGING APPOINTMENTS

Scheduling and managing appointments

Important responsibility

Use office facilities and physician's availability efficiently

Prioritize patients

Your responsibility is to manage all of this while maintaining a calm, efficient, and polite attitude.

APPOINTMENT SCHEDULING SYSTEMS

_____ appointment scheduling

_____ appointment scheduling

MANUAL APPOINTMENT SCHEDULING

The appointment book

Establishing a matrix

THE APPOINTMENT BOOK

Space for noting appointments for 1 year

Organized in various ways

- Single sheet for each day
- Whole week at one time
- Different colors for each day

ESTABLISHING A MATRIX

_____

- Note reason for crossing out time
- Block out time each morning and afternoon for emergencies, late arrivals, other delays

COMPUTERIZED APPOINTMENT SCHEDULING

Saves time

- Toolbars
- Advanced information searches

Once the daily schedule is printed, this important document is referred to as the daily activity sheet or day sheet and is the guide for everyone involved in the flow of patient care.

 CHECKPOINT QUESTION 1

Why is a matrix established?

Answer

_____

_____

_____

TYPES OF SCHEDULING

_____

_____

_____

STRUCTURED APPOINTMENTS

_____

Advantages:

- Good time management
- Optimum use of office facilities

Disadvantage:

- Patient may require more time than allotted

STRUCTURED APPOINTMENTS
(continued)

Buffer time

- Extra time in schedule for emergencies or other demands on time

Methods include:

- Clustering
- Wave
- Modified wave
- Stream
- Double booking

CLUSTERING

Grouping patients with similar problems

Advantages:

- Maximum use of special equipment
- Easy to control schedule
- Efficient use of employees' time

WAVE AND MODIFIED WAVE

Several patients scheduled for first 30 minutes of each hour

Second half-hour left open

Patients seen in order of arrival

Good in large facilities with several departments

FIXED SCHEDULING

Most common method

Reason for visit determines length of appointment

Schedule chronically late patients at end of day

Advise patients to arrive 30 minutes early

STREAMING

Appointments given according to patients' needs

Ensures smooth workflow

Medical assistant must understand procedures for allotting time

DOUBLE BOOKING

Two patients scheduled at same time with same physician

- Beneficial when patients being sent for diagnostic testing

FLEXIBLE HOURS

Better accommodates work and family schedules

Often used by clinics, group practices, family physicians

OPEN HOURS

Patients seen in order of arrival

Common in emergency clinics

Disadvantages:

- Difficult to manage time
- Facilities can become overloaded
- Charts must be pulled and prepared as patients arrive

 CHECKPOINT QUESTION 2

What are the three systems that can be used for scheduling patient office visits?

Answer

_____

_____

_____

FACTORS THAT AFFECT PATIENT SCHEDULING

_____

_____

_____

PATIENTS' NEEDS

With a patient in an emotional state, even the slightest real or imagined miscommunication can lead to a negative response from the patient.

PATIENTS' NEEDS *(continued)*

Before scheduling an appointment, determine:

- Why patient wants to see physician
- How long patient has had symptoms
- Acute or chronic problem
- Convenient time for patient
- Special transportation needs
- Third-party payers' constraints
- Necessary documentation

PROVIDERS' PREFERENCES AND NEEDS

Accommodate for punctual or late providers

Providers' schedule also includes:

- Telephone calls
- Reviewing laboratory and pathology reports
- Dictating charts or notes
- Unscheduled office visitors

PHYSICAL FACILITIES

Affect appointment schedule

You must thoroughly understand the requirements for procedures to be performed in the office to schedule appointments accurately.

 CHECKPOINT QUESTION 3

What are the three factors that can affect appointment scheduling?

Answer

_____

_____

_____

SCHEDULING GUIDELINES

Be pleasant and helpful

Write patient's phone number

Leave some open slots

NEW PATIENTS

The information you exchange at this encounter is crucial, and entering the patient's data correctly is imperative.

NEW PATIENTS *(continued)*

Obtain as much information as possible

Explain payment policy

Offer directions to office

Get permission to call at home or work

Confirm time and date of appointment

Check appointment system

If referral, obtain necessary reports

ESTABLISHED PATIENTS

Check schedule

Offer specific time and date

Write patient's name and phone number

Write appointment reminder card

Double-check schedule

Pleasant word and smile

PREPARING A DAILY OR WEEKLY SCHEDULE

Copies for all providers

Ensure that corrections appear on all copies

Deliver schedule in advance

Include hospital rounds, meetings, and personal engagements

PATIENT REMINDERS

_____

_____

_____

APPOINTMENT CARDS

Name

Day, date, time of return visit

Physician's name and phone number

TELEPHONE REMINDERS

All new patients and patients with appointments scheduled in advance should receive a telephone reminder the day before their appointment.

MAILED REMINDER CARDS

Mail 1 week prior to appointment

Reminders for annual examinations

CHECKPOINT QUESTION 4

What are the three types of patient reminders?

Answer

_____

_____

_____

ADAPTING THE SCHEDULE

Emergencies

Patients who are acutely ill

Walk-in patients

Late patients

Physician delays

Missed appointments

EMERGENCIES

When a patient calls with an emergency, your first responsibility is to _____ _____.

Consult office policy on these situations

List of questions to ask

PATIENTS WHO ARE ACUTELY ILL

Obtain as much information about the patient's medical problem as you can so your message to the physician will allow him or her to decide how soon the patient should be seen.

WALK-IN PATIENTS

Patients who arrive without appointments

Determine reason—medical emergency?

Follow office procedures for walk-in patients

LATE PATIENTS

Cause problems in schedule

Gently but firmly apologize for delay

Routinely late patients

- Advise of office policy for late patients
- Schedule late in day
- Ask patients to call if they are late

PHYSICIAN DELAYS

If patients are waiting in the office, inform them immediately if the physician will be delayed.

Always keep patients informed

Reschedule appointments if necessary

MISSED APPOINTMENTS

Call patient to determine reason

Send written note if necessary

Continued failure to keep appointments should be brought to the attention of the physician, who may want to call the patient personally (particularly if the patient is seriously ill) or send a letter expressing concern for the patient's welfare.

CANCELLATIONS

Cancellations by the office

Cancellations by the patient

CANCELLATIONS BY THE OFFICE

Illness, emergency, or personal time

These cancellations should be noted in the patient's medical record.

Alert at least 1 week prior to appointment

Offer to reschedule

CANCELLATIONS BY THE PATIENT

Ask for reason

Mark in appointment schedule

Offer to reschedule

If appropriate, consult move-up list

MAKING APPOINTMENTS FOR PATIENTS IN OTHER FACILITIES

Referrals and Consultations

Diagnostic Testing

Surgery

REFERRALS AND CONSULTATIONS

Must meet third-party payer's requirements

Provide:

- Physician's name and phone number
- Patient's name, address, and phone number
- Reason

- Urgency
- Referral or consultation?

REFERRALS AND CONSULTATIONS *(continued)*

Record in patient's chart

Offer information to patient

DIAGNOSTIC TESTING

Laboratory tests, radiology, computed tomography, magnetic resonance imaging

Determine exact test

Give referral slip to patient

Explain any advance preparation requirements

Emphasize importance of following instructions

SURGERY

Determine the patient's need for _____ with the insurance carrier.

Call participating facility

- _____
- _____
- _____
- _____

SURGERY *(continued)*

If available, offer preadmission forms

Preadmission testing

Write down all appointment dates, times, locations for patient

 CHECKPOINT QUESTION 5

What information should be readily available when you call to schedule a patient for surgery in another facility?

Answer

When you schedule a patient for surgery, you need the following information:

- ▪ _____
- ▪ _____
- ▪ _____
- ▪ _____
- ▪ _____
- ▪ _____

Chapter 7

Written Communications

WRITTEN COMMUNICATIONS

Must be:

- ▪ _____
- ▪ _____
- ▪ _____

Letters, reports, agendas, meeting minutes

PROFESSIONAL WRITING

Goal:

- ▪ Communicate in a concise, accurate, comprehensible manner

BASIC GRAMMAR AND PUNCTUATION GUIDELINES

Know rules

Apply to your writing

BASIC SPELLING GUIDELINES

Good skills take time to acquire

WHEN THE APPOINTMENT SCHEDULE DOES NOT WORK

Evaluate schedule over time

Since the workflow of the office affects every staff member, involve all employees in your study.

Identify problems

Make adjustments

Words can sound alike but be spelled differently

Consult Appendix E

WHICH HAS A SPELLING ERROR?

"Wound cultures were taken from the left lower leg site?"

OR

"Wound cultures were taken from the left lower leg cite?"

GUIDELINES FOR MEDICAL WRITING

Accuracy

Spelling

Capitalization

Abbreviations and symbols

Plural and possessive

Numbers

ACCURACY

Inaccurate information in some letters can lead to _____ and _____ and _____.

ACCURACY (continued)

You wrote, "The patient was started on the MVP chemotherapy program."

Physician wrote "MVPP"

MVP used in treating *lung cancer*

MVPP used for *Hodgkin's lymphoma*

 CHECKPOINT QUESTION 1

What are three consequences that could arise from in-accurate information in a business letter?

Answer

_____

_____

_____

SPELLING

You can add medical terms to your computer's spell check dictionary, but make sure that any word you add is spelled correctly.

WHICH HAS AN ERROR?

"The patient's mucus was yellow."

OR

"The patient's mucous was yellow."

CAPITALIZATION

Pay particular attention to how words, names, and abbreviations are capitalized.

Intercaps:

- pH
- RhoGam
- rPa
- ReoPro

ABBREVIATIONS AND SYMBOLS

Use abbreviations _____.

Consult:

- Office policy
- Appendix D

ABBREVIATIONS AND SYMBOLS
(continued)

The physician wrote, "The patient had good BS."

You typed, "The patient had good bowel sounds."

The physician meant "BS" to mean breath sounds.

PLURAL AND POSSESSIVE

Which of the following is correct?

- "The patient had multiple bullas."
- "The patient had multiple bullae."

NUMBERS

Spell out 1 to 10

Over 10, express as a numeral

Tips:

- Numbers in an obstetric patient's medical history are not written out
- Watch decimal point placement
- Do not transpose numbers

 WHAT IF?

You are writing a letter and can't find out how to spell a word. What should you do?

LETTER DEVELOPMENT

Understand components

Use correct format

Clear, concise, accurate message

COMPONENTS OF A LETTER

Letterhead

Date

Inside address

Subject line

Salutation

Body

Closing

Signature and typed name

Identification line

Enclosure

Copy

CHECKPOINT QUESTION 2

Whose address is typed as the inside address? What is the purpose of the salutation? What is the purpose of the identification line?

Answer

_____

_____

_____

_____

LETTER FORMATS

_____

_____

_____

FULL BLOCK

Full block is the most formal format and is most commonly used for professional letters.

BLOCK

- Date, subject line, closing, and signature are flush left

SEMIBLOCK

- First sentence of each paragraph is indented five spaces

WRITING A BUSINESS LETTER

Three steps:

- Preparation
- Composition
- Editing

PREPARATION

Good preparation is a key element in writing professional business letters.

MENTAL PREPARATION

Imagine you're talking to recipient

Benefits:

- Eliminate writer's block
- Focus on message
- Enhance organization

MECHANICS OF THE LETTER

_____ = skeleton of letter

_____ = blank space around letter

_____ = typeface

Choose a font that is easy to read and that is appropriate in size.

CHECKPOINT QUESTION 3

Before you begin to type a letter, name three mechanics that you need to select.

Answer

_____

_____

_____

COMPOSITION

*A **clear message** ensures that your reader knows precisely what is expected; an unclear message leaves room for doubt.*

Unclear: Please contact me.

Clear: Please telephone me by Thursday, October 1.

Consultation reports

Explanation of treatments

Thank-you letters

Announcements

COMPOSITION *(continued)*

A concise message is short and to the point.

Concise: "Please enclose a $50 check."

Not concise: "Please enclose a check in an envelope for exactly $50."

MEMORANDUM DEVELOPMENT

A memorandum (often called a memo) is for _____ _____;
it is never sent to patients. It is less formal than a letter and is generally used for brief announcements.

COMPOSITION *(continued)*

Inaccurate messages cause delays and confusion and can lead to poor public relations.

COMPONENTS OF A MEMORANDUM

Standard elements:

- Heading
- Date
- To
- From
- Subject
- Body
- Copy (c)

No salutation or closing

Physician should read and initial before sending

EDITING

Editing is a key step in making your letter a success.

Proofreading:

- Accuracy
- Clarity, conciseness
- Grammar, spelling, punctuation, capitalization

Corrections

- Use spell check with caution

 CHECKPOINT QUESTION 4

What is the purpose of proofreading?

Answer

_____

_____

_____

CHECKPOINT QUESTION 5

What are memorandums used for?

Answer

_____

_____

_____

TYPES OF BUSINESS LETTERS

Welcoming new patients

Test results

SENDING WRITTEN COMMUNICATION

Ensure confidentiality

Use return address

FACSIMILE MACHINES

Facsimile, or fax, machines allow the medical office to send and receive printed material over a phone line.

Cover sheet must be used

- Name, address, phone number of sender
- Name, fax number of recipient
- Number of pages sent
- Date and time sent
- Confidentiality statement

ELECTRONIC MAIL

Electronic mail, or e-mail, allows computer-to-computer communication, whether within the same facility or anywhere throughout the world.

- Confidentiality not guaranteed
- Follow usual steps for letter writing
- Attach letters

UNITED STATES POSTAL SERVICE (USPS)

Envelopes must be correctly prepared so that the optical character readers (OCR) used by the USPS can sort the mail quickly and efficiently.

ADDRESSING ENVELOPES

Standard business envelope is no. 10

Upper left corner used for return address

Recipient address—12 spaces or lines down from top and centered

All words of the address should begin with a capital letter.

Do not hand write

Special notations—2 spaces or lines beneath return address

ADDRESSING ENVELOPES *(continued)*

Additional points:

- Avoid graphics, logos, fancy fonts for ease in reading by OCR

- White or tan envelopes; black type preferred
- Avoid using the "#" sign
- One-eighth inch clearance around address if using window

 CHECKPOINT QUESTION 6

What does an optical character reader do?

Answer

_____

_____

_____

AFFIXING POSTAGE

Stamp

Permit imprint

Postage meter machine

USPS MAILING OPTIONS

Express mail

Priority mail

First-class mail

Standard mail

USPS SPECIAL SERVICES

Certified mail

- Used to provide proof of mailing

Registered mail

- Used to provide proof of mailing and receipt

International mail

OTHER DELIVERY OPTIONS

Airborne Express

Federal Express

United Parcel Service (UPS)

Fees vary

Most offer package tracking, pickup services, guarantees, proof of delivery

RECEIVING AND HANDLING INCOMING MAIL

Sort the mail quickly and promptly to ensure efficient functioning of the office.

TYPES OF INCOMING MAIL

Advertisements

Bills

Consultation letters

Laboratory and radiography reports

Patient correspondence

Professional journals

Samples

Waiting room magazines

OPENING AND SORTING THE MAIL

Any mail marked _____ should be handled first, followed by mail about patient-related issues.

Leave personal mail for physician to open

Handle patient care–related mail appropriately

CHECKPOINT QUESTION 7

What mail must be opened first?

Answer

_____

_____

_____

ANNOTATION

Annotation involves reading a document and highlighting the key points.

COMPOSING AGENDAS AND MINUTES

The purpose of an agenda is to _____

_____

_____.

Minutes

- Type as soon as possible after meeting
- List attendees
- List absentees
- Date and time
- Description of discussion
- Date and time of next meeting

Chapter 8

Medical Records and Record Management

MEDICAL RECORDS AND RECORD MANAGEMENT

Vital to quality patient care

Legal, moral, and ethical standards for proper management

Lawsuits can result if standards disregarded

Many uses:

- Research, quality assurance, patient education
- Documented evidence of patient care

STANDARD MEDICAL RECORDS

Many options for record keeping

Information should be:

- Easily retrievable
- Orderly

- Complete
- Legible
- Accurate
- Brief

Same contents regardless of format (paper vs. electronic)

CONTENTS OF THE RECORD

Patient information

Chief complaint

Present illness

Family and personal history

Review of systems

Progress notes

Radiographic reports

Laboratory results

Diagnosis

Signature of physician and/or medical assistant

Advance directives

Relevant correspondence

CHECKPOINT QUESTION 1

What is the chief complaint?

Answer

_____

_____

_____

ELECTRONIC MEDICAL RECORDS

Computers often used for storing patient data

Scheduling, accounting, tracking

Now used for charting in the clinical area

ELECTRONIC MEDICAL RECORDS
(continued)

Advantages

- Legibility
- Ease of storage and retrieval
- Improved documentation

Disadvantages

- Downtime
- Cost
- Security issues
- Staff training needs

ELECTRONIC MEDICAL RECORD SECURITY

HIPAA ensures patient privacy

Effective April 2003

Suggestions for software programs:

- User friendly commands
- Spell check and free text fields
- Security levels for all functions
- Repels hackers

ELECTRONIC MEDICAL RECORD SECURITY

To maintain security:

- Store backups in a safe place
- Encrypt passwords; use passwords with characters other than letters
- Change log-in passwords every 30 days
- Backup plan for system failure
- Keep terminals, fax machines, etc. out of patients' view

OTHER TECHNOLOGIES FOR MEDICAL RECORD MAINTENANCE

Same security guidelines apply to:

- Personal data device or PDA
- Laptop
- Personal computer (PC)

MEDICAL RECORD ORGANIZATION

Standard chart order

Demographic information kept separate from clinical information

Reverse chronological order

Clinical information formats:

- _____
- _____

MEDICAL RECORD ORGANIZATION *(continued)*

Source-oriented categories:

- Billing and insurance
- Physician orders
- Progress notes
- Laboratory results
- Radiographic results
- Patient education

PROVIDER ENCOUNTERS

Whether the patient is seen by a physician assistant, nurse practitioner, or physician, the visit _____ _____.

NARRATIVE FORMAT

Oldest format

Least structured format

Paragraphs indicate:

- Contact with patient
- What was done
- Outcome

SOAP FORMAT

SOAP = subjective, objective, assessment, plan

SOAP FORMAT *(continued)*

_____

- What patient says
- Use quotations where possible

_____

- What is observed during assessment and examination

_____

- Patient's diagnosis

_____

- List of interventions

POMR FORMAT

POMR = _____

Patient's problems listed with numerical references

Beneficial in group practices

Easy to track treatment and progress

POMR FORMAT *(continued)*

Four components:

Database

- Chief complaint, present illness, physical examination

Problem

- Every problem requiring evaluation

Treatment plan

- Management, workups, therapy

Progress notes

- Corresponding to each problem

CHECKPOINT QUESTION 2

What are three common formats used to document patient–provider encounters?

Answer

_____

_____

_____

DOCUMENTATION FORMS

Medical history forms

Flow sheets

Progress notes

_____

_____

MEDICAL RECORD ENTRIES

The medical record is a legal document that can be subpoenaed in a malpractice suit.

The golden rule in documentation is that _____

_____.

MEDICAL HISTORY FORMS

Often mailed to new patients prior to first visit

Used to gather information on patient

Whether the patient brings the completed form or fills out the history form in the office, you will review the information with the patient to clarify any questions and add additional information gathered in the interview.

MEDICAL RECORD ENTRIES
(continued)

Documentation guidelines:

- Follow office policy
- Ensure correct patient's chart
- Use ink
- Sign complete name and credential
- Record date
- Write legibly
- Check spelling
- Use facility-approved abbreviations only
- Use quotation marks for patient's comments

FLOW SHEETS

Information is recorded in table or graphic form

Eliminate need for long handwritten notes

Color-coded sheets for quick reference

Electronic records easily convert date to charts, graphs, or flow sheets

MEDICAL RECORD ENTRIES
(continued)

Documentation guidelines (continued):

- Do not diagnose
- Document after completing a task
- Document missed appointments
- Document telephone conversations
- Be honest
- Never document for someone else
- Never document false information
- Never delete, erase, Wite-Out information

PROGRESS NOTES

Written statements about patient care

Two columns

- Left column, date and time
- Right column, note

No matter what form is used for documenting, you must always _____
_____.

 CHECKPOINT QUESTION 3

List three advantages of using flow sheets in a medical chart.

Answer

_____

CHARTING COMMUNICATIONS WITH PATIENTS

Communication with patient should be documented (calls, e-mails, and replies)

Make entries immediately after interaction

Order chronologically

When a patient calls or e-mails the office, the conversation must be _____
_____ .

ADDITIONS TO MEDICAL RECORDS

All additions to medical records (e.g., laboratory results, radiographic reports, consultation reports) should be _____
before you put them into the chart.

CHECKPOINT QUESTION 4

What is the golden rule in documentation?

Answer

_____
_____
_____

WORKERS' COMPENSATION RECORDS

Workers' compensation record belongs to

_____

No previous information about patient should be given to insurer

Before treating a patient, obtain verification from employer

Cases kept open for 2 years

MEDICAL RECORD PREPARATION

Gather supplies

- Folders
- Labels

Prepare folders

Prepare "out guides"

- Out guide indicates that a chart has been removed

FILING PROCEDURES

File daily

Four steps:

- Condition—ensure that forms are complete, remove clips, tape, etc.
- Index—separate business records
- Sort—order each group of records
- Store—place record in proper storage area

CHECKPOINT QUESTION 5

Why is it necessary to make a new chart for an established patient who is being seen for an injury sustained at work?

Answer

_____
_____
_____

FILING SYSTEMS

Alphabetic

Numeric

ALPHABETIC FILING

Filing system according to letters

May also include color coding

FILE THESE ALPHABETICALLY

Mary P. Martin

Floyd Pigg, Sr.

Susan Bailey

Ellen Eisel-Parrish

Anita Putrosky

Susan R. Hill

Sister Mary Catherine

Cher

Stephen Dorsky, MD

Mrs. John Moser (Donna)

THE PROPER ORDER IS. . .

_____

_____

_____

_____

_____

_____

_____

_____

NUMERIC FILING

Uses six digits

Read as three groups of two

Straight digit filing

- Numbers read straight from left to right

Terminal digit filing

- Numbers read in pairs from right to left

Provides privacy for patients

Master patient index needed

OTHER FILING SYSTEMS

Other files to be organized:

- Employee files
- Insurance policies
- Accounts payable

Subject filing

Geographic filing

Chronological filing

CHECKPOINT QUESTION 6

What are the two main filing systems? Briefly describe each.

Answer

_____

_____

_____

CLASSIFYING MEDICAL RECORDS

_____

- Patients who have been seen within past few years
- Time frame set by facility

_____

- Patients not seen within designated time frame

_____

- Terminated relationship with office

INACTIVE RECORD STORAGE

Store in:

- Out-of-the-way area
- Physician's home (not always recommended)
- Microfilm or microfiche

CHECKPOINT QUESTION 7

What are the three classifications of medical records? Describe each.

Answer

_____

_____

_____

_____

_____

_____

STORING ACTIVE MEDICAL RECORDS

Shelf files

Drawer files

Rotary or circular files

Storage also a factor in a paperless medical office

RECORD RETENTION

You must observe the _____ in your particular state to know how long medical and business records should be kept in storage.

RECORD RETENTION *(continued)*

Store medical records _____

Permanently store in fireproof cabinet

- Tax records
- Insurance policies
- Liability plans
- Canceled checks (for 3 years)

Store equipment receipts as long as item is in use

 CHECKPOINT QUESTION 8

How long should medical records be kept?

Answer

_____

_____

_____

RELEASING MEDICAL RECORDS

Although the physical medical record legally belongs to the _____, the information belongs to the _____.

Never release original record

Never release information over the telephone.

Fees allowed for copying records

RELEASING MEDICAL RECORDS *(continued)*

Guidelines for releasing information

- Patient must be given opportunity to limit information released
- Patients may release information on a specific disorder or with a time limit
- May not leave out pertinent information
- Mental health, drug and alcohol abuse, and HIV and AIDS information may not be released without specific mention on release form

RELEASING RECORDS TO PATIENTS

Physician decides what information to copy

Parents' consent necessary for minors

 CHECKPOINT QUESTION 9

What is required for a legal disclosure of a patient's HIV status?

Answer

_____

_____

_____

REPORTING OBLIGATIONS

Records are confidential

Public health and safety concerns, legally necessary to report: Vital statistics

- Communicable diseases
- Abuse (child or elder)
- Certain violent injuries

Chapter 9

Transcription

MEDICAL TRANSCRIPTION

Process of _____

In today's computerized world, with a modem and sound privacy protection practices, a transcriptionist could conceivably generate and transmit reports from anywhere in the world.

MEDICAL TRANSCRIPTION *(continued)*

To transcribe well:

- Fast, accurate typist
- Strong medical terminology vocabulary
- Knowledge of grammar, spelling, punctuation
- Excellent listening skills
- Editing skills

THE TRANSCRIPTION PROCESS

Provider writes findings or dictates report

Transcriber plays tape; speed is controlled by foot pedal

Words typed, printed, and proofread

Print copy reviewed by provider

Corrections are made, and a final copy is printed and given to the provider for _____ *and* _____.

OFF-SITE TRANSCRIPTION

Transcription often outsourced

Files delivered in person and online

HIPAA regulations affect online transmission of information

REPORT FORMATTING

Five requirements:

- _____
- _____
- _____
- _____
- _____

Being familiar with the logical sequence and proper sorting of information for each type of document will help you adapt to any prescribed format.

CHECKPOINT QUESTION 1

List five requirements of any professional document.

Answer

_____

_____

_____

_____

_____

TYPES OF MEDICAL REPORTS

The most common documents transcribed in a medical office are _____, _____, *and* _____.

Diagnostic reports

HISTORY AND PHYSICAL EXAMINATION REPORTS

The JCAHO (Joint Commission on Accreditation of Healthcare Organizations) accredits and regulates every aspect of the policies and practices of hospitals and physician offices owned by hospital organizations.

HISTORY AND PHYSICAL EXAMINATION REPORTS *(continued)*

H&P must be on a patient's chart within _____ **hours of admission**

_____ **or** _____

Many physicians also use the H&P format to record a patient's annual physical examination in the office.

HISTORY AND PHYSICAL EXAMINATION REPORTS *(continued)*

Two sections:

- History—_____
- Physical examination—_____

 CHECKPOINT QUESTION 2

List two requirements of JCAHO regarding H&Ps.

Answer

_____

_____

_____

CONSULTATION REPORTS

Detailed account of consulting physician's findings and recommendations

Written in format of H&P

 WHAT IF?

You are transcribing notes and hear an unfamiliar word or phrase on the tape. What should you do?

PROGRESS NOTES

Transcribed notes printed on ongoing sheet or special paper

Must appear in consecutive order

SOAP NOTES

Subjective

Objective

Assessment

Plan

 CHECKPOINT QUESTION 3

Compare subjective and objective information. Give three examples of each.

Answer

_____

_____

_____

_____

_____

HOSPITAL REPORTS

H&Ps, consultation reports, operative reports, pathology reports, discharge summaries, and death summaries are generated primarily in inpatient facilities.

OPERATIVE REPORT

Documents each surgical procedure performed

Done immediately after procedure

Preoperative and postoperative diagnoses, anesthesia, details of procedure, blood loss, sponge and instrument counts, patient condition

PATHOLOGY REPORT

Findings of gross and microscopic examinations

Typical specimens include organs, lesions, tissue

AUTOPSY REPORT

Also called necropsy report or postmortem examination

Generated as autopsy is performed

RADIOLOGY REPORT

Includes:

- Title of procedure
- Contrast medium given
- Interpretation

DISCHARGE SUMMARY

Chronological account of hospital stay

- Reason for admission
- Tests
- Treatments
- Results
- Procedures
- Improvements and setbacks
- Condition upon discharge

Useful report for health care team involved in posthospital care

 CHECKPOINT QUESTION 4

List the information found in a discharge or transfer summary. Why is this an important document?

Answer

_____

_____

_____

_____

_____

_____

TRANSCRIPTION RULES

Follow guidelines of the American Association of Medical Transcription (AAMT)

ABBREVIATIONS

Use caution

- CC means chief complaint
- cc means cubic centimeters

If used, spell out first time used in a report

"When in doubt, spell it out."

CAPITALIZATION

Used for:

- Headings
  - CHIEF COMPLAINT; CC

- Eponyms
  - Down syndrome
- Trade or brand names
  - Valium
- Genus of an organism
  - *Staphylococcus aureus*

CAPITALIZATION *(continued)*

- Department names
  - Forsyth Medical Center Emergency Room
- Proper names of languages, races, religions
  - Hispanic woman
- Acronyms
  - CABG (coronary artery bypass graft)
- To draw attention
  - ALLERGIES: The patient is allergic to. . . .

NUMBERS

Spell out one to nine; 10 and above keyed as numerals

- Two, three; 11, 15

Use numbers consistently

- Dr. Smith saw 14 patients today; one was 2 days old.

Use numerals with symbols

- 100% oxygen

Add zero before and after decimal point

- 8.0×0.6

NUMBERS *(continued)*

Key space between numerals and units of measure

- 10 mg%

Numerals for measurements, laboratory values, age

- BP 110/70

Spell out ordinal numbers

- Felt better the third day after surgery.

Roman numerals for cranial nerves, obstetric history, electrocardiographic leads, types and factors, cancer stages

- Cranial nerves II through XII are intact.

PUNCTUATION

Apostrophes

Commas

Semicolons

Colons

Periods

Quotation marks

Slash marks

Hyphens

APOSTROPHES

Show possession

- Patient's appointment

Form contractions

- She's having flu symptoms

Units of time and money when possessive

- A week's worth of medication

Clarity

- The I's were not dotted

COMMAS

Between items in a series

- Pain is bilateral, severe, and stabbing.

To link two complete sentences

- She is a very sick patient, and I will admit her.

After a conjunctive adverb

- The medical assistant is in great demand; therefore, most schools have a waiting list.

COMMAS *(continued)*

After an introductory phrase or clause

- After she has her chest radiograph, she will come back to the office.

To set off clauses with additional information

- Electroencephalography, a test that assesses the electrical activity in the brain, is a diagnostic tool used by neurologists.

To set off parenthetical expressions

- The pain, according to the patient, measures 10 on the pain scale.

COMMAS *(continued)*

Dates with year, place names, long numbers

- The patient was last seen on May 2, 2003.

Quotations

- The patient said, "I will quit smoking tomorrow."

To prevent confusion

- The physician came in, in order to see the patient.

COLONS

After headings

- FAMILY HISTORY: The patient reports. . .

To introduce a series

- The physician prescribed the following: Keflex, Darvocet-N 100, K-Tabs, and Prinvil.

To separate hours from minutes

- Your appointment is for 10:30 a.m.

After salutation

- Dear Dr. Johnsen:

PERIODS

Ending sentences

With lowercase abbreviations

- a.m.

With abbreviations that shorten a word

- American Association of Medical Assistants, Inc.

After a person's initials

- J. T. Weaver, MD

QUOTATION MARKS

Direct quotation

- The patient stated, "My friend recommended your office to me."

Slang

- The patient stated that he was "blown away" by his improved cholesterol reading.

Titles of articles, short stories

- Please read "Making the Patient Comfortable" in the most recent issue of our professional journal.

SLASH MARKS

Replace "per"

- Give the patient 100% oxygen at 2 liters/minute.

Separate options and alternatives

- This is a pass/fail course.

HYPHENS

Compound words

- Mother-in-law

Avoid confusion or ambiguity

- We will re-treat with a different antibiotic.

Joining two words with identical letters

- Post-traumatic, pre-enteric

Spelling out compound numbers from twenty-one to ninety-nine

HYPHENS (continued)

Compound adjectives before a noun

- 22-gauge needle

Compound adjectives with suffix "free"

- Symptom-free

Compound that includes an acronym

- Post–CABG care

Keying suture sizes

- 2-0 Prolene

GRAMMAR

Correct grammar errors in dictation

Verb tense—most common errors in transcription

Ensure subjects and verbs agree in number and tense

SPELLING

When in doubt, consult reference

- Dictionary
- Spell check

TRANSCRIPTION SYSTEMS

Traditional tape dictation systems

Digital systems

Voice recognition systems

Transcription with word processing software

TRADITIONAL TAPE DICTATION SYSTEMS

Analogue system recording voice onto cassettes

Foot pedal

Tone dial, volume control

Headset

Speaker

Counters

Erase tapes after transcription is final and before discarding worn-out tapes

DIGITAL SYSTEMS

Voice is converted to digits, decoded, and sent via phone lines

Integrates with transcriptionist's computer

Automatically produces information and report format

VOICE RECOGNITION SYSTEMS

Limitations

- There, their, they're
- Accents
- Dialects
- Proper names
- Garbled speech

 WHAT IF?

You are having trouble understanding a particular physician's dictation tapes because of a dialect or foreign accent. How should you handle this situation?

Chapter 10

Computer Applications in the Medical Office

THE COMPUTER

Major role in physician's office

- Administrative applications
  - • _____
  - • _____
  - • _____
  - • _____
- Clinical applications
  - • _____
  - • _____

TRANSCRIPTION WITH WORD PROCESSING SOFTWARE

Macros and templates speed transcription process

Legal experts warn providers not just to report examination results as "normal"

- Describe negative findings

 CHECKPOINT QUESTION 5

Describe the main difference between analogue and digital transcription equipment.

Answer

_____

_____

_____

THE COMPUTER *(continued)*

Hardware

- Central processing unit

CPU cells _____, _____, and _____ data and instruct the computer how to operate a given program.

- Keyboard
- Monitor
- Hard drive
- Printer
- Scanner
- Secondary storage systems

 CHECKPOINT QUESTION 1

What do the CPU cells do?

Answer

_____

_____

_____

PERIPHERALS

Mouse

Battery backup

Modem

CHECKPOINT QUESTION 2

Why should your computer have an Ethernet port or Ethernet interface card?

Answer

_____

_____

_____

CARE AND MAINTENANCE

Cool, dry area out of direct sunlight

Antistatic floor mat or carpet

Dust covers

Antistatic wipes

Free of debris and liquids

Warranty

Data storage

INTERNET BASICS

Used for both administrative and clinical reasons

GETTING STARTED AND CONNECTED

World Wide Web

Electronic mail

CONNECTING TO THE INTERNET

Internet service provider (ISP)

Cable television company

Digital subscriber line (DSL)

If you need to download large files through the Internet, you should use either a _____ or _____.

CHECKPOINT QUESTION 3

Which two types of Internet connections are recommended for downloading large files?

Answer

_____

_____

_____

SECURITY

Never send any _____ over the Internet to a site that does not have a secure sockets layer (SSL).

Lock icon

Set limits for cookies

A _____ is a tiny file left on your computer's hard drive from a website without your permission.

VIRUSES

A virus is a dangerous invader that enters your computer through some source and can destroy your files, software programs, and possibly even the hard drive.
- Do not open suspicious attachments
- Update virus protection software
- New viruses detected daily

DOWNLOADING INFORMATION

Downloading transfers information from _____ to _____ hard drive.

WORKING OFFLINE

Save commonly accessed sites on Web browser

ELECTRONIC MAIL

E-mail promotes good patient care, enhances communication, promotes teamwork, eliminates phone tag, and provides written documentation of messages.

USING E-MAIL

Do not send personal messages

Do not send chain letters

Read e-mail offline

Messages must be professional

Activate encryption

Encryption is a process of scrambling messages so they cannot be read until they reach the recipient.

Use "out-of-office assistant" when necessary

 CHECKPOINT QUESTION 4

What does the encryption feature do?

Answer

_____

_____

_____

ACCESS

Access e-mail through Internet or intranet

Locate and double-click mail icon

Enter password if necessary

COMPOSING MESSAGES

Follow guidelines for writing a business letter

Check spelling, grammar, and punctuation

Short, concise

Flag important messages

Appropriate fonts and size

Generic or plain stationery

Complete subject line

Only one topic

No indents for new paragraphs; skip a line

Permanent signature

ADDRESS BOOKS

Collection of e-mail addresses

- Keep addresses updated
- Organize addresses

ATTACHMENTS

File sent with an e-mail

Guidelines

- Open attachment
- File in appropriate place
- Verify that the correct file is attached before sending e-mail

OPENING E-MAIL

Open your e-mail only

File or delete e-mail after reading it

Open flagged messages first

Forward appropriate messages to supervisor

Block bulk mail or unsubscribe from mailing lists

 CHECKPOINT QUESTION 5

Can you be 100% guaranteed that your e-mail transmissions are safe?

Answer

_____

_____

_____

MEDICAL APPLICATIONS OF THE INTERNET

Surfing that is unorganized and not focused can be time consuming and unproductive.

Since the information that you obtain from the Web will affect patient care, all steps must be taken to ensure that only _____ information is found and used.

Health on the Net (HON) seal

SEARCH ENGINES

Allow you to _____

■ Google, Yahoo, Lycos, Excite, Dogpile

Your key words should be focused to limit the number of responses that you will get.

To narrow your search further, use the advanced search feature.

 CHECKPOINT QUESTION 6

What is a search engine?

Answer

_____

_____

_____

PROFESSIONAL MEDICAL SITES

Use Web address lists at the end of each chapter

Addresses change frequently

Medical specialties have their own sites

Hospital sites

Box 10-4 lists additional health care sites

LITERARY SEARCHES

A literary search involves finding _____ that present new facts or data about a given topic.

■ OVID

■ PubMed
■ CINAHL

CHECKPOINT QUESTION 7

How is a literary search different from a search on an Internet website?

Answer

_____

_____

_____

_____

HEALTH-RELATED CALCULATORS

Due date calendar

■ www.babycenter.com/calculators/duedate

Ovulation calculator

■ www.babycenter.com/calculators/ovulation

Target heart rate calculator

■ www.webmd.com/heartrate

INSURANCE-RELATED SITES

Buying health insurance

■ www.ehealthinsurance.com

Medicare

■ www.medicare.gov

Red-flagged insurance database

■ www.mib.com/html/us_residents.html

PATIENT TEACHING ISSUES

Teach patients to acquire reliable information

Advise them of dangers

Box 10-5 lists good sites for patient education

BUYING MEDICATION ONLINE

If patients want to purchase prescriptions online, advise them to use only sites that are certified by the

_____

_____.

Advise patients to buy only medications prescribed by the physician.

Warn patients to purchase medications from U. S. sites only.

Warn patients about the dangers of self-prescribing, and alert the physician to any communication you have with the patient regarding this practice.

 CHECKPOINT QUESTION 8

Name three safety tips to teach patients about buying medication on the Internet.

Answer

_____

_____

_____

_____

FINANCIAL ASSISTANCE FOR MEDICATIONS

Online resources

- Drug company's home page
- www.medicare.gov/prescription/home.asp
- www.needymedes.com/Mainpage.html
- www.Rxhope.com

MEDICAL RECORDS

Sites for storing personal medical information

Advise patients against storing personal medical information online

Advise patients to download and print forms to complete and store in a safe location

MEDICAL RECORD FORMS

Sites to access medical forms

- Recording personal health histories
  - www.ahima.org/consumer/index.html
- Emergency consent forms for parents
  - www.acep.org/index.cfm/pid/14.htm

Advance directives, medical power of attorney, organ donation

INJURY PREVENTION

_____ *are a leading cause of death of children.*

Sites with information on preventing injuries in children

- American Academy of Pediatrics
  - www.aap.org
- National Safe Kids foundation
  - www.safekids.org

 WHAT IF?

Parents ask you how to keep their child safe on the Internet. What should you say?

INTRANET

_____

_____

Used in large practices

The benefits of an intranet are enhanced communication, quick access to needed information, and increased productivity.

 CHECKPOINT QUESTION 9

How does an intranet differ from the Internet?

Answer

_____

_____

_____

_____

MEDICAL SOFTWARE APPLICATIONS

Never buy or install a new software program or update an existing version without permission from either the office manager or the physician.

Available for both administrative and clinical applications

CLINICAL APPLICATIONS

Clinical software is designed to help the physician, nurse, medical assistant, or other health care professional provide the most efficient, safest, and most reliable health care available.

CLINICAL APPLICATIONS *(continued)*

Virtual patient charts

The advantages to a virtual charting system are that it saves filing space, increases access to patients' charts for all staff members, eliminates hunting for misplaced charts, and keeps the charts better organized and neater.

Up-to-date list of clinical tasks

CLINICAL APPLICATIONS *(continued)*

Prescription management and drug information

A good program that focuses on pharmaceutical information will decrease medication errors, increase patient satisfaction, and provide better patient care, and it can be financially beneficial to the patient and the practice.

Insert laboratory reports or imaging studies into patient records

Telephone triage

CHECKPOINT QUESTION 10

What is a virtual chart?

Answer

_____

_____

_____

ADMINISTRATIVE APPLICATIONS

_____ **used most commonly**

Benefits to the physician's office:

Appointment making and tracking are more efficient with a computer program than with a book format.

Track patient flows

Send insurance claims electronically

Integrate with insurance companies and other businesses

ADMINISTRATIVE APPLICATIONS *(continued)*

Credit card authorization

Check patient insurance eligibility

HIPAA compliance

Send collection letters

Financial management

Payroll

Transcription

Word processing

Managing personnel records

PAGING SYSTEM SOFTWARE

Always double-check to make sure that the physician you are paging is the one on call.

Alpha message is a _____

■ "Call the office regarding lab results."

Paging guidelines:

- Always provide a return number
- Watch spelling
- Concise messages
- Do not give the pager number to anyone

 CHECKPOINT QUESTION 11

What is an alpha page message?

Answer

_____

_____

_____

POWERPOINT

Software program to write and give presentations

Projects slides

Print slides for handouts

MEETING MAKER

Promotes internal coordination of meetings and calendars

Used in large practices with multiple offices and administrative personnel

HANDHELD COMPUTERS

23% of physicians use a handheld computer or PDA

Information entered with a stylus

Synchronizes with desktop computer

PURCHASING A COMPUTER

All key members of the staff should be consulted prior to such a purchase and should be actively involved in selecting the hardware and software.

Determine specific needs

See what other medical offices use

Try out several software packages

Interview and compare vendors

TRAINING OPTIONS

Seek training to achieve the highest benefit from hardware and software

- Vendors
- User's manual
- Help screens
- Tutorials
- Help desk

COMPUTER ETHICS

A computer is essential in the physician's office.

It can lead to invasion of a patient's privacy and unethical behavior.

- Never give out password
- Exit files before leaving computer station

If you are using another person's password to get patient information, you should contact the administrator of the program and get your own code.

COMPUTER ETHICS *(continued)*

Use Internet for professional purposes only

Only read e-mail addressed to you

Sensitive patient data should not be sent via _____ from one office to the other unless it is clearly known that the recipient of the e-mail is the only one with access to it.

Chapter 11

Quality Improvement and Risk Management

QUALITY IMPROVEMENT AND RISK MANAGEMENT

Quality improvement (QI) = _____

_____

Examines how care is delivered

Investigates methods to correct problems

QUALITY IMPROVEMENT PROGRAMS IN THE MEDICAL OFFICE SETTING

Quality improvement programs let an organization scientifically measure the quality of its products and services.

The patient's outcome is _____

_____.

QUALITY IMPROVEMENT PROGRAMS IN THE MEDICAL OFFICE SETTING *(continued)*

QI programs required to report patient outcomes

Legislation may force all health care settings to report outcomes

QUALITY IMPROVEMENT PROGRAMS IN THE MEDICAL OFFICE SETTING *(continued)*

Benefits for health care organizations:

- ▪ _____
- ▪ _____

- ▪ _____
- ▪ _____
- ▪ _____

REGULATORY AGENCIES

The primary regulatory agencies that mandate QI programs are the Joint Commission on Accreditation of Healthcare Organizations (JCAHO), Occupational Safety and Health Administration (OSHA), Centers for Medicare & Medicaid Services (CMS), and state public health departments.

JOINT COMMISSION ON ACCREDITATION OF HEALTHCARE ORGANIZATIONS (JCAHO)

The JCAHO is a private agency that sets health care standards and evaluates an organization's implementation of these standards for health care settings.

Expanded jurisdiction to outpatient and ambulatory care in 1996

JOINT COMMISSION ON ACCREDITATION OF HEALTHCARE ORGANIZATIONS (JCAHO) *(continued)*

Participation in the JCAHO is voluntary for health care organizations; without accreditation, however, the health care organization may not be eligible to participate in particular federal and state funding programs, such as Medicare and Medicaid.

 CHECKPOINT QUESTION 1

What are the benefits to a health care organization of accreditation by the JCAHO?

Answer

_____

_____

_____

_____

- _____
- _____
- _____

JCAHO ACCREDITATION PROCESS

Survey application filed

Facility prepares survey by assessing compliance against standards

JCAHO informs facility of survey date

JCAHO conducts survey

JCAHO mails results within 60 days

Focus, or secondary, survey if necessary

CHECKPOINT QUESTION 3

What is the mission of OSHA?

Answer

_____

_____

_____

JCAHO ACCREDITATION PROCESS
(continued)

Must renew accreditation every _____ years

Must show improvement in several areas:

- Accuracy of patient ID
- Communication effectiveness
- Eliminate errors (wrong procedure, wrong patient)
- Sentinel event policy

A sentinel event is an _____ _____ *to a patient.*

CENTERS FOR MEDICARE & MEDICAID SERVICES

Division of U. S. Department of Health & Human Services

Oversees many programs affecting medical assisting:

- _____
- _____
- _____

CHECKPOINT QUESTION 2

What is a sentinel event?

Answer

_____

_____

_____

_____

CLINICAL LABORATORY IMPROVEMENT AMENDMENTS ACT

Designed to streamline standards and quality of

_____

Laboratory settings must have a complete and comprehensive QI program that studies and corrects problems associated with specimen collection and handling.

OCCUPATIONAL SAFETY AND HEALTH ADMINISTRATION

OSHA's mission is to save lives, prevent injuries, and protect the health of America's workers.

- _____
- _____

HEALTH INSURANCE PORTABILITY AND ACCOUNTABILITY ACT

Four main objectives:

- _____
- _____
- _____
- _____

HEALTH INSURANCE PORTABILITY AND ACCOUNTABILITY ACT
(continued)

Key requirements of HIPAA:

- Privacy officer in each practice
- Post notice in all waiting areas explaining privacy policies
- Ensure patient safety and confidentiality

You will need to focus and guarantee security and privacy of all patient health information.

 ## CHECKPOINT QUESTION 4

What governmental agency would you look to for additional information on HIPAA and CLIA regulations?

Answer

_____

_____

_____

STATE HEALTH DEPARTMENTS

Agency in each state to license and monitor health care organizations

Guidelines for QI programs

Be familiar with state regulations

DEVELOPING A QUALITY IMPROVEMENT PROGRAM

- QI issues to monitor:
  - _____
  - _____
  - _____
  - _____
  - _____
  - _____

SEVEN STEPS FOR A SUCCESSFUL PROGRAM

1. Identify the problem or potential problem.

Problems given top priority are those that are high risk (most likely to occur) and those that are most likely to cause injury to patients, family members, or employees.

SEVEN STEPS FOR A SUCCESSFUL PROGRAM *(continued)*

2. Form a task force.

A task force is a group of employees with different roles in the organization brought together to

_____.

SEVEN STEPS FOR A SUCCESSFUL PROGRAM *(continued)*

3. Assign an expected threshold.

- _____

Thresholds must be realistic and achievable.

SEVEN STEPS FOR A SUCCESSFUL PROGRAM *(continued)*

4. Explore the problem and propose solutions.

5. Implement the solution.

6. Establish a QI monitoring plan.

After implementation, the solution must be evaluated to determine whether it worked and, if so, how well.

7. Obtain feedback.

 ## CHECKPOINT QUESTION 5

How does an organization select problems for a QI program?

Answer

_____

_____

_____

_____

RISK MANAGEMENT

Risk management is an internal process geared to identifying _____ *before they cause injury to patients or employees.*

Problems related to risk factors

- Poor lighting
- Unlocked medication cabinets
- Faulty patient identification procedures

INCIDENT REPORTS

Incident reports, sometimes referred to as occurrence reports, are _____
_____.

- Written by staff member involved in incident
- Reviewed by supervisor
- Sent to central location

 CHECKPOINT QUESTION 6

What is an incident report?

Answer

_____

_____

_____

WHEN TO COMPLETE AN INCIDENT REPORT

Situations of human error or unavoidable accidents

- Medication errors
- Drawing blood from the wrong patient
- Mislabeling of tubes or specimens
- Employee needlesticks
- Workers' compensation injuries

The rule of thumb is, _____
_____.

INFORMATION INCLUDED ON AN INCIDENT REPORT

Name, address, phone number of injured party

Date of birth, sex of injured party

Date, time, location of accident

Brief description of incident

Diagnostic or treatments needed

Patient examination findings

Names, addresses of witnesses

Physician's or supervisor's signature

GUIDELINES FOR COMPLETING AN INCIDENT REPORT

State only _____. *Do not draw conclusions or summarize the event.*

Write legibly

Sign name

Complete within 24 hours of incident

Fill out form completely

Do not photocopy for your record

Do not place in patient's record

 WHAT IF?

You give the wrong medication, and the patient has a bad reaction to it. Would you be better off not documenting the medication error?

TRENDING INCIDENT REPORTS

Completed reports are reviewed and tracked for patterns

- Days of the week
- Common areas of falls
- Medications routinely given incorrectly

Chapter 12

Management of the Medical Office Team

OVERVIEW OF MEDICAL OFFICE MANAGEMENT

Organizational structure

The medical office manager

ORGANIZATIONAL STRUCTURE

The medical office's organizational structure, or chain of command, is depicted in an _____, *a flow sheet that* _____ _____ _____ *and to see where they fit into the team.*

 CHECKPOINT QUESTION 1

What is the purpose of an organizational chart?

Answer

_____

_____

_____

THE MEDICAL OFFICE MANAGER

Officer must be:

- Flexible
- A positive role model
- Honest, fair
- An effective communicator
- Organized
- Focused

THE MEDICAL OFFICE MANAGER
(continued)

Responsibilities include:

- _____
- _____
- _____
- _____
- _____

RESPONSIBILITIES OF THE OFFICE MANAGER

Communication

- With patients
- With staff
- Electronically

COMMUNICATION

You must be a _____, *have good* _____, *and be aware of your own* _____.

COMMUNICATING WITH PATIENTS

Challenging as a manager

- Complaints
- Billing concerns
- Poor care
- Long waits

Be diplomatic

Correct problems quickly

Alleviate negative patient feelings

COMMUNICATING WITH STAFF

- _____
- _____
- _____

STAFF MEETING

Staff meetings must be well organized and should begin and end on time. Agendas should be created prior to the meeting and posted for staff review.

The agenda should be followed as closely as possible.

Private location, away from patients' view

Avoid interruptions

BULLETIN BOARDS

Postings for new policies or procedures

Attractive

Well organized

Updated regularly

COMMUNICATION NOTEBOOK

Write messages to employees

Employees write back to manager

COMMUNICATING ELECTRONICALLY

E-mail:

- Popular
- Easy
- Time-saving

CHECKPOINT QUESTION 2

What are three ways to promote communication with staff members?

Answer

_____

_____

_____

STAFFING ISSUES

Writing job descriptions

Hiring new employees

Evaluating employees

Taking disciplinary actions

Handling terminations

Scheduling

WRITING JOB DESCRIPTIONS

The purpose of a job description is to _____

_____

_____.

One copy to each employee upon hiring

HIRING AND INTERVIEWING EMPLOYEES

Seek applicants

Receive applications

Before interviewing an applicant, _____

_____.

Assess applicant's abilities

- Technical skills
- Fit into organization
- Flexibility

EVALUATING EMPLOYEES

Evaluate annually

Fair, accurate, objective

New employee evaluations

- 1 month after start
- 90 days
- 1 year

TAKING DISCIPLINARY ACTION

Verbal

- Used for first-time minor occurrences
- Note in employee's file

Written

- Serious problems
- Recurring minor problems

Employees should sign any written warning notices.

TERMINATING EMPLOYEES

Terminating employees for unlawful reasons or failing to follow the organization's termination policy can result in _____

_____.

Reasons:

- Tardiness, absenteeism
- Inappropriate dress, behavior
- Alcohol, drug use
- Endangering patients
- Lying or stealing

SCHEDULING

The primary goal of scheduling is to _____.

Secondary goal

- Meet the needs of employees

No matter what scheduling format is used, you are ultimately responsible for ensuring that the appropriate number and type of employees needed are scheduled.

WHAT IF?

You receive a call requesting a reference for an employee who was fired. What should you say?

CHECKPOINT QUESTION 3

What is the medical office manager's primary goal in scheduling?

Answer

_____

_____

_____

_____

POLICY AND PROCEDURES MANUALS

Written rules and regulations

Required by regulatory and accrediting agencies

Written, maintained, and considered one document

POLICY AND PROCEDURES MANUALS *(continued)*

A policy is a _____

_____.

Each policy or procedure is signed by the employees, indicating they have read, understand, and will adhere to the policy or procedure.

TIPS FOR WRITING PERSONNEL MANUALS

Personnel committee

Determine rules and regulations of office

Gather other facilities' manuals

Research laws

Appoint compliance officer

Central location

Review annually

TYPES OF POLICIES AND PROCEDURES

- _____
- _____
- _____
- _____
- _____
- _____
- _____
- _____

SECTION 1: MISSION STATEMENT

A mission statement describes _____

_____

_____.

SECTION 2: ORGANIZATIONAL STRUCTURE

Chain of command

How and when to contact other staff members

Coverage for managers

On-call policies

SECTION 3: HUMAN RESOURCES OR PERSONNEL

Policies relating to:

- Staff responsibilities
- Benefits
- Rules and regulations

SECTION 4: QUALITY IMPROVEMENT AND RISK MANAGEMENT

Who manages program

Steps for developing program

Incident reporting

SECTION 5: CLINICAL PROCEDURES

Patient intervention tasks

Infection control

Patient education

Sample documentation forms

SECTION 6: ADMINISTRATIVE PROCEDURES

Administrative tasks

- Accounting
- Appointment scheduling
- Insurance filing

SECTION 7: INFECTION CONTROL

Protective equipment

Biohazardous waste disposal

Disease identities

Needlesticks and exposures

OSHA documentation

Employee education

 CHECKPOINT QUESTION 4

Which seven elements must be included when writing a policy or procedure?

Answer

_____

_____

_____

_____

DEVELOPING PROMOTIONAL MATERIALS

Education pamphlets

Brochure

Newsletters

Holiday cards

Guidelines

- Spelling, grammar, accuracy
- Clear language
- Avoid abbreviations
- Brightly colored materials

FINANCIAL CONCERNS

Budgets

Payroll

Petty cash

BUDGET

A budget is a _____ that helps an organization estimate its anticipated expenditures and revenues.

- _____ budget
  - Costs to run the office
- _____ budget
  - Large outlays of money

 CHECKPOINT QUESTION 5

What are the two basic types of budgets?

Answer

_____

_____

_____

PAYROLL

Correct pay, on time for all employees

State and federal laws on deductions

Sometimes outsourced

PETTY CASH

Used to purchase small items

Reimburse employees for small items

MAINTENANCE OF INVENTORY AND SUPPLIES

Keep office neat, clean, well organized

Outside agency

SERVICE CONTRACTS

A service contract is an agreement between the medical organization and a service company in which the company agrees to perform regular inspections of and care for a specific piece of equipment.

INVENTORY

Develop inventory system

Responsibility for ordering

Procedure for ordering

Check deliveries

EDUCATION

Staff education

Patient education

Manager education

STAFF EDUCATION

Keep staff updated on:

- Procedures
- Drugs and vaccines

- Coding and billing regulations
- Annual training
  - CPR
  - Infection control
  - Fire safety

STAFF EDUCATION *(continued)*

Select educational topic each month

Select presenter

Present at staff meeting or other appropriate time

Outside professional seminars

PATIENT EDUCATION

Booklets

Posters

Teach staff on patient education

MANAGER EDUCATION

Workshops, conferences, courses

Professional organizations

- Medical Office Management Association
- Professional Association of Health Care Office Management

LEGAL ISSUES REGARDING OFFICE MANAGEMENT

Americans with Disabilities Act

Sexual harassment

Family and Medical Leave Act

Other legal considerations

AMERICANS WITH DISABILITIES ACT

All offices with 15 or more employees

Building accessible to physically challenged people

- Entrance ramps
- Widened restrooms and doors
- Elevated toilet bowls
- Braille signs
- Special telephone services

SEXUAL HARASSMENT

Be alert for signs

Policy for handling complaints

FAMILY AND MEDICAL LEAVE ACT

Allows 12 weeks of leave for family needs

Position must be held for employee

OTHER LEGAL CONSIDERATIONS

CLIA (Clinical Laboratory Improvement Amendments Act) regulations

OSHA regulations

JCAHO regulations

State laws

- Patient care
- Insurance billing
- Payroll management

 CHECKPOINT QUESTION 6

What are some of the legal issues of concern to the medical office manager?

Answer

_____

_____

_____

_____

_____

_____

Chapter 13

Credit and Collections

CREDIT AND COLLECTIONS

Office depends on the _____ generated by patient visits

Collecting fees is essential for success

FEES

Fee schedules

Discussing fees in advance

Forms of payment

Payment by insurance companies

Adjusting fees

FEE SCHEDULES

Physician sets fees for visits, laboratory work, and procedures

UCR concept

- U = usual; fair value of service
- C = customary; competitive rates
- R = reasonable; two criteria combined

RBRVS concept

- Resource-based relative value scale
- Fees based on relative value of service; adjusted for location

FEE SCHEDULES *(continued)*

Physician also considers cost of office operation

List of services and prices must be available for patients

Various fees based on insurance company reimbursement schedules

DISCUSSING FEES IN ADVANCE

It is always a good policy to discuss fees with patients in advance.

Provide brochure listing fees and collections

Always collect _____ from a new patient on the first visit.

Get _____ on first visit

FORMS OF PAYMENT

Cash

Personal check

Credit and debit cards (Visa, MasterCard, Discover)

PAYMENT BY INSURANCE COMPANY

Largest proportion of fees paid by insurers

Patients' information must be current

Always make a copy of _____ and _____ for billing reference.

ADJUSTING FEES

Adjustment = _____

Example: when the office accepts a set insurance rate for a service that is lower than the practice's rate

Difference is adjusted in credit adjustment column on patient's account

ADJUSTING FEES *(continued)*

Professional courtesy fees

- Reduced rate for other health care professionals

Write-offs

- Cancellation of unpaid debt

CHECKPOINT QUESTION 1

To avoid collection problems, what should you get from a new patient on the first visit?

Answer

_____

_____

CREDIT

Extending credit

Legal considerations

EXTENDING CREDIT

Patients not always able to pay entire bill

Credit may be extended

Patients pay their bill over time in _____

LEGAL CONSIDERATIONS

Practice may charge interest

Truth-in-lending must be made available

Cannot be denied based on:

- _____
- _____
- _____
- _____
- _____
- _____
- _____

CHECKPOINT QUESTION 2

On what grounds should credit *not* be denied?

Answer

_____

_____

_____

COLLECTIONS

Collecting _____ payments owed to practice

Costly

Time consuming

Many practices outsource collections

LEGAL CONSIDERATIONS

Collector should exercise reasonable restraint

Guidelines for collecting debt

Collecting from a patient's estate requires diplomacy

COLLECTING A DEBT

Monthly billings

Aging accounts

Collecting overdue accounts

- Overdue notices
- Telephoning the patient
- In-office reminders

MONTHLY BILLINGS

Bills sent monthly to patients with outstanding balances

Variety of billing cycles

If your facility changes a billing cycle, you are legally required to _____ of the change _____ months before the change takes effect.

AGING ACCOUNTS

Calculated from the first date of billing

Aging schedule to track overdue accounts

Good measure of practice's ability to collect fees

- 80% of fees should be collected within 30 days
- Review billing and collection process if necessary

COLLECTING OVERDUE ACCOUNTS

- _____
- _____
- _____

OVERDUE NOTICES

Copy of monthly statement indicating an "overdue notice" or "second notice"

Form letter with overdue amount written in

TELEPHONING THE PATIENT

If written notice brings no response

- Phone the patient
- Ask when payment may be coming
- Document reply

IN-OFFICE REMINDERS

Handle discreetly

Give patient copy of overdue notice

Ask when payment is forthcoming

 WHAT IF?

A patient who has an overdue account wants to schedule an appointment. What should you do?

COLLECTION ALTERNATIVES

Collection agencies

Small claims court

Credit bureaus

 CHECKPOINT QUESTION 3

What are three ways of collecting overdue accounts?

Answer

_____

_____

_____

Chapter 14

Bookkeeping and Banking

BOOKKEEPING AND BANKING

In most medical practices, bookkeeping and banking involve maintaining both patient and office account records, including petty cash, accounts receivable (money owed to the practice), and accounts payable (money owed by the practice).

DAILY BOOKKEEPING

Bookkeeping = _____
_____

In medical office:

- Patient payments
- Patient charges

DAILY BOOKKEEPING (*continued*)

Single-entry bookkeeping system

Assets = liabilities + equity
- Assets = all things of value owned by practice
- Liabilities = monies owed by practice
- Equity = capital invested in practice

Both sides must balance

Each transaction causes a charge (_____)
on one side and a payment (_____) on the other

DAILY BOOKKEEPING (*continued*)

Cash-basis accounting is used in most facilities

- Income considered as such only when
  _____
- Payables considered expenses when
  _____

MANUAL ACCOUNTING

Pegboard bookkeeping system

- Encounter forms and charge slips
- Posting a charge
- Posting a payment
- Posting a credit
- Posting a credit adjustment
- Posting a debit adjustment
- Posting to cash-paid-out section of day sheet

PEGBOARD BOOKKEEPING SYSTEM

Pegboard holds day sheet in place

All transactions recorded on day sheet

One ledger card per patient

After patient transaction, bookkeeper uses ledger card and charge slip to make entry

All entries appear consecutively

Transactions are added at end of the day

DAY SHEET

Keeps track of daily patient transactions

Contains several sections:

- Deposit slip
- Distribution columns
- Payments
- Adjustments
- Posting proofs

DAY SHEET (*continued*)

Deposit slip

- Detachable from day sheet
- At end of day:
  - _____
  - _____

DAY SHEET (*continued*)

Distribution columns

- _____
- Columns assigned according to needs of practice

The distribution columns, regardless of how they are assigned, provide the physician with important information about how the practice _____.

DAY SHEET (continued)

Adjustments

- An entry to change an account
  - _____ in fees
  - Return charges to an account if insufficient funds available

DAY SHEET (continued)

Posting proofs

The posting proofs section is where _____ are entered and the day sheet _____, much as one would balance a checkbook.

Total all columns at end of day

DAY SHEET (continued)

If posting proofs do not balance, locate and correct error

Do not erase or Wite-Out errors, but _____ and _____.

DAY SHEET (continued)

Day sheets track accounts receivable

File completed day sheets in a ledger

Completed day sheets are important legal documents and must be kept for _____ for tax purposes.

CHECKPOINT QUESTION 1

What are five sections of a pegboard day sheet?

Answer

_____

_____

_____

_____

_____

WHAT IF?

You cannot balance the day sheet. What do you do?

LEDGER CARDS

Ledger card = _____

Photocopy of ledger card often used as _____

The ledger card is a legal document and should be kept for the same length of time as the patient's medical record.

LEDGER CARDS (continued)

Ledger cards with _____ are kept separate from _____ ledger cards; this makes it easier to photocopy the monthly bills or find a ledger card when a patient calls about an outstanding bill.

ENCOUNTER FORMS AND CHARGE SLIPS

Preprinted patient statements

- List codes for basic office charges
- Sections for current balance and next appointment

Most have three-part copies:

- First copy for facility
- Second copy to patient for insurance filing
- Third copy to patient for receipt of services

ENCOUNTER FORMS AND CHARGE SLIPS (continued)

Charge slips:

- Smaller version of encounter form
- Used in conjunction with ledger cards

 ### CHECKPOINT QUESTION 2

How do ledger cards and encounter forms differ?

Answer

_____

_____

POSTING A CHARGE

Charge column = record of _____

_____

- Office visits
- Electrocardiograms
- Blood work
- Consultations

POSTING A PAYMENT

_____

- Insurance checks
- Money orders
- Credit card payments
- Cash received

POSTING A CREDIT

Credit = _____

Brackets used to indicate _____

- Example: [25]

Handled two ways:

- Credit subtracted from charges on next patient's visit
- Patient mailed a refund

POSTING A CREDIT ADJUSTMENT

Credits _____

- Professional discounts
- Difference between standard fee and insurance fee
- Accounts turned over to collection agencies

 ### CHECKPOINT QUESTION 3

What do brackets around an amount listed in a column indicate?

Answer

_____

POSTING A DEBIT ADJUSTMENT

_____ **patient's account balance**

- Insufficient funds notice from bank; previous payment no longer valid
- Payment received after account turned over to collection agency
- Refunds to patients

 ### CHECKPOINT QUESTION 4

How does a credit adjustment differ from a debit adjustment?

Answer

_____

_____

_____

POSTING TO CASH-PAID-OUT SECTION OF DAY SHEET

Physician may take cash from receipts

Deposit will be short

Physician should sign cash-paid-out section of day sheet

Also used with payments from insurance carrier that have been adjusted for previous overpayments

COMPUTER ACCOUNTING

Used in most medical offices

Fulfill same functions as pegboard system but:

- Faster
- Easier to locate patient information
- More accurate

Also used to:

- Write checks
- Manage electronic banking
- Manage appointments
- Generate reports

POSTING TO COMPUTER ACCOUNTS

To post payments:

- Enter source and amount of payment
- Allowed amount for service
- Necessary adjustments

COMPUTER ACCOUNTING REPORTS

Easy to generate financial reports

Daily, weekly reports contain same information as

_____

_____ **used to correct errors before printing final reports**

BANKING

Banks and their services

- Checking accounts
- Savings accounts
- Money market accounts

Bank fees

- Monthly service fees
- Overdraft protection
- Returned check fee

Types of checks

BANKS AND THEIR SERVICES

Before choosing a bank, consider:

- Location
- Monthly fees
- Overdraft protection programs
- Interest-bearing accounts
- Returned check fees

CHECKING ACCOUNTS

Allow you to _____

Deposit money collected in the office daily

Maintain checkbook and reorder checks as needed

SAVINGS ACCOUNTS

Typically used for:

- _____
- _____

Higher interest rate than with checking accounts

MONEY MARKET ACCOUNTS

Combination of savings and checking accounts

Higher minimum balance needed

Higher interest rate than with checking accounts

BANK FEES

Fees charged for services

Special services or plans often available for small businesses

MONTHLY SERVICE FEES

Fee charged _____

May be fixed or charged per check

May avoid by maintaining specific minimum balance

OVERDRAFT PROTECTION

Guarantees payment even if insufficient money in account

RETURNED CHECK FEE

Charged for any deposited check that is returned for insufficient funds

Typically charged to _____

List fee in _____ column of patient ledger

TYPES OF CHECKS

Standard business check

Certified check—signed by bank to verify amount is available in account

Cashier's check—sold to a customer for cash or personal check

Traveler's check—safe way to carry cash when traveling

Money orders—guarantee payment to recipient

 CHECKPOINT QUESTION 5

List three types of checks available through banks.

Answer

_____

_____

_____

WRITING CHECKS FOR ACCOUNTS PAYABLE

Accounts payable = _____

- Rent
- Utilities
- Taxes
- Salaries
- Vendors
- Patient refunds
- Petty cash

WRITING CHECKS FOR ACCOUNTS PAYABLE *(continued)*

Computer systems

- Enable you to enter information
- Print checks
- Track transactions

Manual system

- Write legibly; use current date
- Write amount of payment in figures and words
- Record in check registry

WRITING CHECKS FOR ACCOUNTS PAYABLE *(continued)*

Record transaction in proper account or category for tax purposes

- Subtract amount from check register balance

CHECKS AND MAKING DEPOSITS

When checks are received in the office, they are first _____.

To endorse a check requires writing (or rubber stamping) on the back of the check the name and number of the account into which it will be deposited.

RECEIVING CHECKS AND MAKING DEPOSITS *(continued)*

This way, if the payments are lost or stolen, no one else can cash them.

It also ensures that the bank deposits the payments to the correct account.

RECEIVING CHECKS AND MAKING DEPOSITS *(continued)*

Total all checks and cash received after payments are posted

Amount should match _____ on day sheet

Detach deposit slip from day sheet or print slip from computer program

Complete a deposit slip and wrap it around the checks

RECEIVING CHECKS AND MAKING DEPOSITS *(continued)*

Never include _____ *in a deposit that is mailed or placed in a depository.*

Cash deposits should always be hand-delivered, and a teller's receipt should always be obtained.

RECONCILING BANK STATEMENTS

Compare monthly bank statements to your records

Statement includes:

- All checks written
- All deposits
- Electronic transactions
- Service charges

RECONCILING BANK STATEMENTS (continued)

Verify all checks and deposits listed correctly

Back of bank statement contains worksheet for balancing account

 CHECKPOINT QUESTION 6

What information is found on a bank statement?

Answer

_____

_____

PETTY CASH

A petty cash account is a _____
kept in the office specifically for _____,
such as buying postage stamps or office supplies.

Fund should always be the same designated amount

- Place a voucher or receipt in fund when

_____

PETTY CASH (continued)

Petty cash funds should be kept separate from patient cash payments.

Keep fund in _____ **area**

A voucher with an attached receipt should always be placed in the petty cash box, both to provide proof of the purchase and to keep the account balanced.

PETTY CASH (continued)

Replenish _____

- Cash a check in amount of total of vouchers
- Place money in fund
- Remove and file vouchers

 CHECKPOINT QUESTION 7

List six guidelines for managing petty cash.

Answer

_____

_____

_____

_____

_____

_____

Chapter 15

Accounts Payable and Payroll

ACCOUNTS PAYABLE AND PAYROLL

Accounting = _____

Assesses financial history and current financial stakes

Basis for financial management

ACCOUNTS PAYABLE AND PAYROLL *(continued)*

Checks and balances system necessary for effective record management

Examine accounts monthly

Typically, computer accounting integrated with medical software

- Efficient analysis and tracking
- Improved productivity
- Smarter business decisions

ACCOUNTING CYCLE

Finances operate under either:

- _____
  - Consecutive 12-month period with a specific starting date
- _____
  - January through December

ACCOUNTING CYCLE *(continued)*

Income statements examined quarterly by IRS

Annual tax return summarizes quarterly returns

Well-maintained office records not only facilitate IRS returns but also provide data that define the practice's business picture.

ACCOUNTING CYCLE *(continued)*

Records such as receipts should be retained for ____ years, but records such as bank statements, canceled checks, and IRS tax returns should be kept for ____ _____.

RECORD-KEEPING COMPONENTS

Records should include:

- Income
- Accounts receivable
- Total expenditures according to categories
  - Payroll
  - Cash on hand
  - Liabilities

RECORD-KEEPING COMPONENTS *(continued)*

Bookkeeping systems track categories

- Pegboard (manual system)
- Software package (computer-based system)

RECORD-KEEPING COMPONENTS *(continued)*

Summary reports include:

- Payroll reports
- Itemized category reports
- Account balances
- Profit-and-loss statement

ACCOUNTS PAYABLE

Ordering goods and services

Receiving supplies

Paying invoices

ORDERING GOODS AND SERVICES

Factors to consider:

- _____
  - Purchasing cooperatives
  - Vendor discounts
  - Warehouse or catalog merchandisers
- _____
- _____

ORDERING GOODS AND SERVICES
(continued)

It is preferable to pay for supplies by check or credit card rather than by cash, but when cash purchases are necessary, retain a detailed receipt for tax purposes.

Use purchase orders

Record charges

Verify charges against bill

 CHECKPOINT QUESTION 1

When purchasing office supplies, what factors besides price should you consider?

Answer

_____

_____

_____

RECEIVING SUPPLIES

The office staff member who receives the supplies must check the packing slip against the actual contents to ensure that all supplies are in the shipment.

Compare packing slips to bills when issuing checks

PAYING INVOICES

File payable invoices together

Invoices paid:

- Daily
- Weekly
- Biweekly
- Monthly

MANUAL PAYMENT

Use log or record book to enter information about each check

After writing check, detach from stub

If an error is made:

- _____
- _____
- _____

File check stubs with fiscal records for that year

MANUAL PAYMENT *(continued)*

Information on check includes:

- Check number
- Date of issue
- Payee
- Full amount
- Notes on memo line and stub

Attach to invoice for signature

MANUAL PAYMENT *(continued)*

Memos or notations on check stubs can be referenced later if a question arises concerning payment by a particular check.

Manual system requires writing each check and report

Labor-intensive

PEGBOARD PAYMENT

Same pegboard used for accounts receivable

Check register used in place of day sheet

Carbon strips on checks record information on check register (one-write system)

PEGBOARD PAYMENT *(continued)*

Register columns categorize expenses

Entries totaled when register is completed

Also enables bank deposits

Back page used to track payroll

File completed registers in separate log

- Chronological order
- Most recent register first

COMPUTER PAYMENT

Computer system benefits:

- At-a-glance check registers
- Categories and totals
- Payroll records
- Records for bank deposits
- Compile and print financial reports
- Eliminate mathematical errors

COMPUTER PAYMENT *(continued)*

Checks are presented on the computer screen in the same way that a paper check would normally appear.

Information stored

New balance calculated

COMPUTER PAYMENT *(continued)*

The computer can "memorize" checks so that the information on them can be recalled and reprinted without reentering it; this is especially helpful with payroll checks.

Routine data backups are essential

CHECKPOINT QUESTION 2

Whether using a manual, pegboard, or computer accounts payable system, two steps must always occur when ordering and receiving supplies. What are they?

Answer

_____

_____

_____

PAYROLL

Payroll obligations to all employees in practice

Taxes due to federal, state, and local governments

Responsibility of medical assistant

PAYROLL *(continued)*

Outside payroll services

- Specialize in computing, withholding, and paying taxes and payroll for business
- Cost effective
- Accurate
- Current on all tax laws
- Legally liable

MANUAL PAYROLL SYSTEMS

Check stubs indicate payee, amount, and date

Separate log tracks employees' gross payments and tax withholdings

Information must be totaled monthly, quarterly, and annually

PEGBOARD PAYROLL SYSTEMS

Payroll journal

- Employee payroll record form and correlating back page of check register

COMPUTER PAYROLL SYSTEMS

Most programs integrate payroll, accounts receivable, and accounts payable

Computer programs can calculate tax withholdings automatically, record payroll data, and print payroll checks.

Less time-intense than manual or pegboard systems

EMPLOYEE RECORDS

Maintain a personnel file for each employee:

- _____
- _____
- _____
- _____
- _____
- _____
- _____
- _____

TAX WITHHOLDINGS

W-4 forms must be completed on first day of hire

- Stipulates tax withholdings and exemptions

If any of the information contained on an employee's W-4 form changes, the employee must _____ _____, which is placed in the personnel file.

TAX WITHHOLDINGS *(continued)*

Federal taxes include:

- _____
- _____
- _____

Based on salary

TAX WITHHOLDINGS *(continued)*

The employer must match the amount withheld from each employee's paycheck for _____ _____ and _____ taxes.

Employers not required to match federal, state, or local taxes

Deposit all withheld taxes in account at federal depository

TAX WITHHOLDINGS *(continued)*

Other withholdings:

- Health or life insurance premiums
- Disability premiums
- Pension plan contributions
- Garnished wages

 CHECKPOINT QUESTION 3

What must be withheld from an employee's paycheck?

Answer

_____

_____

_____

PAYMENT OF TAXES

Payroll taxes paid according to different schedules

Schedule depends on gross payroll

IRS requires quarterly returns for all federal taxes withheld

State returns usually due according to same quarterly schedule

W-2 FORMS

W-2 form = _____

- Total gross income
- Federal, state, and local taxes withheld
- Taxable fringe benefits
- Total net income

 CHECKPOINT QUESTION 4

What information does the employee list on the W-4 form? What happens if this information changes?

Answer

_____

_____

_____

_____

 WHAT IF?

The medical practice where you work did not pay its payroll taxes. What could happen?

PREPARATION OF REPORTS

Bookkeeper prepares reports for accountant or IRS

Manual, pegboard, or computer systems enable summaries of income, expenses, and payroll

ASSISTING WITH AUDITS

Types of audits:

- In-house to assist accountant in preparing taxes
- Formal audit with IRS

Information needed for audits:

- Bank statements
- Quarterly and annual tax returns
- Receipts for all expenditures
- Canceled checks
- Payroll records

Chapter 16

Health Insurance

HEALTH INSURANCE

Before 1930, access to care based on ability to pay

Plans originally designed to avoid financial burdens

Blue Cross and Blue Shield

- A federation of 42 independent companies
- Insure 30% of Americans

HEALTH INSURANCE *(continued)*

U. S. health insurance funded by employer, employee, and tax contributions

_____ % of Americans enrolled in some type of plan

Medical assistants must understand differences and special terminology with claims

Medical assistants must instruct patients about insurance

HEALTH BENEFIT PLANS

Group health benefit plans

Individual health benefits

Government-sponsored (public) health benefits

- _____
- _____
- _____

GROUP HEALTH BENEFITS

Sponsored by employer, union, or association

Person covered is employee or union member

Eligibility varies between different plans

GROUP HEALTH BENEFITS *(continued)*

Benefits may be insured or self-funded

_____

- Monthly premium paid to insurance company
- Insurance company pays for benefits

_____

- Money invested by insured
- Insurance company processes claims and make payment
- Third-party payer acts as agent

GROUP HEALTH BENEFITS *(continued)*

For a group benefit plan to cover (pay for) eligible expenses, the patient must meet several criteria, called _____.

Criteria defined in policy or plan

May include minimum number of hours worked and a waiting period from date of employment

Dependents' eligibility based on employee's eligibility

GROUP HEALTH BENEFITS *(continued)*

Confirm eligibility through claims administrator with benefits plan

Number usually found on patient's ID card

CHECKPOINT QUESTION 1

What is the difference between an insured benefits plan and one that is self-funded?

Answer

With insured benefits, a monthly premium is paid by _____ to an insurance company. The _____ in turn is obligated to pay for any eligible health benefits. In contrast, self-funded benefits are provided to eligible employees or members by their _____. Claims are processed by a professional claims administrator, such as a third-party administrator.

INDIVIDUAL HEALTH BENEFITS

Individual health benefits policies are purchased by an individual from an insurance company.

Individual pays premium to insurance company

Insurance company pays doctor or hospital

Usually less generous coverage than group plans

Medical assistants must know primary and secondary insurance carriers for patients with multiple coverage

GOVERNMENT-SPONSORED (PUBLIC) HEALTH BENEFITS

Government-sponsored benefit programs are funded and regulated by the federal government or individual states.

Assist citizens without coverage

Programs include:

- _____
- _____
- _____
- _____

MEDICARE

In 1965, the Social Security Act established Medicare to provide health insurance for the elderly. Elderly persons were defined as Social Security recipients age 65 or older.

1972 amendments expanded coverage

MEDICARE *(continued)*

Medicare Part A

- _____ expenses
- No additional charge to eligible persons

Medicare Part B

- _____ fees
- Optional
- Monthly fees, deducted from Social Security payments

MEDICARE *(continued)*

Social Security recipients automatically enrolled in Medicare at age 65 years

Must _____ Part B if not wanted

Deductibles for Parts A and B

MEDICARE *(continued)*

A patient with Medicare coverage who is actively employed and covered by the employer's plan will have secondary Medicare benefits.

Retired person over 65 with additional insurance has primary Medicare benefits

Physicians must submit claims to Medicare on behalf of patients

MEDICARE *(continued)*

Medicare Part B reimburses ____ % after deductible

Medicaid may cover remaining 20% if patient unable to pay

Known as crossover claim

Centers for Medicare & Medicaid Services (CMS) formerly known as Health Care Financing Administration (HCFA)

MEDICARE *(continued)*

CMS oversees _____ aspects of U. S. health care

Current procedural terminology (CPT) coding system must be used for Medicare claims

Ask patients about secondary coverage in addition to Medicare

 CHECKPOINT QUESTION 2

What is the difference between parts A and B of Medicare coverage?

Answer

Persons enrolled in Social Security are automatically enrolled in Medicare Part A, which covers _____ services and expenses only, and Medicare Part B, which covers the _____ charges for inpatient or outpatient care as well as diagnostic services. Part B does not cover _____, _____, _____, or _____. Part A is provided at _____ to Social Security recipients, and Part B carries a _____. If Part B is not wanted, it must be _____.

MEDICAID

Medicaid provides health benefits to low-income or indigent persons of all ages.

Federal government provides funds to each state for costs

Benefits vary between states

MEDICAID *(continued)*

At a minimum, 100% coverage for:

- _____
- _____
- _____
- _____
- _____
- _____

MEDICAID *(continued)*

Most states require co-payment based on income

Recipients receive a new ID card

_____

Medicaid carriers require authorization before services are given

Reimbursement is usually less

Physicians may choose to not accept Medicaid patients

 CHECKPOINT QUESTION 3

How often do Medicaid recipients receive a new card?

Answer

_____

_____

TRICARE/CHAMPVA

TRICARE, the new name for CHAMPUS, is administered by the U. S. Department of Defense and provides medical coverage for dependents of active service personnel, dependents of service personnel who died during active duty, and retired service personnel.

TRICARE/CHAMPVA *(continued)*

TRICARE

- Three-part system with managed care, HMOs, and PPOs
- Participants assigned primary care manager (PCM)

- Patients who live within 40 miles of a uniformed services hospital must use that facility
- Patients who live more than 40 miles from a uniformed services hospital receive care in physician's office or civilian hospital

TRICARE/CHAMPVA *(continued)*

Civilian Health and Medical Program of the Veterans Administration (CHAMPVA)

- Covers dependents of veterans with service-related disabilities
- Administered by VA hospitals
- Patients select their own physician
- Same benefits as private insurance

MANAGED CARE

United States spends most for health care in world

Most obtain health coverage from employer

Managed care programs

- Less expensive
- Different relationship between insurer, provider, and covered individual from that of traditional programs

MANAGED CARE *(continued)*

Traditional systems

- Covered patient seeks care from any provider
- Insurer pays a portion of fees
- Insurer has no relationship with provider

In managed care systems, however, the insurer has a _____ with the provider.

MANAGED CARE *(continued)*

Contract usually establishes prices and conditions for coverage

Most programs contain:

- _____
- _____
- _____
- _____

MANAGED CARE *(continued)*

- _____
- Often called utilization management (UM) or utilization review (UR)
- Insurer must approve admission of patient to hospital for certain conditions
- Goal to ensure care given in most cost-efficient setting
- Conflicts between UR guideline and physician requirements appealed to peer review organization

MANAGED CARE *(continued)*

_____

- Specialty physicians provide care only after referral from primary physician
- Ensures that services are necessary and delivered in most cost-efficient setting

MANAGED CARE *(continued)*

_____

- Consists of providers who have signed contracts with insurer or health maintenance organization (HMO)
- Patients required to use network providers to receive full coverage

MANAGED CARE *(continued)*

_____

- Network provider cannot bill patients for any amounts not paid by insurer (no balance billing)
- Exceptions: co-payments, coinsurance, deductibles
- If payment denied by insurer due to improper organization, patient cannot be billed

MANAGED CARE *(continued)*

Most physicians contract with multiple programs

Consider requirements for each patient

Check ID cards for details on UM or precertification requirements

MANAGED CARE *(continued)*

Until you are very familiar with the requirements of each of your patients' managed care programs, you should call the number on the ID card before a patient is admitted to a hospital (on a nonemergency basis), referred to another physician, or scheduled for specific laboratory, radiological, or other test or evaluation.

MANAGED CARE *(continued)*

Failure to comply with precertification requirements results in a financial penalty for the patient and possibly also for the physician and the hospital.

 CHECKPOINT QUESTION 4

What are the four key elements of a managed care program?

Answer

_____

_____

_____

_____

HEALTH MAINTENANCE ORGANIZATIONS

In contrast to traditional insurance companies, a HMO promises to provide covered services rather than pay for them.

HMO acts as _____ and
_____

HMO policy lists covered services and service providers

HMO contracts with _____
and _____

HEALTH MAINTENANCE ORGANIZATIONS *(continued)*

The _____, rather than the patient, is responsible for the costs of medical services, and

providers bill the _____ rather than the patient when a reimbursable service is rendered to a HMO member.

Deductibles and coinsurance costs do not apply

HEALTH MAINTENANCE ORGANIZATIONS *(continued)*

Kaiser Permanente Health Plan recognized as first HMO

Built medical group to service employees in remote areas

Paid providers per employee vs. fee-for-service

Evolved into current company serving 6 million members

HEALTH MAINTENANCE ORGANIZATIONS *(continued)*

_____ = payment per capita, rather than fee-for-service payment

Independent practice associations (IPA) allowed nongroup physicians to compete

Medical assistant must know types of relationships a practice has with HMOs

Most HMOs require claims even with capitation

Most require collection and transmission of other patient information

 CHECKPOINT QUESTION 5

How does a HMO differ from a traditional health insurance program?

Answer

_____

_____

_____

_____

PREFERRED PROVIDER ORGANIZATIONS

PPOs contract with providers and lease network to health care plans

PPOs not financial involved in plan

Offer "in network" and "out of network" benefits to patients

Patients choose any provider for services

Benefits are better for "in network" or participating providers

PREFERRED PROVIDER ORGANIZATIONS *(continued)*

Medical assistant must understand administrative requirements for physician's PPO relationships

Most PPOs have provider relations representative to answer questions

PPOs typically operated by a group of hospitals, physicians, an insurance company, or other organization

Physicians participate to accommodate patients

PREFERRED PROVIDER ORGANIZATIONS *(continued)*

Participating physicians agree to perform some administrative services:

- Must accept assignment of benefits and file claims for patients
- Agree to accept reimbursement as payment
- Agree not to bill patient
- Agree to comply with precertification requirements

 CHECKPOINT QUESTION 6

What is the primary difference between a HMO and a PPO?

Answer

A primary difference between a HMO and a PPO is that patients with PPO coverage can _____ _____ and _____;

they simply have an incentive in the form of higher benefits when they see an in-network provider.

PHYSICIAN HOSPITAL ORGANIZATIONS

A physician hospital organization (PHO) is a coalition of physicians and a hospital contracting with large employers, insurance carriers, and other benefits groups to provide discounted health services.

OTHER MANAGED CARE PROGRAMS

Patient sees primary caregiver (_____) for all nonemergencies

Physician treats or refers patient to specialist

The gatekeeper provision seeks to reduce the plan cost of specialists.

The gatekeeper approach also encourages patients to establish a relationship with a primary care physician, who is then in a position to manage the patient's care.

THE FUTURE OF MANAGED CARE

Organization of health care changed by managed care environment

Size of medical practices increasing

Hospitals are purchasing physician practices

Small-group or solo physicians are combining

Some forming public companies and raising capital

THE FUTURE OF MANAGED CARE *(continued)*

Physician's role is affected

Physicians now act as patient care managers or gatekeepers

THE FUTURE OF MANAGED CARE
(continued)

Quality measurement increasingly important

HEDIS (Healthplan Employer Data Information Set) reports indicators of health care quality

- Upgraded continuously
- Being adopted by governmental agencies and employers as a prerequisite for HMO participation

THE FUTURE OF MANAGED CARE
(continued)

Increasingly sophisticated patient care protocols

Providers must document efficacy and quality of service through medical records

Automated medical records

- Improve coordination among providers
- Reduce illness
- Improve quality of care

THE FUTURE OF MANAGED CARE
(continued)

Medical assistants affected by managed care

- Increasing cooperation among physician groups
- Expanded responsibilities in managing patient care, specialist care, and hospitalization
- Uniform care protocols and outcomes measurement
- Data collection and management vital to physician's practice

WORKERS' COMPENSATION

Employees in every state are covered by a workers' compensation program administered by the state. Workers' compensation benefits were developed to _____ resulting from a work-related illness or injury.

WORKERS' COMPENSATION
(continued)

Work-related illness or injury claims are returned with instructions to file with workers' compensation administrator

Before service, determine if illness or injury is work-related

If so, account for services separately

Know your state's workers' compensation regulations and procedures

FILING CLAIMS

If the provider requires patients to make full payment at the time of the visit, the physician may still submit a claim on the patient's behalf; however, the patient may need to submit claims to the claims administrator for reimbursement.

Most providers accept assignment of benefits

Medical assistant should obtain all claims information before submitting for payment

FILING CLAIMS *(continued)*

Patient ID card contains claims information

Copy card and file with medical record

Update annually or with each visit

FILING CLAIMS *(continued)*

_____

_____

_____

CMS-1500 is most widely used claim form

Preexisting conditions may be excluded from coverage for a stated period

FILING CLAIMS *(continued)*

The insurance company or managed care plan cannot process claims with incomplete or inaccurate information and will return them to the provider for completion, correction, and resubmission.

Lengthens time before reimbursement

Critical aspect of medical assistant's role

FILING CLAIMS *(continued)*

Frequent causes of denial and corrective actions you can take

Cause:

- ■ Cannot identify patient as covered person

Corrective action:

- ■ _____
  _____

FILING CLAIMS *(continued)*

Cause:

- ■ Coding deemed inappropriate for services provided

Corrective action:

- ■ _____

FILING CLAIMS *(continued)*

Cause:

- ■ Patient no longer covered

Corrective action:

- ■ _____
  _____
- ■ _____
  _____

FILING CLAIMS *(continued)*

Cause:

- ■ Incomplete data

Corrective action:

- ■ _____

FILING CLAIMS *(continued)*

Cause:

- ■ Services not covered

Corrective action:

- ■ _____

 ## WHAT IF?

The reason for a rejection or denial of a claim is not clear. What should you do?

ELECTRONIC CLAIMS SUBMISSION

All claims required to be submitted electronically according to HIPAA (effective 10/03)

Office software includes the CMS-1500 format

ELECTRONIC CLAIMS SUBMISSION *(continued)*

With a computer and a modem, health claims can be filed immediately, reducing the time for the reimbursement cycle.

You will need to work closely with your practice's software vendor to ensure compatibility with the insurance company's computer systems.

ELECTRONIC CLAIMS SUBMISSION *(continued)*

_____ collect and distribute all electronic claims to appropriate administrators

Require that all fields be completed in correct format

Claims submitted electronically that do not meet the plan's criteria will be _____ by the clearinghouse and must be submitted by mail.

ELECTRONIC CLAIMS SUBMISSION *(continued)*

In addition, claims that are particularly complicated or cumbersome, have attachments, or are otherwise unsuitable for electronic submission should be filed on paper with the claims administrator.

EXPLANATION OF BENEFITS

When the claims administrator settles a claim, that is, makes a payment, an explanation of benefits (EOB) is issued to both the provider and the patient.

Tells how payment was made

May include several claims during a particular period

POLICIES IN THE PRACTICE

Medical assistant must be knowledgeable and precise when administering policies:

- Assignment of benefits
- Balance billing

POLICIES IN THE PRACTICE
(continued)

Assignment of benefits

- Patient's signature must be on file
- Patient must pay all charges and file claim if assignment not accepted

POLICIES IN THE PRACTICE
(continued)

Balance billing

- Difference between physician's usual charge and allowable charge by plan
- Prohibited by most managed care contracts
- Not prohibited with other plan types

POLICIES IN THE PRACTICE
(continued)

UCR (usual, customary, and reasonable) data calculated from surveys of amounts physicians charge for services

Adjusted for regional differences

Reimbursements based on maximum allowable charge according to UCR (for non–managed care plan physicians)

May bill patient for difference between amount charged and UCR amount

Chapter 17

Diagnostic Coding

DIAGNOSTIC CODING

Coding = _____

International Classification of Diseases, Ninth Revision

- System of codes
- Covers diseases, injuries, conditions, and procedures

DIAGNOSTIC CODING *(continued)*

Coding is a way to standardize medical information for purposes such as collecting health care statistics, performing a medical care review, and indexing medical records.

It is also used for health insurance claims processing.

DIAGNOSTIC CODING *(continued)*

Because coding is the basis for reimbursement, it is imperative that you code patient visits accurately and precisely.

Incorrect, insufficient, incomplete coding causes:

- _____
- _____

DIAGNOSTIC CODING *(continued)*

Medical necessity = _____
_____

Code assigned to patient's diagnosis proves medical necessity

CHECKPOINT QUESTION 1

What is meant by medical necessity?

Answer

_____

_____

_____

DIAGNOSTIC CODING

International Classification of Diseases, Ninth Revision, Clinical Modification (ICD-9-CM) is a statistical classification system based on the International Classification of Diseases, Ninth Revision (ICD-9), developed by the World Health Organization (WHO).

DIAGNOSTIC CODING *(continued)*

CM = _____

- Addresses intent of codes to describe patient's clinical picture
- Highly precise

DIAGNOSTIC CODING *(continued)*

ICD-9-CM mandated by HIPAA

Contains:

- More than 10,000 diagnostic codes
- More than 1,000 procedural codes

Organized into three volumes

- Volume 1: Tabular List of Diseases
- Volume 2: Alphabetic Index to Diseases
- Volume 3: Tabular List and Alphabetic Index of Procedures

DIAGNOSTIC CODING *(continued)*

National Center for Health Statistics (NCHS) maintains system in Volumes 1 and 2

Centers for Medicare & Medicaid Services (CMS) maintain system in Volume 3

Changes published regularly with approval of WHO

 ## CHECKPOINT QUESTION 2

What are the three volumes of the ICD-9-CM system?

Answer

_____   _____

_____

_____

 ## CHECKPOINT QUESTION 3

What organization must approve any changes in the disease classification system?

Answer

_____

_____

INPATIENT VERSUS OUTPATIENT CODING

Differences between coding for inpatient facilities and outpatient facilities

- Volumes 1 and 2 used to _____ regardless of setting
- Volume 3 used to report _____

INPATIENT VERSUS OUTPATIENT CODING *(continued)*

- UB-92 (uniform bill) reports charges for nursing services, building maintenance, and costs associated with running facility
  • Does not include physician charges
- CMS-1500 (universal claim form) reports physician services regardless of setting

INPATIENT VERSUS OUTPATIENT CODING *(continued)*

Outpatient = patients treated in:

- _____
- _____
- _____
- _____
- _____

Inpatient = _____

INPATIENT VERSUS OUTPATIENT CODING *(continued)*

Coders employed by physician's practice code physician's services regardless of inpatient or outpatient setting

Example:

- Hospital room, meals, and laboratory tests billed and coded by hospital
- Daily visit by physician billed and coded by physician's office

 CHECKPOINT QUESTION 4

Define the terms *inpatient* and *outpatient*.

Answer

_____

_____

_____

_____

ICD-9-CM: THE CODE BOOK

Available from several publishers

All books follow same format but include unique features

Must have solid foundation in medical terminology and human anatomy

Should have references such as medical dictionary and/or software

ICD-9-CM: THE CODE BOOK *(continued)*

New codes published each _____

Use required following January 1

Update books as needed

You must update codes on superbills (preprinted bills listing a variety of procedures) or any other forms you use.

Millions of dollars lost because incorrect codes taken from out-of-date forms

 CHECKPOINT QUESTION 5

How often is the ICD-9-CM updated?

Answer

_____

VOLUME 1: TABULAR LIST OF DISEASES

Classification of diseases and injuries

Organized by etiology and body system

VOLUME 1: TABULAR LIST OF DISEASES *(continued)*

Each chapter contains a range of three-digit codes

- Example: Chapter 16, Symptoms, Signs, and Ill-defined Conditions (780–799)

Chapters are organized into subject areas, describing general disease

- Example: Symptoms (780–789)

VOLUME 1: TABULAR LIST OF DISEASES *(continued)*

Category codes describe specific diseases

- Example: 780, general symptoms

Fourth digit breaks down the category

- Example: 780.0, alteration of consciousness

Fifth digit is highest level of definition

- Example: 780.01, coma

SUPPLEMENTARY CLASSIFICATIONS

V-codes

E-codes

V-CODES

Range from V01 to V82

Index _____

- History of illness
- Immunizations
- Live-born infants

E-CODES

Range from E800 to E999

Classify _____

Do not affect reimbursement

Provide information to industrial medicine, insurance underwriters, national safety programs, and public health agencies

 CHECKPOINT QUESTION 6

List four reasons for using E-codes.

Answer

_____

_____

_____

_____

VOLUME 2: ALPHABETIC INDEX TO DISEASES

Contains many diagnostic terms not found in Volume 1

Always check all indentations in the index under the condition to ensure that you have the one most appropriate to the diagnosis you intend to code.

VOLUME 2: ALPHABETIC INDEX TO DISEASES *(continued)*

Organized into three sections:

- Section 1, Alphabetic Index to Diseases and Injuries
- Section 2, Table of Drugs and Chemicals
- Section 3, Alphabetic Index to External Causes of Injuries and Poisoning

VOLUME 2: ALPHABETIC INDEX TO DISEASES *(continued)*

Section 1, Alphabetic Index to Diseases and Injuries

- Organized by main terms in boldface type
- Reports the reason for patient encounters
- Code numbers follow the main term, referring to the _____
- Always cross-reference Volume 1 to ensure correct code

Never code directly from the alphabetic index.

VOLUME 2: ALPHABETIC INDEX TO DISEASES *(continued)*

Section 2, Table of Drugs and Chemicals

- Extensive listing of drugs, chemicals, and toxic agents
- Also shows:
  - E-codes
  - American Hospital Formulary Service (AHFS) list numbers

VOLUME 2: ALPHABETIC INDEX TO DISEASES *(continued)*

Section 3, Alphabetic Index to External Causes of Injuries and Poisonings

- Codes describing circumstances of injuries, accidents, and violence
- Not used for medical diagnosis

 CHECKPOINT QUESTION 7

What are V-codes used for?

Answer

_____

_____

_____

VOLUME 3: INPATIENT CODING

Volume 3, Tabular List and Alphabetic Index of Procedures

- Used for _____
- Organized by anatomy

- Codes are two-digit categories, with maximum of two decimal digits where necessary
- Most cover surgical procedures

LOCATING THE APPROPRIATE CODE

Using the ICD-9-CM conventions

Main term

Fourth and fifth digits

When more than one code is used

Coding suspected conditions

Documentation requirements

USING THE ICD-9-CM CONVENTIONS

Conventions = _____

Direct and guide coder to appropriate code

Must be strictly followed

MAIN TERM

Look under main term when locating diagnosis with more than one word

- Example: main term in "breast cyst" is cyst
- Find the condition, not the location

FOURTH AND FIFTH DIGITS

Fourth and fifth digits provide more specificity

Example: Diabetes mellitus, 250

- Fourth digit indicates specific complications accompanying diabetes
- Fifth digit indicates insulin dependency

Incomplete codes affect reimbursement and cause data errors

PRIMARY CODES

Primary diagnosis = patient's chief complaint; reason for seeking care

Listed first on CMS-1500

WHEN MORE THAN ONE CODE IS USED

More than one code used with patients having more than one diagnosis

Sequence multiple codes with the proper service or procedure code

 WHAT IF?

You need to code a condition described as acute, chronic, or both. What code should you use?

LATE EFFECTS

Late effects = _____

- Present after treatment for acute illness
- List code number identifying residual (current) condition first
- Then code number identifying cause of original illness second

CODING SUSPECTED CONDITIONS

Inpatient setting: codes listed after patient's testing complete; code with complete information

Outpatient setting: codes listed as the patient visit occurs; limited by information on hand at the time of patient visit

CODING SUSPECTED CONDITIONS (continued)

If diagnosis is unconfirmed, physician may indicate "rule out," "suspected," or "probable"

Patient's symptom at time of visit is only confirmed reason for encounter

Code only for patient's symptom until definitive diagnosis is available

 CHECKPOINT QUESTION 8

Before a definitive diagnosis is made, what is coded?

Answer

_____

_____

_____

DOCUMENTATION REQUIREMENTS

Choose code assigned for service or procedure based on documentation available

Audits verify that codes used match information recorded in patient's chart on date of service

Audits conducted to:

- ■ _____
- ■ _____

 CHECKPOINT QUESTION 9

List two reasons for a chart audit.

Answer

_____

_____

_____

THE FUTURE OF DIAGNOSTIC CODING: INTERNATIONAL CLASSIFICATION OF DISEASES, TENTH REVISION

ICD-10 scheduled to release by 2005

Will include more codes

Will include hospice and home care

New codes will be alphanumeric

Will include new chapters on eye and ear disorders

ICD-9 reference materials will be obsolete

Allows insurance companies to:

- ■ Communicate with each other
- ■ Compare reimbursable amounts
- ■ Speed claims processing

Chapter 18

Outpatient Procedural Coding

PHYSICIAN'S CURRENT PROCEDURAL TERMINOLOGY

Physician's Current Procedural Terminology (CPT) is a comprehensive listing of _____ provided by physicians.

Originally focused on surgical procedures

Updated every December

PHYSICIAN'S CURRENT PROCEDURAL TERMINOLOGY
(continued)

The aim of CPT-4 was to establish a way for interested parties to know what procedures and services had been provided to the patient without reading a lengthy report.

PHYSICIAN'S CURRENT PROCEDURAL TERMINOLOGY
(continued)

CPT-4 system uses five-digit numeric codes and corresponding meanings

Codes describe specific _____, _____, or _____ provided by physicians

Used in both inpatient and outpatient settings

PHYSICIAN'S CURRENT PROCEDURAL TERMINOLOGY
(continued)

CPT-4 divided into six sections:

- ■ Evaluation and management
- ■ Anesthesia
- ■ Surgery

- Radiology
- Pathology and laboratory
- Medicine

READING DESCRCIPTORS

Read up to semicolon; look down for any indentations using same words before the semicolon

GUIDELINES

Sections begin with specific guidelines and applicable procedures and services

Guidelines contain:

- Definitions
- Explanatory notes
- Listing of previously unlisted procedures
- Directions for filing a special report
- Modifiers

UNLISTED PROCEDURES AND SPECIAL REPORTS

CPT provides unlisted codes at the beginning of each section

Used if service performed is not listed in CPT

Provide copy of procedure report with claim when unlisted code used

UNLISTED PROCEDURES AND SPECIAL REPORTS *(continued)*

Report should include:

- Definition of nature, extent, and need of procedure
- Time, effort, and equipment necessary
- Complexity of symptoms
- Final diagnosis
- Physical findings
- Diagnostic and therapeutic procedures
- Concurrent problems
- Follow-up care

EVALUATION AND MANAGEMENT CODES

Five-digit codes beginning with 9

E/M codes describe various _____, _____, and _____ physicians must make in evaluating and treating patients in various settings (e.g., office, outpatient, hospital).

Documentation must enable physician and coder to decide which code to use

EVALUATION AND MANAGEMENT CODES *(continued)*

To code service described, record must indicate key components present

Two of three key components for established patients

Three of three key components for new patients

EVALUATION AND MANAGEMENT CODES *(continued)*

Components = _____

- History
- Physical examination
- Medical decision making
- Counseling
- Coordination of care
- Nature of presenting problem
- Time

EVALUATION AND MANAGEMENT CODES *(continued)*

Key components:

- _____
- _____
- _____

All other components are contributing elements

EVALUATION AND MANAGEMENT CODES *(continued)*

Four classifications of history and physical described in CPT-4:

- Problem-focused
- Expanded problem-focused
- Detailed
- Comprehensive

EVALUATION AND MANAGEMENT CODES *(continued)*

Medical decision making =

_____

Categorized as:

- Straightforward
- Low complexity
- Moderate complexity
- High complexity

EVALUATION AND MANAGEMENT CODES *(continued)*

When time spent with the patient is more than 50% of the typical time for the visit, time becomes the deciding factor in choosing an E/M code.

Other considerations:

- In-hospital care codes
- Emergency department codes

 CHECKPOINT QUESTION 1

To code for a service in the E/M section, two of the three key components must be present for an established patient, and all three must be present for a new patient. What are the three key elements?

Answer

_____

_____

_____

ANESTHESIA CODES

Five-digit codes beginning with 0

Divided by anatomic site and procedure

Two modifiers used in anesthesia:

- Standard modifier in all sections
- Physical status modifier
  - Indicate patient's condition at time of anesthesia (P1 is normal; P5 will not survive without procedure)

SURGERY CODES

Unstarred codes

Starred codes

Integumentary system

Repairs

Cast reapplication

Multiple procedures furnished on the same day

UNSTARRED CODES

Refer to codes that include a surgical package

Surgical package = _____

_____

_____.

Cannot bill separately for preoperative and postoperative components

UNSTARRED CODES *(continued)*

CMS defines surgical package differently for Medicare patients

Additional procedures done to correct or alleviate problems are coded separately

Complications not requiring revisit to operating room are included in price of surgery

STARRED CODES

Used for surgical service

Surgical package does not apply

Code preoperative anesthesia and postoperative components separately

Check with relevant third-party payers for specific rules

INTEGUMENTARY SYSTEM

Codes for which a measurement is necessary

Measure size of defect and specimen

All excisions include simple closure

REPAIRS

Three types:

- Simple
- Intermediate
- Complex

Measure and recorded in centimeters

CAST REAPPLICATION

Cannot assign same code as cast application

Reapplication does not include treatment for fracture

Carries lower reimbursement than original application

MULTIPLE PROCEDURES FURNISHED ON THE SAME DAY

Code separately unless part of overall service

Place on claim form in order from major to minor

 CHECKPOINT QUESTION 2

What items are included in a surgical package?

Answer

_____

_____

_____

_____

RADIOLOGY CODES

Four radiology subsections:

- Diagnostic radiology/diagnostic imaging
- Diagnostic ultrasound
- Radiation oncology
- Nuclear medicine

Five-digit codes starting with 7

Arranged by anatomic site, from top of body to bottom

Descriptors indicate "with contrast" or "without contrast"

RADIOLOGY CODES (*continued*)

Use two codes if physician performs, supervises, and interprets a procedure

Code procedure

Code for supervision and interpretation

PATHOLOGY AND LABORATORY CODES

Five-digit numbers beginning with 8

Divided into sections for panels of tests

Final part of section includes services and procedures by a pathologist

Submit each tissue specimen under a separate code for diagnosis

PATHOLOGY AND LABORATORY CODES (*continued*)

Subsection on automated multichannel tests

Verify that tests performed are included in the lists under this section before coding

MEDICINE CODES

Five-digit numbers beginning with 9

Pay close attention to immunization injections section (90701 to 90749)

Use two codes when immunization injections delivered

- One code for _____
- One code for _____

MEDICINE CODES *(continued)*

Specify what is injected for therapeutic or diagnostic injections

Medicare includes cost of administering injections in price of office and outpatient visits

Supplying drug is considered separate service

MEDICINE CODES *(continued)*

Also includes:

- Cardiac diagnostic testing
- Performing CPR
- Dialysis treatment

CHECKPOINT QUESTION 3

A patient comes in for a tetanus booster, and the physician gives the booster and completes a routine physical examination. How many codes do you use for this visit?

Answer

_____

_____

_____

CPT-4 MODIFIERS

Modifiers = _____

List of modifiers found in Appendix A of CPT-4

Ways to write modifiers:

- Five-digit code with hyphen followed by two-digit modifier (28702-22)
- Code without a hyphen separating the code and modifier (2870222)
- First modifier as -99 if code needs multiple modifiers (28702-9922. . . .)

CHECKPOINT QUESTION 4

Where can a coder find a list of all CPT modifiers?

Answer

_____

_____

HEALTHCARE COMMON PROCEDURE CODING SYSTEM

Healthcare Common Procedure Coding System (HCPCS) developed by CMS to cover items such as:

- Ambulance service
- Wheelchairs
- Injections

HEALTHCARE COMMON PROCEDURE CODING SYSTEM *(continued)*

The HCPCS uses codes contained in _____ (now known as HCPCS Level 1) plus expanded codes developed by CMS and fiscal intermediaries to classify physician and nonphysician patient care services on the national level (now known as HCPCS Level 2).

HEALTHCARE COMMON PROCEDURE CODING SYSTEM *(continued)*

Level 2 HCPCS codes are most commonly referred to as the _____, and Level 1 HCPCS codes are referred to as _____.

HEALTHCARE COMMON PROCEDURE CODING SYSTEM *(continued)*

By 1987, all hospitals and ambulatory surgical centers were required to use HCPCS for all patients receiving government-sponsored benefits

Twofold purpose:

- Blended payment rate to apply to ambulatory surgery in hospital outpatient department
- Provide a database for future payment amounts for all outpatient services

REIMBURSEMENT

Diagnostic related groups

Resource-based relative value scale

HCPCS LEVEL 1 CODES

Codes listed in CPT-4

Used for procedures and services for private and government insurance programs

DIAGNOSTIC RELATED GROUPS

Diagnostic related groups (DRGs) are categories into which inpatients are placed according to the similarity of their _____, _____, and _____.

Used to determine reimbursement for inpatient services to Medicare patients

HCPCS LEVEL 2 CODES: NATIONAL CODES

Released annually in *National Coding Manual*

Five-digit alphanumeric codes beginning with A through V

Some of the codes include:

- Chemotherapeutic drugs
- Dental services
- Injections
- Orthotics
- Vision care

DIAGNOSTIC RELATED GROUPS
(continued)

Fee attached to each DRG based on national average of all Medicare discharges

Adjusted for local factors

Hospital reimbursed fixed amount according to patient's DRG

DIAGNOSTIC RELATED GROUPS
(continued)

Medical assistants must assign correct ICD-9-CM code when scheduling patients for admission

Outpatient code will influence inpatient DRG assignment

Hospital coder selects DRG according to:

- _____
- _____
- _____

HCPCS LEVEL 3 CODES: LOCAL CODES

Developed to address regional codes

Produced and available through state Medicare carrier

Begin with letters W to Z

 CHECKPOINT QUESTION 5

Where do you find codes for dental services?

Answer

_____

_____

RESOURCE-BASED RELATIVE VALUE SCALE

Physician reimbursement for Medicare services based on fee schedule

Schedule sets maximum fee for service based on resource-based relative value scale (RBRVS)

The goal of RBRVS is to reduce Medicare Part B costs and to establish national standards of payment based on CPT-4 codes.

RESOURCE-BASED RELATIVE VALUE SCALE *(continued)*

Fee calculations based on:

- Intensity of service
- Time required
- Skills needed
- Overhead expenses
- Malpractice premiums

Adjusted by geographical practice cost index (GPCI)

RESOURCE-BASED RELATIVE VALUE SCALE

GPCIs determine the relative value unit (RVU)

National conversion factor assigned yearly

Example:

- CPT code 99205
  - RVU = 4.58
  - National conversion factor = 36.7856
- Medicare allowed charge is $168.48

 CHECKPOINT QUESTION 6

Why are DRGs used?

Chapter 19

Medical Asepsis and Infection Control

INTRODUCTION

- Two goals to prevent spread of disease in medical offices

Answer

_____

_____

_____

FRAUD AND CODING

Examples of fraud:

- Billing for services not performed
- Using another patient's coverage to receive reimbursement
- Falsifying records

_____ usually investigates reports of possible fraud

FRAUD AND CODING *(continued)*

CMS is vigilant with audits of medical offices

Audits can cover past years

If fraud uncovered:

- Physician must repay an amount owed plus interest
- May be unable to participate in Medicare-funded programs

FRAUD AND CODING *(continued)*

To avoid costly errors:

- Keep accurate and complete documentation
- Always use most recent code books
- Follow coding rules; keep updated on changes
- Never code anything about which you are unsure

1. Understand and practice medical asepsis at all times
2. Educate patients and _____ about techniques to use at home

MICROORGANISMS, PATHOGENS, AND NORMAL FLORA

- Microorganisms
  - Very small living organisms seen only with a _____
- Normal flora
  - Part of normal environment

- Also found on skin and throughout gastrointestinal, genitourinary, and _____ systems
- Some required for good health

PATHOGENS AND NORMAL FLORA

- Pathogens
  - Disease-producing microorganisms
  - Bacteria, viruses, fungi, _____
- Transient flora
  - Too many normal flora
  - Normal flora transmitted to another area of the body
  - Can become _____ under the right conditions

BODY'S NATURAL DEFENSES

- Skin
- Eyes
- _____
- Gastrointestinal tract
- Respiratory tract
- Genitourinary tract

CHECKPOINT QUESTION I

What are pathogenic microorganisms? How does the body prevent an invasion and subsequent infection naturally?

Answer

_____

_____

_____

_____

_____

CONDITIONS THAT FAVOR THE GROWTH OF PATHOGENS

- Moisture
- Nutrients
- _____

- Darkness
- Neutral pH
- Oxygen

CHECKPOINT QUESTION 2

Given the six conditions that favor the growth of pathogens, explain how you can alter the growth and reproduction of microorganisms by changing these factors.

Answer

_____

_____

_____

_____

_____

THE INFECTION CYCLE

- A series of specific links of a chain involving a causative agent or invading microorganisms
  - Reservoir host
  - Modes of _____
  - Pathogen spreads
  - Portal of entry
  - Susceptible host

CHECKPOINT QUESTION 3

How are the first and fifth links of the infection cycle related?

Answer

_____

_____

_____

_____

MODES OF TRANSMISSION

- Direct transmission
- _____
- Sources of transmission

CHECKPOINT QUESTION 4

The medical office where you work has a policy about not opening windows that do not have screens in examination rooms and the reception area. Why do you think this policy is or is not important?

Answer

_____

_____

_____

_____

_____

PRINCIPLES OF INFECTION CONTROL

- Most transmission of infectious disease can be prevented by strict adherence to guidelines issued by _____

MEDICAL ASEPSIS

- Practices that render an object or area free from _____ microorganisms
- Handwashing is the MOST IMPORTANT medical aseptic technique

HANDWASHING

- Always wash your hands:
  - Before and after patient contact
  - After contact with any blood or body fluids
  - After contact with _____
  - After handling specimens
  - After coughing, sneezing, or nose blowing
  - After using the restroom
  - Before and after lunch, breaks, leaving for the day

OTHER MEDICAL ASEPSIS TECHNIQUES

- Wear _____
- Wash hands before applying gloves and after removing them

- General office cleaning
- Floors should always be considered contaminated

CHECKPOINT QUESTION 5

Explain why wearing exam gloves does not replace handwashing.

Answer

_____

_____

_____

_____

_____

LEVELS OF INFECTION CONTROL

- _____
- Disinfection
- Sanitation

SANITATION

- Science of maintaining a healthful, disease-free, and hazard-free environment
- Thorough cleaning of instruments and _____ with warm soapy water
- Precedes disinfection and sterilization

DISINFECTION

- Inactivates virtually all recognized pathogenic microorganisms, but not all microbial forms

FACTORS THAT AFFECT DISINFECTION

- Prior cleaning of object
- Amount of _____ material on object
- Type of microbial contamination
- Concentration of germicide used
- Length of exposure to _____
- Shape or complexity of object
- Temperature of process

LEVELS OF DISINFECTION

- High level
  - Destroys most forms of _____ life, but not bacterial spores
- Intermediate level
  - Destroys many _____, fungi, and some bacteria
- Low level
  - Destroys many bacteria and some viruses

 ## CHECKPOINT QUESTION 6

What level of disinfection would you use to clean a nondisposable instrument that comes into contact with the vaginal mucosa, such as a vaginal speculum? Why?

Answer

_____

_____

_____

_____

_____

OCCUPATIONAL SAFETY AND HEALTH ADMINISTRATION GUIDELINES FOR THE MEDICAL OFFICE

- Federal agency responsible for ensuring _____ of all workers
- Mandates federal regulations or laws that must be followed by all medical offices
- Other office policies must be in a manual

EXPOSURE RISK FACTORS AND THE EXPOSURE CONTROL PLAN

- Medical offices must provide clear instructions in the _____ for preventing employee exposure or reducing the danger of exposure to biohazardous materials

EXPOSURE RISK FACTORS

- Exposure risk factor for each worker must be calculated

- Clinical medical assistants
  - Have high exposure risk
  - Require access to _____
  - Require immunization against hepatitis B

EXPOSURE CONTROL PLAN

- Policy required by OSHA for offices with ten or more employees
- Plan of action for all who might become exposed to biohazardous material
- Office must provide appropriate equipment and supplies

IN THE EVENT OF EXPOSURE

1. Apply the principles of first aid and notify your supervisor
2. Physician or supervisor provides guidance for post-exposure testing and follow-up procedures
3. Complete and file an incident report
4. Employer must record exposure on an OSHA 300 log

 ## CHECKPOINT QUESTION 7

Explain the difference between exposure risk factors and the exposure control plan.

Answer

_____

_____

_____

_____

_____

STANDARD PRECAUTIONS

- Set of procedures recognized by the CDC to reduce chance of transmitting _____
- Pertain to contact with blood, all body _____ (except sweat), nonintact skin, and mucous membranes
- Wash hands after touching _____ items

STANDARD PRECAUTIONS *(continued)*

- Or use alcohol-based hand rub
- Wear clean, nonsterile exam gloves
- Change gloves between procedures
- Wear PPE
- Take precautions to avoid injury
- Place used sharps in puncture-resistant containers
- Use barrier devices instead of mouth-to-mouth resuscitation

 CHECKPOINT QUESTION 8

How will following standard precautions help to protect you against contracting an infection or communicable disease?

Answer

_____

_____

_____

_____

_____

PERSONAL PROTECTIVE EQUIPMENT (PPE)

- Must be available and used by all health care workers
- Employees responsible for using PPE correctly
  - Remove all PPE before removing gloves
  - After removing gloves, _____

 CHECKPOINT QUESTION 9

What PPE would you need to wear when assisting the physician with a wound irrigation?

Answer

_____

_____

_____

_____

HANDLING ENVIRONMENTAL CONTAMINATION

- All equipment and areas must be

_____

- Any surface contaminated with biohazardous materials should be promptly cleaned
  - Use an approved germicide or a dilute bleach solution
  - Spill kits or appropriate supplies must be available

SPILL KITS

- Spill kits include
  - Clean gloves
  - Eye protection
  - Gel to absorb biohazardous material
  - Scoop
  - Towels
  - Biohazard _____

SOILED LINENS

- Handling soiled linens
  - Wear gloves
  - Handle as little as possible
  - Fold carefully with contaminated surface

  _____

  - Place in biohazard bag

 CHECKPOINT QUESTION 10

How would you respond to an employee in the medical office who is unsure about how to clean up a spilled urine specimen? Is this biohazardous?

Answer

_____

_____

_____

_____

_____

DISPOSING OF INFECTIOUS WASTE

- EPA and OSHA set policies

■ Individual states determine local policies
  • Large generators are certified and maintain records
  • Medical offices are usually small generators

INFECTIOUS WASTE SERVICE

■ Supplies office with appropriate waste containers and picks up filled containers regularly
■ Disposes waste according to EPA and OSHA guidelines
■ Maintains records
■ Medical office retains records for _____ years

GUIDELINES TO KEEP COSTS DOWN

■ Use separate containers for each type of waste
■ Fill sharps containers only to fill lines
■ Use approved biohazard containers
■ Secure containers before moving them

 CHECKPOINT QUESTION 11

After drawing a blood specimen from a patient, you notice that the tube of blood is leaking onto the examination table where you temporarily put it while finishing the procedure. How would you clean up the blood spill?

Answer

_____
_____
_____
_____
_____

THE HEPATITIS B AND HUMAN IMMUNODEFICIENCY VIRUSES

■ Persistent health care concern

HEPATITIS B VIRUS

■ More viable than HIV
■ Easily killed with dilute _____
■ Transmitted via contaminated blood or body fluids
■ Vaccine must be provided to employees at no cost
■ Postexposure plan required

HUMAN IMMUNODEFICIENCY VIRUS

■ Transmitted via contaminated blood or body fluids
■ No vaccine available
■ Postexposure plan is required

 CHECKPOINT QUESTION 12

Which virus is more of a threat to the clinical medical assistant: HIV or HBV?

Answer

_____
_____
_____
_____

Chapter 20

Medical History and Patient Management

_____
_____
_____

CONDUCTING THE PATIENT INTERVIEW

- Primary goal is to obtain accurate and pertinent
  _____

THE MEDICAL HISTORY

- A record containing
  - Patient's past and present _____
  - Health status of related family members
  - Relevant information about patient's social habits
- Assessment
  - Gathering information to determine patient's problem or reason for seeking medical care

PREPARING FOR THE INTERVIEW

- Be familiar with previous medical history of patient
- Conduct interview in a _____
- Use active listening skills
- Use variety of interviewing techniques
- Observe physical and mental status

METHODS OF COLLECTING INFORMATION

- Medical assistant and physician
- Medical assistant using _____
- Patient fills out form, medical assistant checks
- Physician

INTRODUCING YOURSELF

- Develop trust and _____ with patient
- Always begin by
  - Identifying yourself
  - Your title
  - The purpose of the interview

ELEMENTS OF THE MEDICAL HISTORY

- Most forms contain
  - Identifying data (database)
  - _____ (PH)
  - Review of systems (ROS)
  - Family history (FH)
  - Social history

BARRIERS TO COMMUNICATION

- Unfamiliarity with English language
- Hearing _____
- Cognitive abilities

 CHECKPOINT QUESTION 2

Why is it important to review the medical history form before beginning the interview?

Answer

_____
_____
_____
_____

CHECKPOINT QUESTION 1

What is the difference between the past history and the family history?

Answer

_____
_____

CHECKPOINT QUESTION 3

Why should you let the patient know that any information shared during the interview will be kept confidential?

Answer

_____

_____

_____

_____

_____

ASSESSING THE PATIENT

- Signs and symptoms
- Chief complaint and _____
- Educate the patient

SIGNS

- Objective information observed or perceived by someone other than the patient
  - Rash
  - Bleeding
  - _____
  - Vital sign measurements

SYMPTOMS

- Subjective information of disease or changes in the body as sensed by the patient
  - Leg pain
  - _____
  - Nausea
  - Dizziness

CHIEF COMPLAINT AND PRESENT ILLNESS

- Find out exactly why patient has come to see physician
- Use _____ questions
  - Can you describe what has been going on?
- Avoid close-ended questions
  - Do you have pain?

CHIEF COMPLAINT (CC)

- Statement describing the _____ that led the patient to seek medical care
- Document in medical record at each visit

PRESENT ILLNESS (PI)

- Probe for details to further define the patient's present illness
  - Chronology
  - Location
  - _____
  - Self-treatment
  - Quality
  - Duration

 ## CHECKPOINT QUESTION 4

Explain the difference between a sign and a symptom and give one example of each.

Answer

_____

_____

_____

_____

Chapter 21

Anthropometric Measurements and Vital Signs

ANTHROPOMETRIC MEASUREMENTS

- Height
- Weight
- First visit recorded as _____

WEIGHT

- Required for
  - Prenatal patients, infants, children, and elderly
  - Patients prescribed medications that must be calculated according to _____
  - Patients attempting to lose or gain weight

HEIGHT

- Movable ruler on back of balance beam scales
- Graph type ruler mounted on wall
- Inches or centimeters

 CHECKPOINT QUESTION 1

Why is it important to accurately measure vital signs at every patient visit?

Answer

_____

_____

_____

_____

_____

VITAL SIGNS

- Also known as _____
- Measurements of bodily functions essential to maintaining life processes

- Frequently measured and recorded by medical assistant

TEMPERATURE

- Balance between heat produced and heat _____ by the body
- Afebrile
  - Body temperature within normal limits
  - 98.6° Fahrenheit or 37.0° Celsius
- Febrile
  - Body temperature above normal limits

TEMPERATURE *(continued)*

- Heat normally lost through several processes
  - Respiration
  - Elimination
  - Conduction through the _____

THERMOMETERS

- Measure body temperature using either the Fahrenheit or Celsius scale
  - Oral
  - Rectal
  - _____
  - Tympanic
  - Indicate method used

 CHECKPOINT QUESTION 2

How does an oral temperature measurement differ from a rectal measurement? Why?

Answer

_____

_____

_____

_____

_____

FEVER PROCESSES

- Temperature is regulated by hypothalamus
- Factors that may cause temperature to vary
  - Age
  - Illness

- Gender
- Exercise
- _____
- Emotions
- Illness

STAGES OF FEVER

- Onset may be abrupt or gradual
- Course may range from a day to several weeks
  - Sustained
  - Remittent
  - _____
  - Relapsing
- Resolution
  - Crisis
  - Lysis

CHECKPOINT QUESTION 3

Explain why the body temperature of a young child might be different from an adult's.

Answer

_____

_____

_____

_____

_____

GLASS MERCURY THERMOMETERS

- Used for oral, rectal, and axillary temperatures
  - Use disposable sheaths
- Rectal thermometers
  - Rounded or stubbed end
  - Usually color coded _____
- Axillary or oral thermometers
  - Long, slender bulbs
  - Color coded _____

ELECTRONIC THERMOMETERS

- Portable battery-operated units with interchangeable probes
  - Color coded blue for oral or axillary
  - Color coded red for rectal
  - Keep in charging unit between uses

TYMPANIC THERMOMETERS

- Newest type of thermometer
- Also called _____ thermometer
- Battery powered
- End fitted with disposable cover is inserted into ear

DISPOSABLE THERMOMETERS

- Single-use, disposable thermometers
- Fairly accurate but not as reliable as electronic, tympanic, or glass
- Register quickly by indicating color changes on a strip
- Acceptable for _____

CHECKPOINT QUESTION 4

Why is a tympanic membrane temperature more accurate than an axillary temperature?

Answer

_____

_____

_____

_____

_____

PULSE

- Expansion and relaxation of the arteries can be felt at various points on the body

PALPATION AND AUSCULTATION

- Palpation
  - Each expansion of the artery can be felt and is counted as one _____
- Auscultation
  - Hearing each heart beat

PULSE POINTS

- Carotid artery
- _____

- Brachial artery
- Radial artery
- Femoral artery
- Popliteal artery
- Posterior tibial artery
- Dorsalis pedis artery

PULSE CHARACTERISTICS

- _____
- Rhythm
- Volume

FACTORS AFFECTING PULSE RATES

- Age
- Condition
- Time of day
- Gender
- Body type and size
- _____
- Stress or emotions
- Fever
- Medications
- Blood volume

FACTORS AFFECTING PULSE RATES *(continued)*

- Peripheral pulses may also be auscultated with _____ unit
  - Small battery powered or electronic device
  - Consists of a main box with control switches, a probe, and an earpiece unit that plugs into main box
  - Earpiece unit may be detached, so sounds can be heard by everyone in room

FACTORS AFFECTING PULSE RATES *(continued)*

- Using Doppler device
  - Apply coupling or transmission gel
  - Place end of probe on the area
  - With machine "on," hold probe at a 90° angle with light pressure
  - After assessing rate and rhythm of pulse, clean skin and probe with tissue

 CHECKPOINT QUESTION 5

What characteristics of a patient's pulse should be assessed and how should they be recorded in the medical record?

Answer

_____

_____

_____

_____

_____

RESPIRATIONS

- Exchange of gases between the _____ and the blood in the body
- Body expels carbon dioxide (CO_2) and takes in oxygen (O_2)

PROCESS OF RESPIRATION

- Inspiration
  - Oxygen brought into _____
- Expiration
  - Air in lungs is forced out
- Each respiration is counted as one full inspiration and one full expiration

RESPIRATION CHARACTERISTICS

- Rate
  - Number of respirations occurring in 1 minute
- Rhythm
  - Period of time _____ each respiration
- Depth
  - Volume of air being inhaled and exhaled

ABNORMAL SOUNDS

- Sign of disease process
- Crackles
  - _____ sounds
- Wheezes
  - High-pitched sounds

FACTORS AFFECTING RESPIRATION

- Age
- Elevated body temperature
- Tachypnea
- Bradypnea
- _____
- Apnea
- Hyperpnea
- Hyperventilation
- Hypopnea
- Orthopnea

CHECKPOINT QUESTION 6

What happens within the chest cavity when the diaphragm contracts?

Answer

_____

_____

_____

_____

_____

BLOOD PRESSURE

- Pressure of blood in an artery as it is forced against arterial _____
- Measured in contraction and relaxation phases of cardiac cycle or heart beat
- Measured with stethoscope and sphygmomanometer

PHASES OF CARDIAC CYCLE

- Systole
  - _____ phase of cardiac cycle
- Diastole
  - _____ phase of cardiac cycle

CHECKPOINT QUESTION 7

What is happening to the heart during systole? Diastole?

Answer

_____

_____

_____

_____

_____

KOROTKOFF SOUNDS

- Five phases of sounds heard while auscultating blood pressure as described by Russian neurologist, Nicolai Korotkoff

PULSE PRESSURE

- Difference between systolic and _____ readings

AUSCULTATORY GAP

- Loss of any sounds or a drop of up to 30 mm Hg or more during release of air from blood pressure cuff after first sound is heard

FACTORS INFLUENCING BLOOD PRESSURE

- Atherosclerosis
- Arteriosclerosis
- General health
- Dietary habits
- _____ and tobacco use
- Exercise
- Previous heart conditions
- Family history

FACTORS INFLUENCING BLOOD PRESSURE *(continued)*

- Age
- Stress
- Body position
- _____
- Hypertension

CHOOSING CORRECT BLOOD PRESSURE CUFF SIZE

- Assess size of patient's arm
- Width of cuff should be 40% to 50% of circumference of arm

CHECKPOINT QUESTION 8

How are the pulse pressure and the auscultatory gap different?

Answer

_____

_____

_____

_____

Chapter 22

Assisting with the Physical Examination

INTRODUCTION

- Purpose of complete physical examination is to assess patient's general state of health and detect signs and symptoms of _____
- Physical examination gives physician baseline information
- Baseline aids in diagnosis

THREE COMPONENTS OF PATIENT ASSESSMENT

- Medical history
- Physical examination
- Laboratory and diagnostic _____

MEDICAL ASSISTANTS ARE RESPONSIBLE FOR

- Assisting with collecting medical history
- _____ patient for examination
- Assisting physician during examination
- Collecting various specimens for diagnostic testing

BASIC INSTRUMENTS AND SUPPLIES

- Instruments enable examiner to see, hear, or feel areas of body
- Physician uses the instruments

PERCUSSION HAMMER

- Test _____ reflexes
- Strike tendons of the ankle, knee, wrist, and elbow

TUNING FORK

- Tests _____
- Examiner strikes prongs against hand, causing them to vibrate and produce humming sound

NASAL SPECULUM

- Instrument is inserted into nostril to assist in visual inspection of lining of nose, nasal membranes, and _____

OTOSCOPE AND AUDIOSCOPE

- Otoscope permits visualization of the ear canal and _____ membrane
- Audioscope is used to screen patients for hearing loss

OPHTHALMOSCOPE

- Used to examine interior structures of

_____

EXAMINATION LIGHT AND GOOSENECK LAMP

- Examination lights
  - Used for additional lighting and better visualization
- Gooseneck lamp
  - Floor lamp with a movable stand that bends at the neck

STETHOSCOPE

- Used for listening to body sounds
- Heart
- Lungs
- _____
- Also used for taking blood pressure

PENLIGHT OR FLASHLIGHT

- Used to provide additional light to a specific area

 CHECKPOINT QUESTION I

Which instruments are used to test the ears and hearing?

Answer

_____

_____

_____

_____

_____

INSTRUMENTS AND SUPPLIES USED IN SPECIALIZED EXAMINATIONS

- In addition to basic instruments, specialized equipment may be used during physical examination

HEADLIGHT OR MIRROR

- Otorhinolaryngologist may wear a headlight or head mirror
- Light or mirror attached to a headband
  - Provides direct light on area being examined
  - _____ reflects light into the area

LARYNGEAL MIRROR AND LARYNGOSCOPE

- Laryngeal mirror
  - Stainless steel instrument with long, slender handle and small, round mirror

- Used to examine areas of patient's throat and _____
- Laryngoscope handle is similar to handle of an otoscope or ophthalmoscope
  - Can attach blades and small light source

VAGINAL SPECULUM

- Used for pelvic examination and Papanicolaou (_____) smear
- Inserted into vagina to expand the opening
- Ayre spatula or cervical scraper used to collect cells from vaginal cul-de-sac
- Histobrush used to obtain cells for Pap smear

LUBRICANT

- Water-soluble gel used to reduce friction and provide easy insertion of instruments
- Also used for bimanual exams

ANOSCOPE, PROCTOSCOPE, SIGMOIDOSCOPE

- Anoscope
  - Short speculum inserted into rectum to inspect anal canal
- Proctoscope
  - Speculum used to visualize rectum and anus
- Sigmoidoscope
  - Longer instrument used to visualize rectum and sigmoid _____

DURING RECTAL EXAMINATIONS

- Medical assistant should have available
  - Suction machine
  - Cotton-tipped applicators
  - Glass microscope slides
  - _____ containers
  - Laboratory request slips

 CHECKPOINT QUESTION 2

What are the different uses of the anoscope, proctoscope, and sigmoidoscope? What is the purpose of an obturator?

Answer

_____

_____

_____

_____

_____

EXAMINATION TECHNIQUES

- Physician uses four basic techniques to gather information

  1. Inspection
  2. _____
  3. Percussion
  4. Auscultation

INSPECTION

- Looking at areas of body with naked eye and instruments to observe physical features
  - Movements
  - Skin and membrane _____
  - Contour
  - Symmetry or asymmetry

PALPATION

- Touching or moving body areas with fingers or hands
  - Pulse characteristics
  - Presence of growths, swelling, tenderness, pain
  - Organs assessed for size, shape, _____
  - Skin temperature, moisture, texture, elasticity

PERCUSSION

- Tapping or striking body with hand or instrument to produce sounds
  - _____ percussion
  - Indirect percussion

AUSCULTATION

- _____ to sounds of the body
- Using a stethoscope or ear placed directly on patient's body
- Areas of body that can be auscultated
  - Heart
  - Lungs
  - Abdomen
  - Blood vessels

CHECKPOINT QUESTION 3

Which of the examination techniques requires the use of the hands and fingers to feel organs or structures?

Answer

_____

_____

_____

_____

_____

RESPONSIBILITIES OF THE MEDICAL ASSISTANT

- Room preparation
- _____ preparation
- Assisting the physician
- Postexamination duties

ROOM PREPARATION

- Examination room should be
  - Clean
  - Well-lit
  - Ventilated
  - Comfortable temperature for _____
- Examination table
  - Decontaminated
  - Clean paper

ROOM PREPARATION (*continued*)

- Each day
  - Check each examination room for supplies and equipment
  - Check _____

PATIENT PREPARATION

- Call patient from waiting room
- Escort to treatment room
- Create a supportive and _____ atmosphere
- Treat each patient as an individual

IN THE EXAM ROOM

- Give instructions for disrobing and gowning
- _____ room while patient undresses
- Ask patient to sit on examination table
- Drape legs
- Place chart outside
- Notify physician that patient is ready

ASSISTING THE PHYSICIAN

- Hand instruments or supplies to physician
- Direct light appropriately
- Remain in room as necessary
- Assist patient into _____
- Adjust drapes

POSTEXAMINATION DUTIES

- Perform follow-up treatments and procedures as ordered by physician
  - Offer patient help returning to _____ position
  - Ask patient to dress
  - Tell patient what to do after getting dressed
- Accurately document data

CLEANING THE EXAM ROOM

- Clean all used, nondisposable equipment
- Dispose of used disposable equipment and supplies
- Cover examination table with _____
- Prepare room for next patient

CHECKPOINT QUESTION 4

What are your four basic responsibilities in performance of the physical examination?

Answer

_____

_____

_____

_____

_____

PHYSICAL EXAMINATION FORMAT

- Begins with patient seated on exam table with drape sheet over lap and covering legs
- Physician progresses through examination in sequence
- Patient's general _____ observed throughout

HEAD AND NECK

- Physician inspects skull, scalp, hair, face
  - Trachea and lymph nodes _____ for size and symmetry
  - Thyroid gland palpated for size and symmetry
  - Carotid arteries palpated and auscultated

EYES AND EARS

- Medical assistant performs _____ acuity test prior to exam

EYES

- Physician inspects
  - Sclera for normal color
  - Pupils for PERRLA
  - Eye movement
  - Normal movement
  - _____ vision
  - Interior of eye using ophthalmoscope
  - Retina and interlobular blood vessels using ophthalmoscope

EARS

- Physician inspects and palpates for
  - Size
  - Symmetry
  - Lesions
  - _____

EARS *(continued)*

- Uses _____ to examine interior of ear canal
  - Presence of cerumen
  - Tympanic membrane
  - Discoloration
  - Fluids behind the eardrum
- Auditory acuity tested with tuning fork

NOSE AND SINUSES

- ■ Physician inspects
  - External nose for abnormalities
  - Position of nasal septum
  - Nostrils
  - Sense of smell
  - Paranasal _____

MOUTH AND THROAT

- ■ Physician inspects
  - Mucous membranes of mouth and gums
  - Teeth
  - _____
  - Tonsils
  - Throat

MOUTH AND THROAT (continued)

- ■ Physician inspects
  - General dental hygiene
  - _____ gland function
  - Abnormalities in oral cavity including color, ulcerations, nodules

 CHECKPOINT QUESTION 5

What is the tympanic membrane and how does infection affect its appearance?

Answer

_____

_____

_____

_____

_____

CHEST, BREASTS, AND ABDOMEN

- ■ Physician observes
  - General appearance and _____
  - Respiratory rate and pattern
  - Any obvious masses or swelling

CHEST

- ■ Physician palpates
  - Axillary _____ nodes
  - Area over heart

- ■ Physician auscultates lungs for abnormal sounds
- ■ Physician inspects and palpates posterior chest including muscles of back and spine

BREASTS

- ■ Physician palpates
  - Breasts and nipples in female and _____ patients
  - Tissue up to clavicle, under axilla, and to bottom of rib cage

ABDOMEN

- ■ Physician
  - Inspects abdomen
  - Auscultates the _____
  - Percusses and palpates abdominal organs
  - Palpates lower abdominal area and groin

 CHECKPOINT QUESTION 6

Why is the patient supine for palpation of the breasts?

Answer

_____

_____

_____

_____

_____

MALE GENITALIA AND RECTUM

- ■ Physician inspects
  - Genitalia for symmetry, lesions, swelling, masses, hair distribution
  - Scrotum for testicular size, contour, and consistency
  - Inguinal ring for _____
  - Anus for lesions or hemorrhoids
  - Rectum and prostate gland

FEMALE GENITALIA

- ■ Physician examines
  - Female genitalia and rectum in the lithotomy position

- External genitalia for lesions, edema, cysts, discharge, hair distribution
- Vaginal mucosa and _____ using speculum
- Internal reproductive organs

FEMALE RECTUM

- Rectovaginal examination may be necessary
- Physician inspects and palpates rectum for lesions, hemorrhoids, sphincter tone
- _____ specimen may be obtained

LEGS

- Physician
  - Inspects legs
  - Palpates peripheral _____

REFLEXES

- Examiner uses percussion _____ to test patient's reflexes by striking the biceps, triceps, patellar, Achilles, and planter tendons

POSTURE, GAIT, COORDINATION, BALANCE, AND STRENGTH

- Physician inspects
  - General posture and spine
  - Gait and coordination
  - Balance
  - _____ and strength

CHECKPOINT QUESTION 7

What is the purpose of the rectovaginal and bimanual pelvic examinations?

Answer

_____

_____

_____

_____

_____

GENERAL HEALTH GUIDELINES AND CHECKUPS

- For patients aged 20 to 40 years, physical examinations are scheduled every _____ years
- For patients over 40, annual examinations are required

GENERAL HEALTH GUIDELINES FOR WOMEN

- First Pap smear between ages of 18 and 20 and then annually
- Breast examination by physician recommended every 3 years for women ages 20 to 40
- _____ of breasts performed monthly
- Baseline mammogram between ages of 35 and 40
- Mammogram every 2 years from 40 to 50 years of age, annually after 50

GENERAL HEALTH GUIDELINES FOR 40+

- Baseline _____ at age 40
- Rectal examination and fecal occult blood annually
- Proctoscopic examination (colonoscopy) age 50 and every 3 to 5 years thereafter
- Adult immunizations

CHECKPOINT QUESTION 8

- Why are monthly self-breast examinations important for females between the ages of 20 to 40 years?

Answer

_____

_____

_____

_____

Chapter 23

Surgical Instruments and Sterilization

INTRODUCTION

■ Goal of surgical asepsis
  • To free an item or area from all microorganisms, both pathogens and

    _____
  • Prevents microorganisms from entering the patient's environment

MEDICAL ASSISTANT RESPONSIBILITIES

■ Be familiar with surgical instruments
■ Understand surgical _____
■ Use disinfection and sterilization techniques
■ Use equipment for sterilization, treatment, and diagnostic purposes
■ Maintain accurate records and inventory

PRINCIPLES AND PRACTICES OF SURGICAL ASEPSIS

■ Surgical asepsis requires the absence of _____, infection, or infectious material on instruments, equipment, or supplies

STERILIZATION

■ Complete elimination or destruction of all forms of _____ including spore forms
■ Principle sterilizing agents
  • Steam under pressure
  • Dry heat
  • Certain gases (ethylene oxide)
  • Liquid chemicals

 CHECKPOINT QUESTION 1

What are the differences between sanitization, disinfection, and sterilization?

Answer

_____

_____

_____

_____

_____

_____

STERILIZATION EQUIPMENT

■ Medical assistant responsibilities
  • Be familiar with uses and operation of each piece of equipment
  • Schedule periodic preventive _____ or servicing of equipment
  • Maintain adequate supplies for general operational needs

THE AUTOCLAVE

■ Most frequently used piece of equipment for sterilizing instruments
■ Uses distilled water converted to _____ heated to 250°F or higher to sterilize

THE AUTOCLAVE (continued)

■ Used to sterilize
  • Minor _____ instruments
  • Surgical storage trays and containers
  • Some surgical equipment

THE AUTOCLAVE (continued)

■ Is not used for
  • Instruments or equipment that would be damaged from _____
  • Items that would not be damaged from water but may be destroyed from the heat

 CHECKPOINT QUESTION 2

What is an autoclave and how does it work?

Answer

_____

_____

_____

_____

_____

STERILIZATION INDICATORS

- Packs to register that proper pressure and _____ were attained
- Best method of sterilization is the culture test

CHECKPOINT QUESTION 3

What is the difference between a sterilization indicator and autoclave tape?

Answer

_____

_____

_____

_____

_____

LOADING THE AUTOCLAVE

- Load the autoclave _____ to allow steam to circulate
- Place empty, wrapped containers or bowls on their sides with lids wrapped separately
- Place all packs vertically (on their sides)

CHECKPOINT QUESTION 4

Why is the loading of the autoclave important? How would you load it?

Answer

_____

_____

_____

_____

_____

OPERATING THE AUTOCLAVE

- All components must be correct for items to reach a state of sterility

- Fill reservoir tank with _____ water
- Follow manufacturer's instructions for load content
- Set timer once proper temperature has been attained

END OF AUTOCLAVE CYCLE

- Timer will sound
- Open door slightly to allow load to _____
- Once items are dry
  - Remove packages
  - Store them in a clean, dry, dust-free area
  - Considered sterile for 30 days

MAINTENANCE OF AUTOCLAVE

- Medical assistant is responsible for performing maintenance on autoclave at regular intervals
  - Post schedule for _____
  - Clean lint trap
  - Wash out interior of chamber with cloth or soft brush
  - Check function of all components

CHECKPOINT QUESTION 5

Why is it important to set the timer on the autoclave during a cycle only after the correct temperature has been reached?

Answer

_____

_____

_____

_____

_____

SURGICAL INSTRUMENTS

- Tools and devices designed to perform a specific function such as cutting, _____, grasping, holding, retracting, or suturing
- Medical assistants must know proper use and care of the instruments

FORCEPS

- Used to grasp, handle, compress, pull, or join _____, equipment or supplies
  - Hemostat clamp
  - Kelly clamp
  - Sterilizer forceps
  - Needle holder
  - Spring or thumb forceps

SCISSORS

- Used for dissecting superficial, deep, or delicate tissues and for cutting sutures and bandages
  - Straight scissors
  - Curved scissors
  - _____ scissors
  - Bandage scissors

SCALPELS AND BLADES

- Small surgical _____ with straight handle and sharp straight or convex blade edge
  - Straight or pointed blades
  - Curved blades
  - Reusable handles

TOWEL CLAMPS

- Used to maintain integrity of sterile field by holding sterile _____ in place

PROBES AND DIRECTORS

- Probes show angle and _____ of the operative area
- Directors guide knife or instrument once the procedure has begun

RETRACTORS

- Hold open layers of tissue, exposing the areas beneath
  - Retractors may be plain or _____
  - May be held by assistant or screwed open to be self-retaining

 CHECKPOINT QUESTION 6

What types of instruments are used to remove tissue during a biopsy procedure?

Answer

_____

_____

_____

_____

_____

CARE AND HANDLING OF SURGICAL INSTRUMENTS

- Guidelines
  1. Do not toss or drop instruments into basins or sinks
  2. Avoid _____ instruments into a pile
  3. Always store sharp instruments separately and dispose of properly

CARE AND HANDLING OF SURGICAL INSTRUMENTS *(continued)*

  4. Keep ratcheted instruments in open position when not in use
  5. Rinse gross _____ from instruments as quickly as possible
  6. Check instruments before sterilization to ensure that they are in good working order

CARE AND HANDLING OF SURGICAL INSTRUMENTS *(continued)*

  7. Use instruments only for purpose for which they were designed
  8. _____ instruments before they are sterilized

 CHECKPOINT QUESTION 7

Why should you avoid dropping surgical instruments and what should you do if one drops accidentally?

Answer

_____

_____

_____

_____

_____

STORAGE AND RECORDKEEPING

- ■ When using and maintaining sterile instruments, equipment, and supplies, staff are responsible for
  - Correctly storing items
  - Keeping accurate records of warranties and _____ agreements
  - Keep reordering information on hand

STORAGE

- ■ Use specific storage or supply areas for keeping sterile and nonsterile instruments and equipment
- ■ Keep area clean and _____
- ■ Keep sterile and soiled items separate

RECORDKEEPING

- ■ Records should include
  - Date and time of sterilization cycle
  - General description of contents of load
  - Exposure time and temperature
  - Name or initials of operator

- Results of sterilization indicator
- _____ date of load (usually 30 days)

CHECKPOINT QUESTION 8

What six items should be included on a sterilization record?

Answer

_____

_____

_____

_____

_____

MAINTAINING SURGICAL SUPPLIES

- ■ Keep an up-to-date _____ of all supplies including purchases and replacements
- ■ Equipment Records
  - Date of purchase
  - Model and serial number
  - Time period for recommended service
  - Date that service was requested
  - Name of individual requesting service
  - Reason for request
  - Description of services performed and parts replaced
  - Name of person performing the service and date work was completed
  - Signature and title of person who acknowledged completion of work

Chapter 24

Assisting with Minor Office Surgery

CLINICAL MEDICAL ASSISTANT RESPONSIBILITIES INCLUDE

- _____ physician's instructions to patient
- Identifying the patient and gathering proper equipment and supplies
- Obtaining and witnessing the informed consent document

CLINICAL MEDICAL ASSISTANT RESPONSIBILITIES INCLUDE (continued)

- Preparing the treatment room, instrument, supplies and equipment
- Assisting physician during _____
- Applying dressing and bandage to surgical wounds

CLINICAL MEDICAL ASSISTANT RESPONSIBILITIES INCLUDE (continued)

- Instructing patient about postoperative wound care
- Assisting patient as needed before, during, and after procedure
- Assisting with postoperative patient _____ such as prescriptions, medications, and scheduling return visits

CLINICAL MEDICAL ASSISTANT RESPONSIBILITIES INCLUDE (continued)

- Removing and caring for instruments, equipment, and supplies including properly disposing of disposable items, "sharps," and contaminated or unused supplies
- Preparing _____ for next patient

PREPARING AND MAINTAINING A STERILE FIELD

- Do not let sterile packages become damp or wet
- Always _____ a sterile field
- Hold all sterile items above waist level

PREPARING AND MAINTAINING A STERILE FIELD (continued)

- Place sterile items in middle of sterile field
- Do not spill any liquids onto sterile field
- Do not cough, sneeze, or _____ over sterile field

PREPARING AND MAINTAINING A STERILE FIELD (continued)

- Never reach over the sterile field
- Do not pass soiled supplies over sterile field
- If sterile field has been _____, alert physician

STERILE SURGICAL PACKS

- Prepackaged sterile setups
- Commercially packaged, disposable surgical packs

OPENING STERILE SURGICAL PACKS

- Open sterile items with _____
  - Unsterile area is the outside surface of outside wrapper
- Sterile area includes inside surface of outside wrapper, inside wrapper, and contents of package
  - Must not come into contact with any surface

OPENING STERILE SURGICAL PACKS

- Items are considered contaminated and should be repackaged and resterilized
  - When moisture is present
  - If items are dropped
  - If date is beyond _____ days or expiration date
  - If sterilization indicator has not changed color
  - If wrapper is torn or damaged

- When thought to have been touched by unsterile item

CHECKPOINT QUESTION 1

What are the nine guidelines that must be followed to maintain a sterile field?

Answer

_____

_____

_____

_____

_____

STERILE TRANSFER FORCEPS

- Used to _____ or to place sterile items onto sterile field
- Follow office policy and procedures regarding the guidelines for resterilizing forceps

ADDING PEEL-BACK PACKAGES AND POURING STERILE SOLUTIONS

- Additional items needed during surgery
- Commercial packages contain small or single items
- Must be opened properly
- Contents are _____

ADDING PEEL-BACK PACKAGES

- Three ways to add packages to sterile field
  1. Use sterile transfer _____
  2. Use a sterile gloved hand
  3. Flip contents onto a sterile field

POURING STERILE SOLUTIONS

- Solutions must be added as needed
- Procedures may require sterile water or antiseptic solution
- Sterile solutions are poured into sterile _____ and added to sterile field by using sterile transfer forceps

CHECKPOINT QUESTION 2

What are three ways that contents of peel-back packages can be added to the sterile field?

Answer

_____

_____

_____

_____

PREPARING THE PATIENT FOR MINOR OFFICE SURGERY

- Patient instructions and consent
- Positioning and draping
- Preparing patient's skin

PATIENT INSTRUCTIONS AND CONSENT

- Physician informs patient of details of procedure and risks
- Medical assistant
  - Gives written instruction for preparation
  - Has patient sign _____ documents
  - Answers questions
  - Encourages patient to call office

POSITIONING AND DRAPING

- Before positioning, ask patient to _____
- Offer to help patient remove necessary clothing
- Expose only the necessary area
- Provide sheets or blanket as necessary

POSITIONING

- _____ patient into comfortable position on exam table
- Provide pillows for comfort and support
- After procedure, assist patient from the table
- Offer assistance with patient's clothes

DRAPING

- Type of procedure determines type of drapes
  - Disposable paper drapes
  - Drape sheets and towels
  - _____ drapes
- Use standard precautions when removing contaminated drapes

PREPARING THE PATIENT'S SKIN

- Goal is to remove as many _____ from the skin as possible
  - Apply antiseptic solution to the area
  - Remove gross contaminants
  - Remove hair as necessary

 CHECKPOINT QUESTION 3

What is a fenestrated drape?

Answer

_____

_____

_____

_____

_____

ASSISTING THE PHYSICIAN

- Local anesthetics
- Wound closure
- Specimen collection
- Electrosurgery
- Laser surgery

LOCAL ANESTHETICS

- Commonly used in medical offices
- Two methods used
  - Draw anesthetic into _____ for physician
  - Use sterile syringe and needle included in sterile field setup
  - Show physician the label
  - Clean rubber stopper
  - Hold vial for physician

WOUND CLOSURE

- Closure ensures rapid healing with minimal scarring
- Accomplished by
  - Needles and sutures
  - Skin _____
  - Steri-Strips
- Sutures used to close wounds to bring tissue layers into close approximation

NEEDLES

- Chosen for type of surgery
- Classified by
  - _____
  - Point
  - Eye
- Know physician's preferences

SUTURES

- Come in various _____ and lengths
- Absorbable sutures are readily broken down by body processes
- Nonabsorbable sutures remain in the body permanently or are removed after healing

SKIN STAPLES

- Another form of nonabsorbable suture
- Commonly made of _____
- Must be removed when wound has healed completely

 CHECKPOINT QUESTION 4

How do swaged needles differ from threaded ones?

Answer

_____

_____

_____

_____

_____

STERI-STRIPS

- Adhesive skin closures
- Used for small wounds with little tension
- Usually left in place until they fall off
- Never pull strips away from wound

SPECIMEN COLLECTION

- Specimens include
  - Samples of tissue
  - Wound _____
  - Foreign bodies

SPECIMEN CONTAINERS

- Medical assistant must choose proper container and _____
- Have stock of containers on hand
- Hold open container steady as physician drops specimen into preservative
- Attach label to specimen container with patient's name and date

LABORATORY

- Complete laboratory request form to send with specimen
- _____ specimens to pathology laboratory as quickly as possible

ELECTROSURGERY

- Uses high-frequency, alternating electric current to destroy or cut and remove tissue
  - Fulguration
  - Electrodesiccation
  - _____
  - Electrosection

DURING ELECTROSURGERY

- Medical assistant's responsibilities
  - Ensure patient's safety and comfort
  - Pass _____ to physician as needed
  - Pass electrode in functional position

ELECTROSURGERY SAFETY MEASURES

- Ensure that all working parts are in good repair
- Ensure that all _____ is removed from patient
- Ensure that patient is grounded
- Apply conducting gel to the pad and to patient's skin

ELECTROSURGICAL MACHINES

- Periodic maintenance by office staff
- Routine inspections by trained technicians
- Keep surfaces clean and _____
- Cover machines when not in use

 CHECKPOINT QUESTION 5

Which type of electrosurgery is used for incision or excision of tissue?

Answer

_____

_____

_____

_____

_____

LASER SURGERY

- Lasers are devices that focus high intensity _____ in a narrow beam to create extreme heat and energy
- Common types of lasers
  - Argon laser
  - Carbon dioxide laser
  - Nd:YAG

LASER SURGERY PROCEDURES

- Complete training program before assisting
- Everyone in room required to wear _____
- Follow recommended maintenance procedures

CHECKPOINT QUESTION 6

What is one important safety feature worth noting when assisting with a laser procedure?

Answer

_____

_____

_____

_____

_____

POSTSURGICAL PROCEDURES

- Applying and removing _____ dressing
- Cleaning exam table and operative area

STERILE DRESSINGS

- Handle using sterile techniques
- Considered contaminated if damp, if wrapper is _____, or if removed improperly from wrapper

USES FOR STERILE DRESSINGS

- Used directly over a wound to
  - Cover and protect from contamination
  - _____ drainage
  - Exert pressure to control bleeding
  - Hide disfigurement
  - Hold medications against a wound

REMOVING STERILE DRESSINGS

- Always wear clean _____
- Carefully observe for any drainage or exudates
- Note this in patient's chart

CHECKPOINT QUESTION 7

What is the difference between a dressing and a bandage?

Answer

_____

_____

_____

_____

_____

CLEANING THE EXAMINATION TABLE AND OPERATIVE AREA

- Sanitize/sterilize used equipment
- Discard used disposable equipment
- Clean examination room
- Remove papers and sheets and discard appropriately
- Applying gloves; wipe down all surfaces with approved _____
- Replace table sheet paper

COMMONLY PERFORMED OFFICE SURGICAL PROCEDURES

- Excision of a skin _____
- Incision and drainage of abscesses

EXCISION OF A LESION

- May be performed by
  - Electrocautery
  - Lasers
  - _____
  - Standard surgical equipment

INCISION AND DRAINAGE

- Abscess
  - Localized collection of _____ in a cavity surrounded by inflamed tissue
  - Site is incised
  - Infected material drains away

ASSISTING WITH SUTURE AND STAPLE REMOVAL

- Inform patients that they might feel a _____ sensation
- Cleanse area with antiseptic solution
- Using sterile gloves or sterile transfer forceps, clean area in a circular motion
- Discard wipe after each sweep
- Use sterile suture or staple remover kit

Chapter 25

Pharmacology

INTRODUCTION

- Pharmacology is the study of _____, their actions, dosages, side effects
- Clinical medical assistants administer medications under supervision of physician

MEDICATION NAMES

- _____ name
- Generic name
- Trade name

 CHECKPOINT QUESTION 1

What is the difference between a drug's chemical name and trade name?

Answer

_____

_____

_____

_____

_____

LEGAL REGULATIONS

- Consumers in the United States are protected by several federal regulations regarding the production, prescribing, or _____ of medications

FOOD AND DRUG ADMINISTRATION (FDA)

- Established to regulate the manufacture and _____ of drugs and food products and to ensure accuracy in the ingredients listed on the labels of food and drug products

DRUG ENFORCEMENT AGENCY

- Controlled Substances Act
  - Regulates the manufacture and distribution of drugs whose use may result in dependency or _____
- Bureau of Narcotics and Dangerous Drugs (BNDD)
  - Registers those who manufacture, prescribe, administer or dispense controlled substances

REGISTRATION WITH DRUG ENFORCEMENT AGENCY

- Physician must register with the DEA
- As medical assistant, you may be responsible for maintaining or reminding physician about professional records and _____ including registration with DEA

SCHEDULE OF CONTROLLED SUBSTANCES

- DEA responsible for revising list of drugs included in Schedule of Controlled Substances
- List includes drugs identified as having potential for abuse and _____
  - Drug dependence
  - Psychological, physical, or both
- Patients must be monitored for signs of dependency

CONTROLLED SUBSTANCES INVENTORY

- List controlled substances on a special _____ form in office
- Record every time a controlled substance leaves the medical office
- Inventory forms must be kept for 2 years

SECURING CONTROLLED SUBSTANCES

- Controlled substances must be _____ in a safe or in a secure box
- Number of persons with access to keys should be limited
- If drugs are lost or stolen, local law enforcement agency must be notified immediately

CHECKPOINT QUESTION 2

What information needs to be documented when a controlled substance is administered in the medical office?

Answer

_____

_____

_____

_____

_____

SOURCES OF DRUGS

- ■ Plants
- ■ Minerals
- ■ Animals
- ■ _____

DRUG ACTIONS AND INTERACTIONS

- ■ Pharmacodynamics
- ■ _____
- ■ Drug interactions
- ■ Side effects and allergies

PHARMACODYNAMICS

- ■ Study of how drugs act within the body including actions on specific cells, tissues, or organs
- ■ All drugs cause cellular change and some degree of physiologic change
  - • Local effect
  - • _____ effect

PHARMACOKINETICS

- ■ Study of the action of drugs within the body based on
  - • Route of administration
  - • Rate of absorption
  - • _____
  - • Elimination of drug from the body

PROCESS OF PHARMACOKINESIS

- ■ Absorption
- ■ Distribution
- ■ _____
- ■ Excretion

DRUG INTERACTIONS

- ■ When two or more drugs are taken simultaneously, one drug may increase, decrease, or _____ the effects of the other
  - • Prescribed drugs
  - • OTC drugs
  - • Herbal or natural supplements
  - • Alcohol

TYPES OF INTERACTIONS

- ■ _____
- ■ Antagonism
- ■ Potentiation
- ■ Physicians prescribing two or more drugs may be using interactions to cause a desired effect

SIDE EFFECTS AND ALLERGIES

- ■ When taking medical history, always ask about _____ to medications and note prominently on medical record

DRUG ALLERGIES

- ■ Reactions such as hives, dyspnea, or wheezing after receiving a medication
- ■ May be immediate or delayed up to 2 hours or longer
- ■ _____
  - • Life threatening allergic reaction

SIDE EFFECTS

- ■ Reactions to medications that are predictable
  - • Noted by the _____
  - • May occur in some patients who take the medication

CHECKPOINT QUESTION 3

How does synergism differ from antagonism?

Answer

_____

_____

_____

_____

_____

SOURCES OF INFORMATION

- *Physician's Desk Reference*
  (_____)
- *United States Pharmacopeia Dispensing Information (USPDI)*
- *American Hospital Formulary Service (AHFS)*
- *Compendium of Drug Therapy*

PRESCRIPTIONS

- Medications may be
  - Administered

Chapter 26

Preparing and Administering Medications

MEDICATION ADMINISTRATION BASICS

- As a clinical medical assistant
  - Be familiar with medications ordered by physician and procedures necessary to administer them
  - Look up any drugs you are not familiar with
- Be familiar with
  - _____
  - Abbreviations
  - Symbols and sign

- Dispensed
- Prescribed
- Medical assistant may be permitted to complete _____ and obtain physician's signature
- All medications must be documented in medical record

CHECKPOINT QUESTION 4

What does the superscription on the prescription indicate and how does this differ from the subscription?

Answer

_____

_____

_____

_____

SAFETY GUIDELINES

- To ensure safety, follow these guidelines
  - Know the policies of your office
  - Give only medications ordered in _____
  - Check with the physician if you have doubts

SAFETY GUIDELINES *(continued)*

- Avoid distractions while preparing and administering medications
- Work in a quiet, well-lit area
- Check the _____ when taking medication from shelf, when preparing it, and when replacing it on shelf

SAFETY GUIDELINES *(continued)*

- Place the order and the medication side by side to compare for accuracy

- Check the _____ of medication and routes for administration
- Read labels carefully
- Check patient's medical record for allergies
- Check medication's expiration date

SAFETY GUIDELINES *(continued)*

- Be alert for indications that medication's properties have changed
- _____ exactly
- Have sharps containers as close as possible

SAFETY GUIDELINES *(continued)*

- Put on gloves for all procedures that might result in contact with blood or body fluids
- Stay with the patient while oral medication is being taken
- Never return a medication to the container after it is poured or removed
- Never recap, bend, or break a used _____

SAFETY GUIDELINES *(continued)*

- Never give a medication poured or drawn up by someone else
- Never leave the medication cabinet _____ when not in use
- Never give keys for the medication cabinet to an unauthorized person

CHECKPOINT QUESTION 1

When are the "three checks" for safe medication administration performed?

Answer

_____

_____

_____

_____

_____

SEVEN RIGHTS FOR CORRECT MEDICATION ADMINISTRATION

- Right _____

- Right time
- Right dose
- Right _____
- Right drug
- Right technique
- Right _____

SYSTEMS OF MEASUREMENT

- Most common system used is _____ system
- Apothecary system still used by some physicians
- Household system is sometimes used by patients

METRIC SYSTEM

- Based on multiples of ten
- _____ used; not fractions
- Base unit of length is the meter (m)
- Base unit of weight is the gram (g or gm)
- Base unit of volume is the liter (L or l)

PREFIXES

- Micro (0.000001)
- Milli (0.001)
- _____ (0.01)
- Deci (0.1)
- Kilo (1000.0)

APOTHECARY SYSTEM

- Liquid measurements include
  - Drop (gt)
  - Drops (gtt)
  - Minim (min, m)
  - Fluid dram (fl dr)
  - _____ (fl oz)
  - Pint (pt)
  - Quart (qt)
  - Gallon (gal)

APOTHECARY SYSTEM *(continued)*

- Solid measurements include
  - Grain (gr)
  - _____ (dr)
  - Ounce (oz)
  - Pound (lb)

HOUSEHOLD SYSTEM

- _____ (tsp)
- Tablespoon (Tbsp)
- Ounce (oz)
- Cup (c)
- Pint (pt)
- Quart (qt)
- Pound (lb)

 CHECKPOINT QUESTION 2

What are three systems of measurement and which one should be avoided? Why?

Answer

_____

_____

_____

_____

_____

CONVERTING BETWEEN SYSTEMS OF MEASUREMENT

- While working in clinical setting, medical assistants may find it necessary to _____ from one system to another

APOTHECARY OR HOUSEHOLD TO METRIC

- To change
  - Grains to grams, divide number of grains ordered by _____
  - Grains to milligrams, multiply grains by _____
  - Ounces to cubic centimeters or millimeters, multiply ounces by _____

APOTHECARY OR HOUSEHOLD TO METRIC *(continued)*

- To change
  - Cubic centimeters (or mL) to fluid ounces, divide the cc (or mL) by _____

- Kilograms to pounds, multiply kilograms by _____
- Pounds to kilograms, divide the pounds by _____

METRIC TO METRIC

- To change
  - Grams to milligrams, _____ grams by 1000 or move the decimal point three places to the right
  - Milligrams to grams, _____ the milligrams by 1000 or move the decimal point three places to the left
  - Milligrams to micrograms, _____ the milligrams by 1000 or move the decimal three places to the right

METRIC TO METRIC *(continued)*

- To change
  - Micrograms to milligrams, _____ the micrograms by 1000 or move the decimal three places to the left
  - Liters to milliliters, _____ the liters by 1000 or move the decimal three places to the right
  - Milliliters to liters, _____ the milliliters by 1000 or move the decimal three places to the left

CALCULATING ADULT DOSAGES

- Administration of medication is an exact science
- Errors in calculations could prove fatal
- Dosages are most frequently calculated for adults by
  - _____ method
  - Formula method
- Measurements must be in the same system and same unit of measurement before calculation can be made

RATIO AND PROPORTION

- Ratio method to calculate dosages
  - Use amount of medication ordered and information on medication label to create a ratio
  - Once ratio has been determined, the _____ can be calculated
  - Dose on hand:Known quantity = Dose desired:Unknown quantity

FORMULA METHOD

- Formula method is written as
  (Desired ÷ On hand) × _____

CHECKPOINT QUESTION 3

Before calculating dosages, what must be done with the measurements?

Answer

_____

_____

_____

_____

_____

CALCULATING PEDIATRIC DOSAGES

- Calculating dosage by _____ (BSA) using chart
- Young's rule
- Clark's rule
- Fried's rule

CHECKPOINT QUESTION 4

What is the most accurate method used to calculate a pediatric dosage?

Answer

_____

_____

_____

_____

_____

ROUTES OF MEDICATION ADMINISTRATION

- Physician chooses after considering many factors
  - Cost
  - Safety

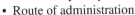

- _____ by which drug will be absorbed by body
- Route of administration

ORAL, SUBLINGUAL, AND BUCCAL ROUTES

- Oral
  - Tablets, capsules, pills, liquids taken by _____
  - Usually absorbed through walls of the gastrointestinal tract
- Sublingual
  - Placed under the _____; must not be swallowed
  - Absorbed directly into bloodstream

ORAL, SUBLINGUAL, AND BUCCAL ROUTES *(continued)*

- Buccal
  - Placed in the _____ between cheek and gum
  - Absorption through vascular oral mucosa

CHECKPOINT QUESTION 5

What are the disadvantages of the oral route for medication administration?

Answer

_____

_____

_____

_____

_____

PARENTERAL ADMINISTRATION

- Administration by _____ used
  - If patient cannot take medications orally
  - If drug cannot be absorbed through gastrointestinal system
  - For more rapid absorption of drug
- Medication cannot be retrieved once injected
- Possible for infections to develop

EQUIPMENT FOR INJECTIONS

- Ampules, vials, cartridges
- Needles and syringes

AMPULES

- Small _____ containers
- Break at the neck
- Aspirate solution into syringe
- Once open, all medication must be used or discarded

VIALS

- Glass or plastic container sealed with
  _____
- Single dose or multiple dose
- May hold solution or powder
- Powders must be reconstituted

CARTRIDGES

- Prefilled syringes contain premeasured medication in _____ cartridge with needle attached
- Placed in a holder for administration
- After use, discard cartridge into sharps biohazard container

NEEDLES AND SYRINGE

- Variety used for injections
  - Type of injection
  - Size of _____

SYRINGES

- 3 mL hypodermic syringe is most common
- 5 or 10 mL usually used for _____ only
- All consist of plunger, body or barrel, flange, and tip

NEEDLES

- Lengths vary from 3/8 inch to 1 1/2 inch
- _____ varies from 18 to 30

- Choose needle appropriate for route of injection
- Insulin syringe used strictly for administering subcutaneously to diabetic patients

 CHECKPOINT QUESTION 6

What are ampules and vials and how do they differ?

Answer

_____

_____

_____

_____

_____

TYPES OF INJECTIONS

- Intradermal
- Subcutaneous
- _____
- Z-track method

 CHECKPOINT QUESTION 7

Name the types of injections and the possible sites for each type.

Answer

_____

_____

_____

_____

_____

OTHER MEDICATION ROUTES

- Rectal
- Vaginal
- _____
- Inhalation
- Intravenous

Chapter 27
Diagnostic Imaging

PRINCIPLES OF RADIOLOGY

- Commonly used diagnostic and therapeutic procedures
  - X-ray imaging
  - Computed tomography scans
  - _____
  - Magnetic resonance imaging
  - Nuclear medicine

X-RAYS

- High-energy waves that cannot be seen, heard, felt, tasted, or smelled
- Have the ability to _____ the human body
- Penetrating waves create two-dimensional shadowlike images on film

X-RAYS MACHINES

- Sophisticated and technologically advanced
- Many work with computers to produce digital images
- _____ units are capable of visualizing motion with body

OUTPATIENT X-RAYS

- Some medical offices have on-site x-ray equipment
- Medical assistant may be permitted to take and process simple _____

 CHECKPOINT QUESTION I

What are x-rays?

Answer

_____

_____

_____

_____

_____

PATIENT POSITIONING

- X-ray examinations usually require a minimum of _____ exposures taken at 90° to each other
- These angles are basis for standard positioning

EXAMINATION SEQUENCING

- Most radiographic procedures can be performed in any order
- Certain procedures must follow specific sequences
  - Patients with _____ symptoms
  - Barium studies

 CHECKPOINT QUESTION 2

Why is it important to schedule a barium enema before an upper GI or barium swallow?

Answer

_____

_____

_____

_____

_____

RADIATION SAFETY

- X-rays have potential to cause cellular or genetic damage
- At highest risk
  - _____ women
  - Children
  - Reproductive organs of adults

RADIATION SAFETY PROCEDURES FOR PATIENTS

- Reduce exposure amounts as much as possible
- Avoid unnecessary examinations
- Limit area of body exposed
- _____ sensitive body parts
- Evaluate potential pregnancy status

RADIATION SAFETY PROCEDURES FOR CLINICAL STAFF

- Limit amount of time exposed to x-rays
- Stay far away from x-rays
- Use available _____
- Avoid holding patients during exposure
- Wear individual dosimeters
- Ensure proper working condition of equipment

DIAGNOSTIC PROCEDURES

- Routine radiographic examinations
- Named for part of body involved
- Performed for viewing _____ structure or abnormalities

MAMMOGRAPHY

- Specialized x-ray examination of the _____
- Screening tool for breast cancer
- Breast compressed in specialized device
- Has become vital adjunct to biopsy procedures

CONTRAST MEDIA EXAMINATIONS

- Radiographic contrast media helps differentiate between body structures
- Used to evaluate structure and _____

CONTRAST MEDIA

- Introduced into body in several ways
  - _____
  - Intravenously
  - Through a catheter
- Medical assistant must ensure that patients understand preparation instructions

 CHECKPOINT QUESTION 3

How do contrast media help in differentiating between body structures?

Answer

_____

_____

_____

_____

_____

FLUOROSCOPY

- Use x-rays to observe _____ within the body
  - Barium sulfate through the digestive tract
  - Iodinated compounds showing the beating of the heart

COMPUTED TOMOGRAPHY (CT, CAT SCAN)

- Tomography
  - X-ray tube and film move in relation to one another, blurring all structures except those in focal plane.
- CT uses x-rays from a tube circling the patient, analyzed by computers to create _____ images

SONOGRAPHY (ULTRASOUND)

- High-frequency _____ waves, not x-rays, create cross-sectional still or real-time images
- Used to demonstrate heart function or abdominal or pelvic structures
- Used in prenatal testing to visualize developing fetus

MAGNETIC RESONANCE IMAGING (MRI)

- Combination of high-intensity _____ fields, radio waves, and computer analysis creates cross-sectional images
- Used to study central nervous system, joint structure
- Patient must be prepared for lengthy procedure in enclosed machine

 CHECKPOINT QUESTION 4

How does fluoroscopy differ from computed tomography and sonography?

Answer

_____

_____

_____

_____

_____

INTERVENTIONAL RADIOLOGIC PROCEDURES

- Designed to treat specific disease conditions
  - Percutaneous transluminal coronary angioplasty
  - Laser angioplasties
  - Vascular _____
  - Embolizations

CHECKPOINT QUESTION 5

How could PTCA be a life-saving measure?

Answer

_____

_____

_____

_____

_____

RADIATION THERAPY

- High-energy radiation is used to destroy _____ cells
- Treatments must be planned carefully by radiologist
- Most patients have some side effects

THE MEDICAL ASSISTANT'S ROLE IN RADIOLOGIC PROCEDURES

- Help alleviate _____ patients feel
- Give patients information about examinations
- Make patients feel comfortable enough to ask questions
- Answer questions in terms patient can understand

PATIENT EDUCATION

- Explain what to expect in simple language, not technical medical terms
- Explain preparations for examinations
- Explain what to do _____ procedure

ASSISTING WITH EXAMINATIONS

- Give patient _____ for what clothing to remove
- Assist with clothing removal
- Help position patient for the procedure
- Perform specific procedures
- Place film into automatic processor
- Reload new film
- Distribute radiographs and report

HANDLING AND STORING RADIOGRAPHIC FILMS

- Unexposed film must be protected from moisture, heat, and light
- Store in a cool, dry place, preferably a lead-lined box
- Film packets must be opened in a _____
- Place film in cassette for use outside of darkroom

CHECKPOINT QUESTION 6

How can the medical assistant help with radiologic examinations?

Answer

_____

_____

_____

_____

_____

TRANSFER OF RADIOGRAPHIC INFORMATION

- Radiographic images remain part of permanent record

- Digital images saved on disk
- X-ray films belong to site where study was performed
- Examining physician or radiologist writes summary of the examination
- Medical assistant obtains patient's _____ to have summary sent to office physician

TELERADIOLOGY

- Use of computed imaging and information systems
- Provides new benefits in medicine
- Digital _____ can be transmitted via telephone lines to distant locations
- Allows for consultation with experts on difficult cases

Chapter 28

Medical Office Emergencies

- Location of nearest hospital emergency department
- Telephone number of poison control center
- Procedures for emergency situations
- List of personnel trained in _____
- Emergency medical kit

EMERGENCY MEDICAL KIT

- Proper equipment and supplies should be readily available
- Keep in designated location
- _____ contents periodically

MEDICAL OFFICE EMERGENCY PROCEDURES

- Immediate care given to sick or _____ persons
- When properly performed, it can mean
  - Difference between life and death, rapid recovery and long hospitalization
  - Or temporary disability and permanent disability

THE EMERGENCY MEDICAL SERVICES (EMS) SYSTEM

- In medical office, notify EMS for
  - Heart attack
  - Shock
  - Severe _____ difficulties
- Provide immediate care to patient
- Direct other staff to notify physician

MEDICAL OFFICE EMERGENCY PROCEDURES (continued)

- Involves
  - _____ emergency
  - Performing basic first aid measures
  - Furnishing temporary assistance or basic life support until advanced life support can be obtained
- Effective January 1, 2005
  - American Association of Medical Assistants will require certified medical assistants to demonstrate proof of current CPR certification for recertification

THE EMERGENCY MEDICAL SERVICES SYSTEM (continued)

- Give EMS personnel
  - Patient symptoms
  - Nature of emergency
  - _____ treatment

THE EMERGENCY MEDICAL SERVICES SYSTEM (continued)

- Document emergency situations
  1. Basic patient identification
  2. Chief complaint if known
  3. Times of events
  4. _____ signs

EMERGENCY ACTION PLAN

- Local emergency telephone number (usually 911)

5. Specific emergency management techniques
6. Observations of patient's condition
7. Past medical history

CHECKPOINT QUESTION 1

List the items you should attempt to document before the ambulance arrives in an emergency situation?

Answer

_____

_____

_____

_____

_____

PATIENT ASSESSMENT

■ Two primary objectives
  1. Identify and correct any _____ problems
  2. Provide necessary care
■ Each step must be managed effectively before proceeding to the next
■ Survey scene quickly to identify potential hazards or clues to patient's medical illness

RECOGNIZING THE EMERGENCY

■ Do not assume that the obvious injuries are the only ones present
■ Less noticeable or _____ injuries may also have occurred during an accident
■ Look for causes of injury

THE PRIMARY ASSESSMENT

■ Quickly assess
  • Responsiveness
  • Airway
  • Breathing
  • _____

CHECKPOINT QUESTION 2

What is the purpose of the primary assessment?

Answer

_____

_____

_____

_____

_____

THE SECONDARY ASSESSMENT

■ Ask the patient questions to obtain additional information
■ Perform more thorough physical evaluation
  1. General appearance
  2. Level of _____ (AVPU system)
  3. Vital signs
  4. Skin

THE PHYSICAL EXAMINATION

■ Performed after completing primary and secondary surveys
■ _____ survey
■ Physician performs this examination

HEAD AND NECK

■ If a cervical spine injury is suspected, immobilize spine immediately
■ Inspect face for
  • _____
  • Bruising
  • Bleeding
  • Drainage from nose or ears
■ Examine mouth
■ Check pupils

CHEST AND BACK

■ Evaluate anterior chest _____ status
■ Thoroughly evaluate patients with cardiac or respiratory complaints
■ Palpate chest and back to reveal areas that indicate rib fractures

ABDOMEN

■ Evaluate on all patients, but particularly those with
  • Gastrointestinal symptoms
  • Suspicion of blood or fluid loss

- Inspect abdomen for
  - Scars
  - Bruises
  - Masses
- _____ abdomen may indicate hemorrhage with abdominal cavity

ARMS AND LEGS

- Last step of head-to-toe survey
- Inspect for
  - Swelling
  - Deformity
  - _____
- Note any tremors in hands

ARMS AND LEGS (continued)

- Determine neurologic status of
  - _____
  - Movement
  - Range of motion
  - Sensation
- Determine muscle strength in upper extremities
- Assess sensation

CHECKPOINT QUESTION 3

What are the diagnostic signs that are evaluated in the secondary assessment?

Answer

_____

_____

_____

_____

_____

TYPE OF EMERGENCIES

- Shock
- Bleeding
- Burns
- Musculoskeletal injuries
- Cardiovascular emergencies
- Neurologic emergencies

- Allergic and anaphylactic reactions
- _____
- Heat and cold related emergencies
- Behavioral and psychiatric emergencies

SHOCK

- Lack of oxygen to cells of the body, including the brain cells, due to decrease in blood pressure
  - Hypovolemic shock
  - Cardiogenic shock
  - Neurogenic shock
  - Anaphylactic shock
  - _____ shock

MANAGEMENT OF THE PATIENT IN SHOCK

- Observe and maintain open airway and adequate breathing
- Control bleeding
- Administer _____
- Immobilize patient if spinal injuries may be present

MANAGEMENT OF THE PATIENT IN SHOCK (continued)

- Splint fractures
- Prevent loss of _____
- Assist physician with starting intravenous line
- Elevate feet and legs
- Transport to closest hospital

CHECKPOINT QUESTION 4

What does the term shock mean?

Answer

_____

_____

_____

_____

_____

BLEEDING

- Closed wound
  - Skin is not broken
  - Apply _____ to reduce and prevent swelling
- Open wound
  - Skin is broken
  - Follow standard precautions

MANAGEMENT OF BLEEDING AND SOFT-TISSUE INJURIES

- Control bleeding by applying direct _____
- Elevate the wound above the level of the heart
- Cover wound with sterile gauze
- Preserve severed parts
- Immobilize—do not remove—impaled objects

BURNS

- Four major sources of burn injury
  1. Thermal
  2. Electrical
  3. Chemical
  4. _____

CLASSIFICATION OF BURN INJURIES

- Superficial
- Partial-thickness
- _____ thickness

CALCULATION OF BODY SURFACE AREA

- Most commonly estimated by rule of _____
- Calculates percentage of total body surface of individual sections of body

MANAGEMENT OF THE BURN VICTIM

- Eliminate source of burn
- Notify physician and call EMS
- Assess patient's airway, breathing, circulation; begin _____
- Remove jewelry and clothing
- Wrap patient in clean, dry sheet

- Administer oxygen
- Treat for shock
- Transport to hospital

 CHECKPOINT QUESTION 5

What are the four major sources of burn injuries?

Answer

_____

_____

_____

_____

_____

MUSCULOSKELETAL INJURIES

- Injuries to muscles, bones, and joints are common problems
- Muscles, tendons, and ligaments torn or _____
- Fractures and dislocations associated with external forces

MANAGEMENT OF MUSCULOSKELETAL INJURIES

- Difficult to distinguish between strains, sprains, fractures, and dislocations
- Assume a fracture and _____ with a splint
- Apply ice to reduce swelling

TYPES OF SPLINTS

- Commercially available splints
  - Traction
  - Air
  - Wire ladder
  - Padded board
- Examine extremity for impaired _____
  - Observe skin color
  - Locate a pulse in artery distal to affected extremity
  - Watch for increased swelling
- If circulation becomes impaired, remove or loosen splint

CARDIOVASCULAR EMERGENCIES

- Early symptoms of _____
  - Chest pain not relieved by rest
  - Complaint of pressure in chest or upper back
  - Nausea or indigestion
  - Chest pain that radiates up into neck and jaw or down one arm
  - Anxiety

CARDIOVASCULAR EMERGENCIES
(continued)

- Early treatment includes
  - Basic life support
  - Early _____
  - Advanced life support
- Patient's survival chances improved if
  - Cardiopulmonary resuscitation initiated promptly
  - Patient is rapidly and successfully defibrillated

NEUROLOGIC EMERGENCIES

- _____ caused by abnormal discharge of electrical activity in brain
  - Erratic muscle movements
  - Strange sensations
  - Complete loss of consciousness
- Thorough patient history is important

MANAGEMENT OF SEIZURE PATIENT

- Assess patient's _____, airway, breathing, and circulation
- Do not force objects between teeth
- Clear and maintain airway
- Assist patient into recovery position
- Protect patient from injury
- Protect neck and cervical spine in necessary

ALLERGIC AND ANAPHYLACTIC REACTIONS

- Anaphylaxis
  - _____ allergic reaction
  - Generalized reaction
  - Can occur within minutes to hours after exposure to allergen

COMMON ALLERGENS

- Includes drugs, insect venom, food, and pollen
- Ask every patient about allergies at every visit
- 1%–2% who receive _____ have allergic reaction
- 1 in 50,000 injections of penicillin results in death due to anaphylaxis

SIGNS AND SYMPTOMS

- Severe itching
- Feeling of warmth
- _____ in throat or chest
- Rash
- Signs of shock

MANAGEMENT OF ALLERGIC AND ANAPHYLACTIC REACTIONS

- Mild reactions
  - Administer oxygen or medications
- Respiratory involvement
  - Physician may order _____
- Severe reaction
  - More aggressive therapy
  - Intravenous line
  - Monitor cardiac rhythm
  - Restore respiratory and circulatory function

MANAGEMENT OF ALLERGIC AND ANAPHYLACTIC REACTIONS
(continued)

- Do not leave patient
- Assist patient to _____ position
- Assess patient's respiratory and circulatory status
- Observe skin color and warmth
- Cover with blanket
- Start intravenous line and administer oxygen
- Document vital signs, medications, treatments
- Communication relevant information to EMS

 CHECKPOINT QUESTION 6

What is the primary cause of death in anaphylaxis?

Answer

_____

_____

_____

_____

_____

POISONING

- Most toxic exposures occur in the _____
- Almost 50% occur in children between the ages of 1 and 3
- 90% of all reported poisonings are accidental

POISON CONTROL CENTER

- American Association of Poison Control Centers (_____) has established standards and regional poison control centers throughout the country
- Valuable resource
- Post phone number near all phones

MANAGEMENT OF POISONING EMERGENCIES

- Few toxic substances have specific _____
- Treat signs and symptoms
- Assess organ systems involved
- Obtain patient information *before* calling poison control
- Never give syrup of ipecac unless directed by the poison control center

HEAT AND COLD RELATED EMERGENCIES

- Human beings control core body temperature within a range of several degrees
- Severe conditions can disrupt normal _____ mechanisms of body
  - Hyperthermia
  - Hypothermia

HYPERTHERMIA

- General condition of _____ body heat
- Heat cramps
- Signal need for cooling and rest
- Heat exhaustion
- Heat stroke
  - True emergency

- May result in brain damage or death
- Requires rapid cooling of the body

HYPOTHERMIA

- Abnormally low body temperature
- Signs and symptoms
  - Cool, pale skin
  - Lethargy and _____
  - Shallow and slow respirations
  - Slow, faint pulse rate

BASIC MANAGEMENT OF HYPOTHERMIA

- Handle patient _____
- Remove wet clothing
- Cover patient
- Give warm oral fluids
- Avoid caffeine and alcohol

FROSTBITE

- Exposure to cold can cause tissues to freeze, resulting in _____
- Fingers, toes, ears, and nose most vulnerable

SUPERFICIAL FROSTBITE

- Firm and _____ gray or yellow skin
- Skin loses sensation after hurting or tingling
- Warm affected part with another body part

DEEP FROSTBITE

- Most often afflicts hands and feet
- Skin becomes _____ and entire area feels hard to the touch
- Must be managed in hospital
- Notify EMS

BEHAVIORAL AND PSYCHIATRIC EMERGENCIES

- _____, disturbed moods, thoughts, or actions
- Guidelines for handling
  - Notify physician and EMS as directed
  - Offer reassurance and general support to patient and others present
  - Document information including vital signs and patient behavior

Chapter 29

Dermatology

COMMON DISORDERS OF THE INTEGUMENTARY SYSTEM

- _____ (integument) largest organ of body
- Clear skin indicates general state of wellness
- Pallor, cyanosis, or dry scale-like skin indicates poor general health

COMMON DISORDERS OF THE INTEGUMENTARY SYSTEM *(continued)*

- Skin has many functions
  - Maintains _____
  - Protects underlying tissues and organs
  - Protects body from mechanical injury, damaging substances, and ultraviolet rays of sun
- Unbroken skin prevents entrance of microorganisms

 CHECKPOINT QUESTION I

How does the integument help to prevent infection?

Answer

_____

_____

_____

_____

_____

SKIN INFECTIONS

- Many integumentary disorders manifested by _____ or abnormalities in skin tissue
- Lesions may be primary or secondary resulting from primary lesions
- Medical assistant should always wear protective equipment

BACTERIAL INFECTIONS

- _____
- Folliculitis
- Furuncle
- _____
- Cellulitis

 CHECKPOINT QUESTION 2

Which three bacterial infections develop in the hair follicles? Briefly describe each.

Answer

_____

_____

_____

_____

_____

VIRAL SKIN INFECTIONS

- Herpes _____
- Herpes _____
- Verruca

 CHECKPOINT QUESTION 3

Which viral skin infection is linked to a common childhood disorder? Explain.

Answer

_____

_____

_____

_____

_____

FUNGAL SKIN INFECTIONS

- Tinea capitas
- Tinea _____
- Tinea cruris
- Tinea pedis
- Tinea ungulum
- Tinea _____

CHECKPOINT QUESTION 4

What is the difference between tinea capitas and tinea pedis?

Answer

_____

_____

_____

_____

_____

PARASITIC SKIN INFECTIONS

- _____
- Pediculosis

INFLAMMATORY REACTIONS

- _____
- Seborrheic dermatitis
- Urticaria
- _____
- Psoriasis

CHECKPOINT QUESTION 5

What is urticaria and which layer of the skin does it affect?

Answer

_____

_____

_____

_____

_____

DISORDERS OF WOUND HEALING

- _____ an overproduction of scar tissue
- Complication of wound healing

DISORDERS CAUSED BY PRESSURE

- Callus and corn
- Decubitus _____
- Intertrigo

ALOPECIA

- _____ may occur from
  - Physical trauma
  - Systemic diseases
  - Bacteria or fungal infections
  - Chemotherapy
  - Excessive radiation
  - Hormonal imbalances
  - Genetic predisposition
  - Cannot be reversed

DISORDERS OF PIGMENTATION

- _____
- Vitiligo
- Leukoderma
- Nevus

CHECKPOINT QUESTION 6

What are four disorders of pigmentation? Briefly describe.

Answer

_____

_____

_____

_____

_____

SKIN CANCERS

- _____ cell carcinoma
- _____ cell carcinoma
- Malignant melanoma

CHECKPOINT QUESTION 7

Which is more likely to metastasize—basal cell or squamous cell carcinoma?

Answer

_____

_____

_____

_____

_____

DIAGNOSTIC PROCEDURES

- Physical examination of the skin
- Wound _____
- Skin biopsy
- Urine melanin
- Wood's light analysis

PHYSICAL EXAMINATION OF THE SKIN

- Performed mostly by inspection
- Many lesions can be diagnosed by
  - Characteristic size
  - Shape
  - _____ on skin
- Laboratory studies may be necessary to confirm diagnosis

PHYSICAL EXAMINATION OF THE SKIN *(continued)*

- Before the exam, medical assistant will
  - Assemble the equipment
  - Verify informed _____
  - Direct specimens to laboratory
  - Observe standard precautions

PHYSICAL EXAMINATION OF THE SKIN *(continued)*

- During the exam, medical assistant will
  - Ensure adequate _____
  - Assist in obtaining wound cultures
  - Maintain _____
  - Apply topical medications, sterile dressings, and bandages

PHYSICAL EXAMINATION OF THE SKIN *(continued)*

- After exam, medical assistant will instruct patient about caring for skin condition at home
  - Keeping bandages clean and dry
  - Returning to office to have sutures removed
  - How long to avoid getting area wet
  - Applying _____ medications

WOUND CULTURES

- Consist of
  - Obtaining sample of wound exudate
  - Applying specimen to growth _____
  - Allowing microorganisms to grow
- Sample of propagated culture
  - Placed on in laboratory
  - Observed under microscope to diagnose bacterial or fungal infections

OBTAINING WOUND CULTURES

- Wash hands and put on gloves
- Remove and dispose of dressings
- Assess wound for signs of _____
- Obtain a wound collection device

OBTAINING WOUND CULTURES *(continued)*

- Open and prepare the sterile culture tube
- Clean the wound, apply sterile _____
- Remove gloves, wash hands, document procedure

SKIN BIOPSY

- Three types performed by the physician
  - _____ method
  - Punch method
  - Shave biopsy method

URINE MELANIN

- Melanin is not normally present in urine unless patient has malignant melanoma
  - Urine test
  - Specimen sent to laboratory
  - Allowed to sit for 24 hours
  - Examined under microscope for presence of _____

WOOD'S LIGHT ANALYSIS

- _____ light used to detect fungal and bacterial infections, scabies, alterations in pigment
  - Abnormalities appear as fluorescent colors
  - Can be diagnosed by physician and treated accordingly

 CHECKPOINT QUESTION 8

Why is a skin biopsy performed?

Answer

_____

_____

_____

_____

BANDAGING

- Bandages used for many purposes
  - Applying pressure to control bleeding
  - Holding a dressing in place
  - Protecting dressings and wounds from _____
  - Immobilizing an injured body part
  - Supporting an injured body part

Chapter 30

Orthopedics

THE MUSCULOSKELETAL SYSTEM AND COMMON DISORDERS

- Muscles allow movement of body parts through _____ and _____
- Bones support body and act in response to contractions and relaxations
- Joints hold two or more bones together

TYPES OF BANDAGES

- Roller bandages
- _____ bandages
- Tubular gauze bandages

BANDAGE APPLICATION GUIDELINES

- Properly applied, bandages should
  - Feel comfortably _____
  - Be fastened securely enough to remain in place until removed

BANDAGE APPLICATION GUIDELINES *(continued)*

- Observe principles of medical asepsis
- Keep area and bandage dry and clean
- Never place bandages directly over _____
- Never allow skin surfaces of two body parts to touch each other within a bandage

BANDAGE APPLICATION GUIDELINES *(continued)*

- Pad joints and any bony prominences
- Bandage affected part in normal position
- Apply bandages beginning at _____ part and extending to _____ part of body
- Talk with patient during bandaging
- When bandaging hands and feet, leave fingers and toes exposed whenever possible

MOST COMMON DISORDERS

- _____
- Dislocations
- Fractures
- Joint disruptions
- _____

REACTIONS TO COMMON DISORDERS *(continued)*

- Pain
- _____
- Inflammation
- Deformity
- Limitation of range and function

SPRAINS AND STRAINS

- ■ _____ is injury to a joint capsule and its supporting ligaments
- ■ _____ is injury to a muscle and its supporting tendons
- ■ Damage may result in joint instability
- ■ Common symptoms are inflammation and pain

TREATMENT FOR SPRAINS

- ■ Mild
  - • Apply _____ at time of injury
  - • Exercise
  - • Therapeutic devices and compression wraps
- ■ Moderate
  - • Prevent further injury
  - • Healing may take 6 to 8 weeks
- ■ Severe
  - • Often require surgery
  - • Recovery may take longer than 8 weeks

DISLOCATIONS

- ■ _____ occurs when the end of a bone is displaced from its articular surface
- ■ Can be caused by
  - • Trauma
  - • Disease
  - • May be congenital

DISLOCATIONS (continued)

- ■ Common sites
  - • Shoulders
  - • _____
  - • Fingers
  - • Hips
  - • _____

SUBLUXATION

- ■ Partial _____ where bone is pulled out of socket
- ■ Can result from
  - • Weakness
  - • Decreased muscle tone
  - • Gravity
  - • Neurologic deficit

SUBLUXATION (continued)

- ■ Common symptoms
  - • Pain
  - • Pressure
  - • Limited movement
  - • Deformity
  - • _____ and loss of pulse

CHECKPOINT QUESTION 1

How does a luxation differ from a subluxation?

Answer

_____

_____

_____

_____

_____

FRACTURES

- ■ Break or _____ in a bone
- ■ Causes of fractures
  - • Falls or other trauma
  - • Disease
  - • Tumors
  - • Unusual stress

SYMPTOMS OF FRACTURES

- ■ Swelling
- ■ _____
- ■ Lack of movement or unusual movement
- ■ Contusions
- ■ Deformity of body part involved

TREATMENT OF FRACTURES

- ■ _____ (realigning the bones)
- ■ Casting, splinting, wrapping, and taping
- ■ Surgery may be required

CASTS

- ■ Used to immobilize fractures and to facilitate healing in the proper _____

- Plaster casts are traditional
  - Rather soft until fully dry
  - Must be kept dry at all times
- Fiberglass casts are rapidly becoming material of choice

ASSISTING WITH PLASTER OR FIBERGLASS CAST APPLICATION

- Position patient comfortably
- Drape
- _____ part to be casted
- Apply bandage or dressing to lesions
- Assemble supplies
- Assist physician as directed
- Clean skin outside of cast

PLASTER OR FIBERGLASS CAST REMOVAL

- Cast cutter is used
- Wear _____
- Assure patient skin will not be cut
- Warn patient that skin will be pale and dry, muscle will be weak

HEALING OF FRACTURES

- Most important criterion healing is adequate _____
- Blood secretes callus
- Amputation may be necessary
- Prothesis enables function

 CHECKPOINT QUESTION 2

What is the difference between an open and closed reduction?

Answer

_____
_____
_____
_____
_____

BURSITIS

- Inflammation of _____
- Common sites
  - Shoulder
  - Elbow
  - Hip
  - Knee
  - Heel
- Most common symptom
  - Pain during range of movement

BURSITIS *(continued)*

- Treatment
  - Antiinflammatory medications
  - Rest
  - Heat or cold applications
  - _____
  - Activities within pain-free range
  - Physical therapy

OSTEOARTHRITIS

- Degenerative joint disease caused by wear and tear on the _____ joints
- Treatment
  - Antiinflammatory medications
  - Corticosteroid injections
  - Ambulatory aids

RHEUMATOID ARTHRITIS

- Systemic _____ disease that attacks the synovial membrane lining of the joint
- Treatment
  - Similar to osteoarthritis
  - Protection of painful joints
  - In severe cases, joint may be surgically replaced

 CHECKPOINT QUESTION 3

How does osteoarthritis differ from rheumatoid arthritis?

Answer

_____
_____
_____
_____
_____

TENDONITIS

- Muscles attached to bones by tendons
- Tendonitis is _____ of these structures
- Most common sites
  - Shoulder
  - Rotator cuff

TENDONITIS *(continued)*

- Treatment
  - Antiinflammatory medications
  - Rest
  - _____ applications
  - Ultrasound
  - Iontophoresis
  - Massage
  - Transverse friction massage

FIBROMYALGIA

- Condition that causes widespread pain, muscular stiffness, _____ difficulty sleeping
- Treatment
  - Relieving symptoms
  - Nonsteroidal antiinflammatory medications
  - Exercise
  - Rest
  - Personal counseling

SPINE DISORDERS

- Vertebral column
  - Made up of 33 vertebrae and numerous joints
  - Vertebra separated by 23 intervertebral disks
- Strong _____ and structures support and protect the spine

ABNORMAL SPINAL CURVATURES

- Exaggerated or abnormal curvatures of spine affect
  - _____
  - Alignment of shoulders and hips
- Treatment
  - Braces
  - Transcutaneous muscle stimulation
  - Surgery

HERNIATED INTERVERTEBRAL DISK

- Soft center of disk ruptures through tough outer layer
- Common symptoms
  - Severe back pain
  - _____
  - Spasms
  - Weakness
  - Limitation of movement

HERNIATED INTERVERTEBRAL DISK *(continued)*

- Treatment
  - Physical therapy for traction
  - _____
  - Mild extension exercises
  - Surgery

 CHECKPOINT QUESTION 4

What are three abnormal curvatures of the spine? Briefly describe each.

Answer

_____

_____

_____

_____

_____

DISORDERS OF THE UPPER EXTREMITY

- Structures of upper extremity
  - _____
  - Elbow
  - _____
  - Hand

ROTARY CUFF INJURY

- Rotator cuff formed by _____ of four muscles

- Injuries cause
  - Severe pain
  - Weakness
  - Loss of function
- Surgical intervention often necessary

ADHESIVE CAPSULITIS (FROZEN SHOULDER)

- Shortening of muscles and joint structures
- _____ develop when joint is immobilized causing the collagen fibers to stick to each other
- Treatment
  - Antiinflammatory medications
  - Heat or cold applications
  - Physical therapy

LATERAL EPICONDYLITIS (TENNIS ELBOW)

- Sprain or strain of tendons of origin of wrist and finger _____ muscles
- Symptoms include
  - Extreme pain with extension of wrist

LATERAL EPICONDYLITIS (TENNIS ELBOW) (continued)

- Treatment
  - Ice applications
  - _____
  - Iontophoresis
  - Avoiding movements that cause pain
  - Use of a forearm strap distal to elbow joint
  - Transverse friction massage
  - Gentle _____ exercise
  - Surgery

CARPAL TUNNEL SYNDROME

- _____ motion injury
- Compression of median nerve at wrist
- Symptoms
  - Numbness in the thumb, index and middle fingers
  - Pain and weakness
  - Often pain awakens patient at night

CARPAL TUNNEL SYNDROME (continued)

- Treatment
  - Antiinflammatory medications
  - _____
  - Surgery

DUPUYTREN'S CONTRACTURE

- _____ deformities of the fingers
- Treatment
  - Surgery
  - Corticosteroid injections
  - Stretching of tight structures

DISORDERS OF THE LOWER EXTREMITIES

- Structures of lower extremities
  - Hip
  - _____
  - Ankle
  - _____

CHONDROMALACIA PATELLA

- Degenerative disorder affecting the _____ that covers back of patella
- Treatment
  - Rest
  - Physical therapy
  - Bracing or taping knee
  - Antiinflammatory medications
  - _____ therapy
  - Exercises
  - Arthroscopy

PLANTAR FASCIITIS

- Inflammation of the plantar fascia _____
- Treatment
  - Foot orthotic device
  - Physical therapy
  - Ice therapy
  - Massage
  - Ultrasound
  - Nonsteroidal antiinflammatory medications
  - Night splint
  - Surgery

GOUT

- Metabolic disease involving overproduction of
  _____
- Treatment
  - Nonsteroidal antiinflammatory medications
  - Avoidance of purine-rich foods and alcohol-related products
  - Medication to prevent uric acid formation

MUSCULAR DYSTROPHY

- _____ disorders characterized by varying degrees of progressive wasting of skeletal muscles
- No known cure
- To relieve symptoms
  - Exercise
  - Physical therapy
  - Use of splints or braces

OSTEOPOROSIS

- Bones are deficient in _____ making them brittle and vulnerable to fractures
- Treatment
  - Preventing fractures
  - Hormone therapy
  - Calcium and vitamin D supplements

BONE TUMORS

- Bone tissue is rarely primary site for malignancies, but is frequently secondary site for _____
- Surgical treatment
  - Excision of the tumor
  - Or amputation if bone is an extremity
  - Chemotherapy and radiation are usually indicated

COMMON DIAGNOSTIC PROCEDURES

- _____
- Diagnostic studies

PHYSICAL EXAMINATION

- Physician
  - Assesses structure, function, movement, _____
- Patient history

DIAGNOSTIC STUDIES

- Radiology
- Diagnostic imaging
- _____
- Myelograms
- Bone scars
- Computed tomography (CT)

DIAGNOSTIC STUDIES (continued)

- Magnetic resonance imaging (MRI)
- Electromyography (EMG)
- Nerve conduction velocity (NCV)
- _____
- Bone or muscle biopsy

CHECKPOINT QUESTION 5

What are ten procedures that can be used to diagnose musculoskeletal disorders?

Answer

_____

_____

_____

_____

_____

THE ROLE OF THE MEDICAL ASSISTANT

- Warm and cold applications
- _____ assist devices

WARM AND COLD APPLICATIONS

- Medical assistant may instruct patient in administering treatment at home
  - Patient should understand purpose for procedure
  - How to perform procedure
  - Expected results
  - Precautions or _____

PRECAUTIONS

- Do not apply heat or cold _____ than recommended
- Monitor heat temperatures

 ## CHECKPOINT QUESTION 6

How does the body respond to prolonged exposure to temperature extremes?

Answer

_____

_____

_____

_____

_____

AMBULATORY ASSIST DEVICES

- Patients who require assistance to maintain mobility may use
  - Crutches
  - Canes
  - _____
  - Wheelchairs
- Medical assistant often teaches patient how to use these ambulatory aids safely

CRUTCHES

- Axillary crutch
- _____ or Canadian crutch

CANES

- Standard cane for slight assistance
- _____ or quad cane for greater stability
- To measure proper cane length
  - Have patient stand erect

- Cane should be level with greater trochanter
- Patient's elbow should be bent at a 30° angle

CANES *(continued)*

- To walk with a cane, patient should
  1. Position cane on _____ side
  2. Advance cane and affected leg together
  3. Bring unaffected leg forward to a position just ahead of cane
  4. Repeat the steps

WALKERS

- Comfortable aids for elderly or others with weakness or poor coordination
- To use a walker
  1. Stand erect and move walker ahead about _____ inches
  2. With hands on walker grips, step into walker
  3. Move walker ahead again
  4. Repeat the steps

 ## CHECKPOINT QUESTION 7

On which side of the body is the cane positioned?

Answer

_____

_____

_____

_____

_____

Chapter 31

Ophthalmology and Otolaryngology

INTRODUCTION

- _____ specialize in disorders of the eyes
- Otolaryngologists specialize in disorders of the ears, nose, and throat

COMMON DISORDERS OF THE EYE

- Eye is complex, highly developed organ
- Many components may malfunction or become infected or diseased

CATARACT

- _____ or clouding, of the lens that leads to decreased visual acuity
- Symptoms
  - Gradual blurring and loss of vision
  - Milky opacity at the pupil
- Treatment
  - _____ removal of opaque lens
  - Intraocular lens implanted or vision is corrected by contact lenses or special glasses

STY OR HORDEOLUM

- Infection of any of the _____ glands of the eyelids
- Symptoms
  - Redness
  - Swelling
  - Pain
- Warm compresses
- Topical antibiotic drops or ointments

CONJUNCTIVITIS

- Infection of the mucous membrane covering the _____

- Signs and symptoms
  - Tearing
  - Occasionally exudates and pain
- Treatment
  - Antibiotic ophthalmic drops or ointment

CONJUNCTIVITIS (continued)

- Highly contagious
  - Infected child should not go to _____
  - Wash hands frequently
  - Avoid rubbing eyes
  - Discard all eye make-up
  - Wash all towels, washcloths, and pillowcases after use

 CHECKPOINT QUESTION 1

What is the difference between a sty and conjunctivitis?

Answer

_____

_____

_____

_____

_____

CORNEAL ULCER

- _____ away of the corneal surface, leaving scar tissue that may lead to visual disturbances or blindness
- Signs and symptoms
  - Tearing
  - Pain on blinking
  - Sensitivity to light
- Treatment
  - Rest
  - Antibiotic therapy

RETINOPATHY

- General term for any disease or disorder affecting the _____
- Symptoms
  - Small intraocular hemorrhages
  - Night blindness
  - Loss of central visual fields
  - Loss of vision sudden or gradual

RETINOPATHY (continued)

- ■ Treatment
  - • Based on treating underlying cause
  - • Some forms respond well to treatment
  - • Others progress to full _____

GLAUCOMA

- ■ Group of disorders that result in increased _____
- ■ Symptoms of gradual form
  - • Mild or no pain
  - • Visualizing halos around lights
  - • Loss of peripheral vision

GLAUCOMA (continued)

- ■ Symptoms of _____ form
  - • Acute and sudden blockage
  - • Severe eye pain
  - • Blurred vision
  - • Headache
  - • Nausea
  - • Vomiting
  - • Blindness may result within days

GLAUCOMA (continued)

- ■ Treatment for _____ glaucoma
  - • Medications or diuretics that decrease intraocular pressure
- ■ Treatment for acute glaucoma
  - • Iridectomy

REFRACTIVE ERRORS

- ■ Primary types and symptoms
  - • _____, cannot focus on objects near face
  - • _____, objects must be near face for focus
  - • _____, peering through wavy glass
  - • _____, lens no longer accommodates near vision

REFRACTIVE ERRORS (continued)

- ■ Treatment
  - • Corrective lenses
  - • Reshaping the lens with lasers

 ## CHECKPOINT QUESTION 2

What are four common refractive errors? Briefly explain each.

Answer

_____

_____

_____

_____

_____

STRABISMUS

- ■ Misalignment of eye movements, usually caused by muscle incoordination
  - • _____
  - • _____
  - • _____
  - • _____
- ■ Treatment
  - • Patching unaffected eye
  - • Surgery

COLOR DEFICIT

- ■ Absence of or a defect in color perception
- ■ Red, green, or blue perception impaired or absent
- ■ Affects more _____ than _____
- ■ Color deficit has no cure or correction

DIAGNOSTIC STUDIES OF THE EYE

- ■ Basic exam equipment
  - • _____
  - • Lighted instrument used to visually examine the inner surfaces of eye

VISUAL ACUITY TESTING

- ■ Visual acuity commonly assessed using the _____ eye chart
- ■ Hung 20 feet away from patient at eye level
- ■ Normal vision (20/20) means patient can read at 20 feet what normal eye should see at a distance of 20 feet
- ■ Picture chart used for children

CHECKPOINT QUESTION 3

When is the "E" chart used to test visual acuity?

Answer

_____

_____

_____

_____

_____

COLOR DEFICIT TESTING

- ■ _____ method consists of a series of 14 color plates with many four-colored dots forming a pattern of contrasting color within arrangement of dots
- ■ Patients with deficient color perception unable to see pattern

TONOMETRY AND GONIOSCOPY

- ■ Tonometer used to measure _____ or tension
- ■ _____ performed using gonioscope to measure angle of anterior chamber between iris and cornea

THERAPEUTIC PROCEDURES OF THE EYE

- ■ Instilling eye medications
- ■ Eye _____

INSTILLING EYE MEDICATIONS

- ■ Medical assistants frequently responsible for
  - • Instilling ophthalmic medications in the office
  - • _____ patients about the procedure for home use

COMMON DISORDERS OF THE EAR

- ■ Ear is divided into three sections
  - • _____
  - • _____
  - • _____

CERUMINOSIS

- ■ Impacted _____
- ■ Symptoms
  - • Gradual hearing loss
  - • Tinnitus
- ■ Treatment
  - • Wax softened by warm ear drops or _____ removed by ear curet or gently washed with an irrigating device

CONDUCTIVE AND PERCEPTUAL HEARING LOSS

- ■ _____ loss, sound waves are not appropriately transmitted to the level of the cochlea
- ■ _____ loss, transmission from the oval window through to the receptors in the brain

CONDUCTIVE AND PERCEPTUAL HEARING LOSS *(continued)*

- ■ Many patients present with both, called _____
- ■ Treatment
  - • Aimed at addressing underlying cause
  - • Stapedectomy
  - • Cochlear implants
  - • Hearing aids

CHECKPOINT QUESTION 4

What is the difference between conductive and perceptual hearing loss?

Answer

_____

_____

_____

_____

_____

MÉNIÈRE'S DISEASE

- ■ Degenerative condition upsets body's ability to maintain equilibrium in addition to a loss of hearing

- Symptoms
  - _____
  - Sensorineural hearing loss
  - _____
  - Nausea and vomiting
- No curative treatment
  - Palliative medications

OTITIS EXTERNA

- Inflammation or infection of _____
- Symptoms
  - Pain on movement of adjoining structures
- Treatment
  - Antibiotics, topical or systemic
  - Warm compresses
  - Medications to relieve pain

OTITIS EXTERNA (continued)

- Prevention
  - Apply alcohol solution after swimming
  - Wear _____ while swimming
  - Avoid using objects to clean inside ear canal

OTITIS MEDIA

- Inflammation or infection of _____
- Disorder is more common in infants and children
- Symptoms
  - Severe pain
  - Fever of varying degrees
  - Mild to moderate hearing loss
  - Infants may be fussy and tug at their ears

OTITIS MEDIA (continued)

- Treatment
  - _____ for bacterial infections
  - Analgesics
  - Decongestants
  - Myringotomy

OTOSCLEROSIS

- Disorder of ossicles of the inner ear, especially _____
- Treatment
  - Hearing aids
  - Implantation of a stapedial prosthesis

DIAGNOSTIC STUDIES OF THE EAR

- Visual examination
- Audiometry and _____
- Tuning fork test

VISUAL EXAMINATION

- Using an otoscope, physician views auditory canal and _____
- Disposable otoscopes are available
- Nondisposable otoscopes use disposable specula covers

AUDIOMETRY AND TYMPANOMETRY

- Audiometer used to detect _____
  - Produces pure tones heard through earphones
  - Results are recorded by the audiometer on a graph
- Tympanometry uses _____ rather than tones

THE TUNING FORK TESTS

- _____ test
  - Lightly tap tuning fork, placing end on mastoid bone, then moving to external auditory meatus
- _____ test
  - Gently tap tuning fork, placing on midline of forehead

THERAPEUTIC PROCEDURES OF THE EAR

- Ear irrigations
- Ear _____

EAR IRRIGATIONS

- Performed to
  - Relieve pain
  - Remove debris or _____
  - Apply medication solutions

EAR INSTILLATIONS

- Include
  - Local _____ for pain of otitis externa or otitis media
  - Topical antibiotics for otitis externa

CHECKPOINT QUESTION 5

What is an audiometer used for and how does it work?

Answer

_____

_____

_____

_____

_____

COMMON DISORDERS OF THE NOSE AND THROAT

- Allergic rhinitis
- _____
- Nasal polyps
- Sinusitis
- Pharyngitis and _____
- Laryngitis

ALLERGIC RHINITIS

- Inflammation of _____ of nasal passages
- Symptoms
  - Paroxysmal sneezing
  - Intense rhinorrhea
  - Congestion
  - Watery reddened eyes
- Treatment
  - Antihistamine medications
  - Desensitization therapy

EPISTAXIS

- Generally occurs from _____ to nasal membranes
  - May be secondary to other disorders
- Treatment
  - Patient sits upright with the head slightly forward

- Compress the nares against the septum for 5 to 10 minutes with ice or cold, wet compress
- Advise patient to remain still and not to blow nose
- For severe epistaxis, physician may insert nasal packing or _____

NASAL POLYPS

- Small hanging pendulous tissues that obstruct _____
- Symptoms
  - Feeling of fullness or congestion
  - Nasal discharge
- Treatment
  - Corticosteroids

SINUSITIS

- Inflammation of one or more of the _____
- Acute sinusitis results from upper respiratory infection
  - Fairly easily resolved
- Chronic sinusitis more persistent
  - Difficult to control

SINUSITIS *(continued)*

- Symptoms
  - Signs of upper respiratory infection
  - Purulent nasal discharge
  - Facial pain over sinus areas
- Treatment
  - Antihistamines
  - _____ nose drops
  - Steroidal nasal sprays
  - Antibiotics

CHECKPOINT QUESTION 6

What factors may contribute to epistaxis?

Answer

_____

_____

_____

_____

_____

PHARYNGITIS AND TONSILLITIS

- Inflammation of the _____ of the throat and/or the tonsils
- Symptoms
  - Sore throat
  - Difficulty swallowing
- Treatment
  - Antibiotics
  - Surgery

LARYNGITIS

- Inflammation of _____
- Symptoms
  - Hoarseness
  - Cough
  - Difficulty speaking
- Treatment
  - Resolves on its own
  - Rest the voice
  - Cool mist humidifiers

DIAGNOSTIC STUDIES OF THE NOSE AND THROAT

- _____
  - Nasal speculum to inspect nose
  - Penlight and tongue depressor to view throat

- X-rays
- Cultures
- Palpation

THERAPEUTIC PROCEDURES OF THE NOSE AND THROAT

- _____ for suspected pharyngitis or tonsillitis
- Gently swab throat with sterile culture swab to obtain specimen
- Specimen is processed in medical office or sent to laboratory

CHECKPOINT QUESTION 7

Why is it necessary to use a sterile swab to obtain the throat culture specimen?

Answer

_____

_____

_____

_____

Chapter 32

Pulmonary Medicine

INTRODUCTION

- Respiratory system
  - Provides body with _____
  - Eliminates _____
  - Helps protect body from environmental contaminants

COMMON RESPIRATORY DISORDERS

- _____ respiratory disorders
- _____ respiratory disorders

UPPER RESPIRATORY DISORDERS

- Caused by
  - Infectious _____
  - Allergic reactions that produce inflammation
- Also considered upper respiratory disorders
  - Acute rhinitis
  - Sinusitis
  - Pharyngitis
  - Tonsillitis
  - Laryngitis

LOWER RESPIRATORY DISORDERS

- _____
  - Bronchitis
  - Pneumonia
- _____
  - Asthma
  - Chronic bronchitis
  - Emphysema

BRONCHITIS

- Inflammation of mucous membranes of
  _____
- Most prominent symptom
  - Productive cough
- Treatment
  - Antibiotics
  - Smoking cessation
  - Rest
  - Increased fluid intake
  - Cough suppressants

PNEUMONIA

- Bacterial or viral infection in the
  _____
- Diagnostic tests include
  - Analysis of sputum specimen
  - Chest x-ray

BACTERIAL PNEUMONIA

- Symptoms
  - More sudden and _____ in onset
  - Fever, cough, chills, dyspnea
- Treatment
  - Antibiotics
  - Bed rest
  - Symptomatic medications

VIRAL PNEUMONIA

- Symptoms
  - More _____ in onset
- Treatment
  - Bed rest
  - Hospitalization

CHECKPOINT QUESTION 1

What are the characteristic symptoms of bacterial and viral pneumonia?

Answer

_____

_____

_____

_____

_____

ASTHMA

- Reversible inflammatory process involving the bronchi and _____
- Symptoms
  - Dyspnea
  - Coughing
  - Wheezing
  - Cyanosis
- Treatment
  - Considered a
    _____
  - Many medications available
  - Nebulized breathing treatment with a bronchodilator

CHECKPOINT QUESTION 2

What are factors that may trigger an asthma attack?

Answer

_____

_____

_____

_____

_____

CHRONIC OBSTRUCTIVE PULMONARY DISEASE (COPD)

- Chronic _____
- Caused by smoking over long period of time

CHRONIC BRONCHITIS

- Chronic inflammation and swelling of
  _____ with excessive
  mucus production, obstruction of bronchi, and
  trapping of air behind mucus plugs
- Prone to develop respiratory infections

EMPHYSEMA

- Walls of damaged alveoli become
  _____ and _____

PATIENTS DIAGNOSED WITH COPD

- Process not usually _____
  _____
- Progression can be slowed
  - Prescribed exercise regimen
  - Proper use of medications
  - Good nutrition
  - Home oxygen therapy

 CHECKPOINT QUESTION 3

What two disease processes are present in a patient with chronic obstructive pulmonary disease (COPD)?

Answer

_____

_____

_____

_____

TUBERCULOSIS

- Infectious disease caused by
  _____
- Symptoms
  - Productive cough
  - Night sweats
  - Malaise
- Treatment
  - Antibiotic therapy that lasts for months

COMMON CANCERS OF THE RESPIRATORY SYSTEM

- _____ cancer
- _____ cancer

LARYNGEAL CANCER

- Most commonly seen in _____
  and alcoholics
- Symptoms
  - Hoarseness that lasts longer than 3 weeks
  - Feeling a "lump" in the throat
  - Pain and burning in throat when drinking
    citrus juice or hot liquids
- Treatment
  - Radiation
  - Laryngectomy

LUNG CANCER

- Most common cause of _____
  in men and women
  - 80% lung cancer patients are smokers
- Symptoms present late in the disease
  - Chronic cough
  - Wheezing
  - Dyspnea
  - Hemoptysis
  - Chest pain
- Treatment
  - Surgery, radiation, chemotherapy
  - May improve patient's prognosis

 CHECKPOINT QUESTION 4

What factor appears to contribute to both laryngeal cancer and lung cancer?

Answer

_____

_____

_____

_____

_____

COMMON DIAGNOSTIC AND THERAPEUTIC PROCEDURES

- Physical examination of the respiratory system
- _____ and cytology

- Chest x-ray
- Bronchoscopy
- Pulmonary function tests
- Arterial blood gases
- Pulse oximetry

PHYSICAL EXAMINATION OF THE RESPIRATORY SYSTEM

- Consists of four parts
  - _____
  - _____
  - _____
  - _____
- Patient should be sitting up and all clothing removed from waist up

 CHECKPOINT QUESTION 5

What are the four parts of the chest examination?

Answer

_____

_____

_____

_____

_____

SPUTUM CULTURE AND CYTOLOGY

- Sputum cultures obtained to aid with diagnosis and treatment
- Obtain specimen that patient has coughed up and expectorated from _____
- Medical assistant processes specimen and prepares laboratory request

CHEST X-RAY

- Help in diagnosis of pulmonary problems
- Two views often ordered
  - Posterior to anterior (_____) view
  - Lateral view
- Medical assistant may need to schedule x-ray and request results

BRONCHOSCOPY

- Endoscopic procedure where lighted scope is inserted into _____ for direct visualization
- Requires patient's written consent
- Usually performed in outpatient surgical setting
- Also used therapeutically

PULMONARY FUNCTION TESTS

- Performed using a _____ that measures the amount of air a patient can move in and out of lungs
- Physician gains information concerning mild, moderate, or severe obstructive or restrictive disease

ARTERIAL BLOOD GASES (ABG)

- Measures pH and the pressures of _____ _____ in arterial blood
- Results can indicate
  - Whether lungs are adequately exchanging gases
  - Metabolic acid-base problems
  - Not routinely performed in medical office

PULSE OXIMETRY

- Pulse oximeter used to determine percentage of _____ of capillary blood cells
- Obtain as baseline for patient's
  - With chronic respiratory conditions
  - Experiencing respiratory symptoms

 CHECKPOINT QUESTION 6

What are the ways the physician can obtain information to help diagnose respiratory disorders?

Answer

_____

_____

_____

_____

_____

Chapter 33

Cardiology

COMMON CARDIOVASCULAR DISORDERS

- Cardiovascular system consists of the heart and blood vessels including the _____
  _____

SYMPTOMS OF CARDIAC DISORDERS

- _____
- Dyspnea
- Fatigue
- _____
- Nausea and vomiting
- Irregular heartbeat

SYMPTOMS OF CARDIAC DISORDERS (continued)

- Changes in peripheral circulation
- _____
- Skin ulcers that do not heal
- Pain that increases with ambulation and decreases with rest
- Changes in skin color

DISORDERS OF THE HEART

- _____
- Congestive heart failure
- Myocardial infarction
- Cardiac _____
- Congenital and valvular heart disease

CARDITIS

- Inflammation of layers of the
  _____
  - Pericarditis
  - Myocarditis
  - Endocarditis

- Signs and symptoms
  - Sharp pain
  - Dyspnea
  - Neck venous distention
  - Pallor
  - Hypertension

CARDITIS (continued)

- Treatment
  - Relieve symptoms
  - Correct underlying cause
  - Administer medications

 CHECKPOINT QUESTION 1

How does the pain in pericarditis differ from pain that occurs during a myocardial infarction?

Answer

_____
_____
_____
_____
_____

CONGESTIVE HEART FAILURE (CHF)

- Condition in which the heart is unable to _____ effectively
- Symptoms
  - Edema of lower extremities
  - Dyspnea
- No cure for CHF
- Treatment
  - Relieve symptoms
  - Prevent permanent damage
  - Administrate medications

MYOCARDIAL INFARCTION

- Death of any part of the heart
- Symptoms
  - Pain that last longer than 20–30 minutes unrelieved by rest
  - _____
  - Diaphoresis

- Weakness
- Vomiting
- _____

MYOCARDIAL INFARCTION
(continued)

- ■ Symptoms (continued)
  - Feeling of viselike grip around chest cavity
  - Cool, clammy, pale skin
  - _____
  - Indigestion
- ■ Procedures
  - Percutaneous transluminal coronary angioplasty (PTCA)
  - Coronary artery bypass graft (CABG)

CARDIAC ARRHYTHMIA

- ■ Abnormal heart rhythm
  - _____
  - _____
  - _____
- ■ Symptoms
  - Dizziness
  - Unconsciousness
  - Cardiac arrest

CARDIAC ARRHYTHMIA *(continued)*

- ■ Treatment
  - Automatic external defibrillators (_____)
  - Cardiopulmonary resuscitation (_____)

CHECKPOINT QUESTION 2

Which two cardiac arrhythmias are cardiac emergencies and require immediate intervention by the medical assistant?

Answer

_____
_____
_____
_____
_____

CONGENITAL AND VALVULAR HEART DISEASE

- ■ Disease of heart valves
  - Atrial septal defect
  - Ventricular septal defect
  - Patent ductus arteriosus
  - Coarctation of the aorta
  - Aortic or pulmonic _____
  - Bicuspid aortic valve
  - Mitral valve _____
  - Tetralogy of Fallot
  - Rheumatic heart disease

CONGENITAL AND VALVULAR HEART DISEASE *(continued)*

- ■ Symptoms
  - _____
  - Shortness of breath
  - Limited ability for physical exertion
  - Pulmonary edema, dyspnea, productive cough

CONGENITAL AND VALVULAR HEART DISEASE *(continued)*

- ■ Treatment depends on type and severity
- ■ Severe cases
  - Low sodium diets
  - Prophylactic antibiotics
  - _____

CHECKPOINT QUESTION 3

What microorganism may be responsible for rheumatic heart disease and cardiac valvular damage?

Answer

_____
_____
_____
_____
_____

DISORDERS OF THE BLOOD VESSELS

- ■ _____
- ■ Hypertension

■ Varicose veins
■ Venous thrombosis and pulmonary embolism
■ Cerebrovascular accident
■ _____
■ Anemia

■ Symptoms
  • Diastolic blood pressure higher than 120 mm Hg
  • Blurred vision
  • Headache
  • Possibly confusion

ATHEROSCLEROSIS

■ Collection of _____ made of calcium and cholesterol inside walls of vessels
■ Signs and symptoms
  • Pain or numbness
  • Loss of normal blood flow
  • Loss of palpable pulse
  • Coronary artery disease

HYPERTENSION *(continued)*

■ Treatment
  • Low-sodium, _____ diet
  • Exercise program
  • Weight reduction if needed
  • Antihypertensive and lipid reducing medications
  • Diuretic medications

ATHEROSCLEROSIS *(continued)*

■ Treatment for severe condition
  • _____ using lipid lowering medications
  • Surgery to remove plaque or improve blood flow through artery
■ Medical assistant's responsibilities
  • Coordinate diagnostic procedures
  • Educate patients
  • Provide emotional support

CHECKPOINT QUESTION 5

Which two disorders may result from untreated hypertension?

Answer

_____

_____

_____

_____

_____

CHECKPOINT QUESTION 4

What are four predisposing factors for heart disease?

Answer

_____

_____

_____

_____

_____

VARICOSE VEINS

■ Superficial veins of the legs become swollen and _____
■ Symptoms
  • Swelling
  • Aching
  • Feeling of heaviness in legs
  • May be asymptomatic

HYPERTENSION

■ Resting systolic blood pressure above _____ mm Hg, diastolic pressure above _____ mm Hg
  • Essential hypertension
  • Malignant hypertension

VARICOSE VEINS *(continued)*

■ Treatment
  • Avoid standing or _____ for long periods of time
  • Wear elastic support stockings
  • Elevate legs
  • Surgery

VENOUS THROMBOSIS AND PULMONARY EMBOLISM

- ■ _____ in peripheral or pulmonary veins
- ■ Symptoms
  - • Dyspnea
  - • Syncope
  - • Severe pleuritic chest pain
- ■ Treatment
  - • Bed rest with elevation of affected extremity
  - • Anticoagulant medications
  - • Surgery

 CHECKPOINT QUESTION 6

What disease occurs when the superficial veins in the legs become swollen and distended?

Answer

_____

_____

_____

_____

_____

CEREBROVASCULAR ACCIDENT

- ■ Damage to blood vessels in the _____
- ■ Symptoms
  - • Weakness or paralysis
  - • Involvement of language and comprehension
- ■ Treatment
  - • Reduce further damage to tissue
  - • Regain use of affected extremities
  - • Rehabilitation

TRANSIENT ISCHEMIC ATTACK (TIA)

- ■ _____ are a warning sign for impending CVA
- ■ Symptoms
  - • Mild numbness or tingling
  - • Difficulty swallowing
  - • Coughing and choking
  - • Slurred speech
  - • Unilateral visual disturbances
  - • Dizziness
  - • Patients should be sent to emergency room

ANEURYSM

- ■ _____ effect in weakened blood vessel walls
  - • Dissecting
  - • Sacculated
  - • Berry
- ■ Symptoms
  - • Pain or pressure at the site
- ■ Treatment
  - • Surgical resection is the only option

ANEMIA

- ■ Deficiencies in _____ or numbers of red blood cells
- ■ Symptoms
  - • Cardiovascular alterations
  - • Anorexia and weight loss
  - • Dyspnea on exertion
  - • _____
- ■ Treatment
  - • Increasing dietary iron
  - • Blood transfusions
  - • Injection of vitamin B_{12}

COMMON DIAGNOSTIC AND THERAPEUTIC PROCEDURES

- ■ Invasive techniques
- ■ Noninvasive techniques
- ■ Performed in medical office
  - • Auscultating heart and chest cavity
  - • Chest x-ray
  - • 12-lead _____
- ■ Performed in outpatient surgical center or hospital
  - • Sophisticated procedures such as cardiac catheterization

PHYSICAL EXAMINATION OF THE CARDIOVASCULAR SYSTEM

- ■ Medical assistant's responsibilities
  - • Obtain vital information
  - • Obtain complete list of patient's medications
  - • Obtain brief social and _____

 CHECKPOINT QUESTION 7

What is a murmur?

Answer

_____

_____

_____

_____

_____

ELECTROCARDIOGRAM (ECG)

- Graphic record of electrical current as it progresses through heart
- Medical assistant's responsibilities
  - Explain procedure
  - Apply _____
  - Handle ECG paper carefully

ECG LEADS

- Standard system of electrode placement
  - 12 leads
  - 4 color-coded wires
- Position 4 limb electrodes in _____ areas
- Each lead provides specific measurements

CHECKPOINT QUESTION 8

Which three waves represent a cardiac cycle on an ECG?

Answer

_____

_____

_____

_____

_____

ECG INTERPRETATION

- Interpreted by physician
  - _____
  - _____
  - _____
- Medical assistant's responsibility
  - Obtain ECG of good quality

HOLTER MONITOR

- Small, portable device worn for long periods of time to record _____
- Medical assistant's responsibility
  - Instruct patient to keep diary of daily activities

CHEST X-RAY

- Provides valuable basic information about the anatomic location and _____ of the heart, great vessels, and lungs

CARDIAC STRESS TEST

- Measures response of cardiac muscle to increased demands of oxygen
- Medical assistant's responsibilities
  - Attach electrodes
  - Monitor, record blood pressure
  - Watch patient for signs of _____
  - Have emergency resuscitation equipment available

CHECKPOINT QUESTION 9

What is the purpose of a cardiac stress test?

Answer

_____

_____

_____

_____

_____

ECHOCARDIOGRAPHY

- Harmless _____ that create an image of heart on a screen
- Medical assistant's responsibilities
  - Schedule outpatient procedure
  - Give patient instructions

CARDIAC CATHETERIZATION AND CORONARY ARTERIOGRAPHY

- _____ procedure used to help diagnose or treat conditions affecting the coronary arterial circulation
- Procedure not done in medical office

Chapter 34

Gastroenterology

Answer

_____

_____

_____

_____

_____

INTRODUCTION

- The gastrointestinal (GI) system is responsible for
  - Ingestion
  - Digestion
  - _____
  - Elimination of food

COMMON GASTROINTESTINAL DISORDERS

- Mouth disorders
- _____ disorders
- Stomach disorders
- Intestinal disorders
- Functional disorders
- _____ disorders
- Gallbladder disorders
- Pancreatic disorders

MOUTH DISORDERS

- Caries
  - Tooth decay
- Stomatitis
  - Inflammation of oral mucosa
- _____
  - Inflammation of the gingiva
- Oral cancers

MOUTH DISORDERS

- Medical assistant's responsibilities
  - Medical history
  - Patient education
  - Making referrals per physician

 CHECKPOINT QUESTION 1

What are the two most common causes of stomatitis?

ESOPHAGEAL DISORDERS

- Hiatal hernia
- Esophageal _____
- Esophageal cancers

HIATAL HERNIA

- Defect in the _____ that allows portion of stomach to slide up into the chest cavity
- Symptoms
  - Indigestion
  - Epigastric pain
- Treatment
  - Diet modifications
  - _____
  - Weight loss
  - Elevating head of bed
  - Drug therapy

ESOPHAGEAL VARICES

- Result from _____ within the esophageal veins
- Before rupture occurs, treatment is sclerotherapy
- In the event of esophageal hemorrhage, patient should be transported to emergency room

ESOPHAGEAL CANCERS

- Most common among older men and is usually fatal
- Symptoms
  - _____
  - Vomiting
  - Weight loss
- Treatment
  - Surgery
  - Chemotherapy
  - Radiation

CHECKPOINT QUESTION 2

What is a hiatal hernia and how can it affect the esoph-agus?

Answer

_____

_____

_____

_____

_____

STOMACH DISORDERS

- ■ _____
- ■ _____
- ■ _____

GASTRITIS

- ■ Inflammation of _____ of stomach
- ■ Signs and symptoms
  - • Evidence of GI bleeding
  - • Epigastric discomfort
  - • Nausea
  - • Vomiting
- ■ Treatment
  - • Eliminating irritant
  - • Restoring proper gastric acidity
  - • Antibiotics

PEPTIC ULCERS

- ■ Ulcers within GI tract
- ■ Symptoms
  - • Abdominal pain, especially after _____
  - • Melena
  - • Hematemesis
- ■ Treatment
  - • Avoid irritants
  - • Limit production of hydrogen
  - • Antibiotics
  - • Surgery

GASTRIC CANCER

- ■ Spreads rapidly to adjacent organs and throughout the _____ cavity

- ■ Signs and symptoms
  - • Chronic indigestion
  - • Weight loss
  - • Anorexia
  - • _____
  - • Fatigue
  - • Hematemesis
  - • Dark, bloody stools

GASTRIC CANCER (continued)

- ■ Treatment
  - • Surgery
  - • Chemotherapy
  - • Radiation

INTESTINAL DISORDERS

- ■ Gastroenteritis
- ■ Duodenal ulcers
- ■ _____ syndromes

GASTROENTERITIS

- ■ Generalized inflammation of stomach, _____ or colon
- ■ Symptoms
  - • Abdominal
  - • Nausea
  - • Vomiting
  - • Diarrhea
  - • Fever

GASTROENTERITIS (continued)

- ■ Treatment is _____
  - • Limiting food intake
  - • Treating nausea, vomiting, and diarrhea
  - • Maintaining fluid balance
  - • Intravenous fluids
  - • Antibiotics or antiparasitic medications

DUODENAL ULCERS

- ■ Ulcerative lesions caused by exposure to _____
- ■ Treatment
  - • Limiting or avoiding irritating factors
  - • Lowering stomach acid by reducing gastric acidity
  - • Surgery

MALABSORPTION SYNDROMES

- Prevent the normal absorption of nutrients through walls of small intestines
- Signs
  - Pale, frothy stools
  - _____ high in fat content
- Treatment
  - Addressing suspected causing
  - Avoiding or replacing substances malabsorbed
  - Supplemental vitamins

CHECKPOINT QUESTION 3

How are peptic and duodenal ulcers different?

Answer

_____

_____

_____

_____

_____

CROHN'S DISEASE

- Inflammation of deep lining of the
  _____
- Symptoms
  - Diarrhea and cramping
  - Constipation
  - Anorexia
  - Fever

CROHN'S DISEASE (continued)

- Treatment
  - Restoration of _____
  - Corticosteroids
  - Rest
  - _____ diet
  - Surgery

ULCERATIVE COLITIS

- Inflammatory bowel disease affecting
  _____ of the colon

- Symptoms
  - Weakness
  - Anorexia
  - Nausea
  - Vomiting
- Treatment
  - Controlling inflammation
  - Preventing loss of fluids and nutrients
  - _____
  - Surgery

IRRITABLE BOWEL SYNDROME

- Bouts of _____ alternating with _____
- Treatment
  - Stress management
  - Identifying offending food irritants

CHECKPOINT QUESTION 4

Which inflammatory bowel disease can lead to life-threatening bowel obstruction? How?

Answer

_____

_____

_____

_____

_____

DIVERTICULOSIS

- _____ of bowel wall causing small out-pouches in lining of intestinal wall
- Symptoms
  - Fever
  - Abdominal pain
- Treatment
  - _____ diet
  - Stool softeners
  - Bland diet

POLYPS

- Masses of benign mucous membrane tissue lining the _____

- Usually slow growing, but may become cancerous
- Treatment
  - If removed early, cancer may be prevented

HERNIAS

- Organs or intestines protrude through weakened _____
  - Inguinal
  - Ventral
  - Umbilical
- Sign
  - Protrusion over the area where hernia is present

HERNIAS *(continued)*

- Treatment
  - Surgery
  - Eating _____ meals
  - No food before bedtime

APPENDICITIS

- Inflammation and infection of appendix
- Symptoms
  - Severe abdominal pain with tenderness over

    _____

  - Vomiting
  - Fever
  - Elevated white blood count
- Treatment
  - Surgery

HEMORRHOIDS

- External or internal _____ in the rectum
- Symptoms
  - Bleeding during defecation
  - Rectal pain and itching
- Treatment
  - Regulate diet to control constipation
  - Local pain relief
  - Stool softeners
  - Surgical _____

COLORECTAL CANCERS

- Often fatal, cause is unknown
- Symptoms

- Vague
  _____

  with occasional bloody stools
- Treatment
  - Surgical removal of affected area
  - Chemotherapy
  - Radiation

FUNCTIONAL DISORDERS

- _____
- _____
- _____

CONSTIPATION

- _____ has fecal material present that stays in the colon too long making it hard and dry
- To avoid constipation
  - Increase oral fluid intake
  - Eat foods high in fiber
  - Maintain regular bowel habits
- Treatment
  - Stool softeners
  - OTC fiber products

DIARRHEA

- Loose, watery stools
- Treatment
  - Medications to slow _____
  - Bland diet

INTESTINAL GAS

- Produced by bacterial decomposition of
  _____
- Symptoms
  - Feeling of fullness
  - Eructation
  - Flatulence
- Treatment
  - Avoid offending foods
  - OTC and prescription medications

 ## CHECKPOINT QUESTION 5

- What causes hemorrhoids?

Answer

_____

_____

_____

_____

_____

LIVER DISORDERS

- Cardinal signs of liver dysfunction
  - _____
  - _____
  - _____
- Diagnostic tests
  - Liver function tests
  - X-rays and barium studies
  - Radioisotope liver scans
  - Percutaneous peritoneoscopy and biopsy
  - Surgical laparotomy and liver biopsy

HEPATITIS

- Inflammation or infection of the liver
  - Hepatitis A
  - Hepatitis B
  - Hepatitis C
  - Hepatitis D
  - Hepatitis E
- Symptoms
  - Fatigue
  - _____
  - Flu-like symptoms with fever

HEPATITIS *(continued)*

- Symptoms (continued)
  - Jaundice
  - _____
  - Light stools
- Treatment
  - No cure once infection occurs
  - Rest and take in a supportive diet
  - Interferon-A

CHECKPOINT QUESTION 6

How does the cause of viral hepatitis differ from that of toxic hepatitis?

Answer

_____

_____

_____

_____

_____

CIRRHOSIS OR FIBROSIS

- Chronic disease characterized by destruction of liver cells and formation of _____ or fibers
- Symptoms
  - Vague GI discomfort
  - Respiratory efficiency decreases
  - Bleeding
  - Dermal pruritus
  - Jaundice
  - Hepatomegaly

CIRRHOSIS AND FIBROSIS *(continued)*

- Treatment
  - Avoiding hepatotoxins or abstinence from _____
  - Good diet
  - Vitamin supplements
  - Supportive care

LIVER CANCER

- Liver is rarely a primary site for cancer
- Frequent site for metastasis
- Symptoms
  - Weight loss
  - Weakness
  - _____
  - Jaundice

LIVER CANCER *(continued)*

- Treatment
  - _____
  - Chemotherapy
  - Liver transplant

GALLBLADDER DISORDERS

- Cholelithiasis and _____
- Gallbladder cancer

CHOLELITHIASIS AND CHOLECYSTITIS

- Cholelithiasis is formation of _____ made of cholesterol and bilirubin
- Cholecystitis is acute or chronic _____ of the gallbladder
- Symptoms
  - Acute right upper abdominal quadrant pain
  - Indigestion
  - Nausea
  - Intolerance
  - Jaundice

CHOLELITHIASIS AND CHOLECYSTITIS (continued)

- Treatment
  - Pain medication
  - Avoiding _____ foods
  - Surgical removal of stones
  - Lithotripsy

GALLBLADDER CANCER

- Rare and difficult to diagnose
- Symptoms
  - Right upper quadrant pain
  - Nausea
  - Vomiting
  - Weight loss
  - Anorexia
- Treatment
  - Surgical _____

CHECKPOINT QUESTION 7

How are cholelithiasis and cholecystitis different?

Answer

_____

_____

_____

_____

_____

PANCREATIC DISORDERS

- _____
- Pancreatic cancer

PANCREATITIS

- Inflammation of the pancreas
- Symptoms
  - Vomiting
  - Steady epigastric pain _____
    _____
- Treatment
  - Pain relief
  - Medication to reduce pancreatic secretions while organ recovers

PANCREATIC CANCER

- Malignancy usually causes death within _____ of diagnosis
- Symptoms
  - Weight loss
  - Back and abdominal pain
  - Diarrhea
  - Jaundice

PANCREATIC CANCER (continued)

- Treatment
  - Surgical removal of pancreas
  - Chemotherapy
  - _____

COMMON DIAGNOSTIC AND THERAPEUTIC PROCEDURES

- History and physical examination of gastrointestinal system
- Blood tests
- Radiologic studies
- _____
- Fecal tests

HISTORY OF THE GI SYSTEM

- History must include
  - Occupation
  - Family history
  - Recent travel to _____ countries
  - Current medications

HISTORY OF THE GI SYSTEM
(continued)

- Patient concerns might include
  - _____
  - GI bleeding
  - Weight gain or loss
  - Social history of alcohol use
  - Laxative and enema use

HISTORY OF THE GI SYSTEM
(continued)

- Physician will assess
  - Skin turgor (elasticity)
  - Jaundice
  - _____
  - Bruising
  - Breath odor
  - Size and shape of abdomen
  - Presence and quality of
    _____
- Abdominal contents will be palpated by physician during examination

BLOOD TESTS

- White and red blood cell counts
- Erythrocyte sedimentation rate
- Liver function tests
- Pancreatic _____ studies

RADIOLOGIC STUDIES

- Consist of instilling _____ into the GI tract orally or rectally to outline the organs and identify abnormalities
  - Fluoroscope
  - Barium swallow
  - Small bowel series
  - Barium enema
  - Cholecystography
  - Percutaneous transhepatic cholangiography

RADIOLOGIC STUDIES *(continued)*

- Role of medical assistant
  - Determining requirements for referrals or precertification
  - Schedule procedure in outpatient facility
  - _____ patient on preparations
  - Route report to physician

NUCLEAR IMAGING

- _____ are injected into body and images are taken using nuclear scanning device
- Role of medical assistant
  - Coordinate any third-party payer requirements
  - Schedule test at a nuclear imaging center or hospital
  - Follow up with patient when results are returned

ULTRASONOGRAPHY

- Use of high frequency _____ to diagnose disorders of internal structures
- Role of medical assistant
  - Very little if any patient preparation
  - Schedule in the imaging department of outpatient or inpatient facilities

ENDOSCOPIC STUDIES

- Physician passes soft, _____ down esophagus into stomach and small intestine or up into colon for direct visualization
  - Endoscopic retrograde cholangiopancreatography
  - Anoscopy
  - Sigmoidoscopy examination

ENDOSCOPIC STUDIES *(continued)*

- Some physicians prefer that bowel be free of feces
  - May order a light meal the evening before exam
  - Evening _____ may be ordered
  - Enema
  - Light breakfast may be allowed
- Other physicians prefer to view mucosa as it normally appears
- Follow procedure manual

 CHECKPOINT QUESTION 8

What does anoscopy involve and how does it differ from sigmoidoscopy?

Answer

_____

_____

_____

_____

_____

FECAL TESTS

- As part of routine examination, physician may order _____ to test for occult blood
- Follow standard precautions when collecting stool specimens
- Medical assistant's responsibilities
  - Instruct patient in procedure
  - Assist in collection of stool specimen
  - Ensure patient understanding and compliance

SCREENING FOR OCCULT BLOOD

- Most physicians routinely screen patients over the age of 50 for occult blood
- Testing stool for occult blood

- Patient uses a test pack or kit
- Usually collected by _____ at home

SCREENING FOR OCCULT BLOOD
(continued)

- Positive test
  - Blood detected
  - Physician orders further diagnostic testing since there are numerous reasons for blood in stool including
    - Hemorrhoids
    - Polyps
    - Diverticula
    - _____
    - Colorectal cancer

SCREENING FOR OCCULT BLOOD
(continued)

- Medical assistant's responsibilities
  - Instruct patient how to use kit
  - Instruct patient to follow prescribed _____

Chapter 35

Neurology

INTRODUCTION

- Nervous system is chief communication and command center for all parts of body
- Two divisions of nervous system
  - _____
    (CNS) includes
    - Brain
    - Spinal cord
  - _____
    (PNS) contains
    - Nerves that transmit impulses

COMMON NERVOUS SYSTEM DISORDERS

- Infectious disorders
- _____ disorders
- Seizure disorders
- Developmental disorders
- _____
- Brain tumors
- Headaches

INFECTIOUS DISORDERS

- _____
- Encephalitis
- Herpes zoster
- Poliomyelitis
- _____
- Rabies
- Reye syndrome

MENINGITIS

- Inflammation of the _____ covering the spinal cord and brain
- Viral meningitis is usually not life-threatening and is often short-lived
- Bacterial meningitis is often severe and may be fatal

MENINGITIS (continued)

- Symptoms
  - Nausea
  - Vomiting
  - _____
  - Headaches
  - Stiff neck
  - Photophobia
  - Rash

MENINGITIS (continued)

- Treatment for _____ meningitis
  - Fluids
  - Bed rest
- Treatment for _____ meningitis
  - Antibiotics
  - Generally requires hospitalization

MENINGITIS (continued)

- Medical assistant's responsibilities
  - Complete infectious diseases form
  - Individuals (family, friends, co-workers) may require _____ treatment to prevent contracting disease

 CHECKPOINT QUESTION 1

How does the treatment of viral meningitis differ from that of bacterial meningitis?

Answer

_____

_____

_____

_____

_____

ENCEPHALITIS

- Inflammation of the _____
- Symptoms
  - Drowsiness
  - Headaches
  - Fever
  - Seizures and coma may occur in later stages
- Treatment
  - Hospitalization for intravenous fluid therapy and supportive care
- Local health department should be notified

HERPES ZOSTER

- Virus that spreads down length of a _____ causing redness, swelling, pain
- Treatment
  - Analgesics or nerve blocks for pain
  - Topically, calamine lotion may be applied to skin to reduce itching
  - Antiviral medications

POLIOMYELITIS

- Highly contagious _____ that affects brain and spinal cord
- Symptoms
  - Stiff neck, fever, headaches, and sore throat
  - Nausea, vomiting, diarrhea
  - Paralysis may develop
  - Muscles atrophy

POLIOMYELITIS (continued)

- Treatment
  - Acute stage, palliative and supportive
  - After acute stage, _____
  - Emotional support

POSTPPOLIOMYELITIS MUSCULAR ATROPHY (PPMA) SYNDROME

- _____ of disease documented in some individuals who had polio as children
- Symptoms
  - Similar to those that signaled onset of original disease
- Treatment
  - Outpatient basis with supportive care
  - No cure available
  - Emotional support

TETANUS

- Infection of nervous tissue caused by

  _____
- All deep, dirty wounds should be treated as high risk for tetanus
- Symptoms
  - Spasms of voluntary muscles
  - Restlessness
  - Stiff neck
  - Seizures
  - Dysphagia
  - Facial and oral muscles contract

TETANUS (continued)

- If untreated
  - Respiratory muscles become _____

    _____
  - Disease typically fatal
- Prevention is best defense against tetanus
  - Clean wounds immediately
  - Remove dead tissue
  - Antibiotics

 CHECKPOINT QUESTION 2

What are the initial signs of a tetanus infection?

Answer

_____

_____

_____

_____

_____

RABIES

- Virus that spreads to the organs of _____

  _____
- Animals that commonly transmit rabies
  - Skunks
  - Squirrels
  - Raccoons
  - Bats
  - Dogs
  - Cats
  - Coyotes
  - Foxes

- Initial symptoms
  - Fever
  - General malaise
  - Body aches

RABIES (continued)

- As disease progresses
  - Mental derangement
  - Paralysis
  - _____
  - Drooling
- Immediate treatment of wound is first priority
  - Antibiotics
  - Prophylactic vaccine therapy
- All animal bites must be reported to animal control center

REYE SYNDROME

- Nervous system illness typically occurs in children after _____
- Initial symptoms
  - Vomiting
  - Lethargy
- As brain swelling continues
  - Confusion
  - Seizures
  - Coma

REYE SYNDROME (continued)

- Treatment
  - _____
  - Aggressive antibiotics
  - Supportive care

DEGENERATIVE DISORDERS

- Multiple sclerosis (_____)
- Amyotrophic lateral sclerosis (_____)

MULTIPLE SCLEROSIS (MS)

- _____

  covering neurons
- Symptoms
  - Progressive loss of muscle control
  - Loss of balance

- Shaking tremors
- Poor muscle coordination
- Dysphasia
- Tingling and numbness

MULTIPLE SCLEROSIS (continued)

- As disease progresses
  - Bladder dysfunction
  - Visual disturbances
  - Nystagmus
- Treatment
  - Palliative
  - Physical therapy
  - Prosthetic appliances
  - _____
  - Steroids

AMYOTROPHIC LATERAL SCLEROSIS (ALS)

- Terminal disease with no known cause that causes a _____ of motor neurons
- Begins with loss of muscle mobility
  - Forearms
  - Hands
  - Legs

AMYOTROPHIC LATERAL SCLEROSIS (continued)

- Progresses to
  - Facial muscles
- Treatment
  - Patient _____
  - Family education

SEIZURE DISORDERS

- Seizures are involuntary contractions of voluntary muscles caused by a rapid succession of electrical impulses through the brain
- Seizures have many causes
- _____ is most common form

SEIZURE DISORDERS (continued)

- _____ seizures
  - Usually occur only childhood
  - Child may appear to fall asleep or drift away momentarily
  - Some muscle twitching may occur
- _____ seizures
  - Also called tonic-clonic seizures
  - More involved than petit mal seizures

SEIZURE DISORDERS (continued)

- Treatment
  - During seizure, prevent
    _____ to patient
  - Epilepsy is treated with pharmacological agents that must be taken regularly

FEBRILE SEIZURES

- Occur most commonly in children between the ages of 6 months and 3 years who are febrile
- Must have complete physical and neurologic examination to rule out
  _____ origin
- Treatment
  - Gently return child's body temperature to more manageable level
  - Cool compresses
  - Do not give aspirin products

FOCAL (JACKSONIAN) SEIZURES

- Begins as small localized seizure that spreads to _____
- Cause of focal seizures must be researched to prevent progression to generalized seizures

 CHECKPOINT QUESTION 3

How do petit mal seizures differ from grand mal seizures?

Answer

_____

_____

_____

_____

_____

DEVELOPMENTAL DISORDERS

- _____
- _____
- _____

NEURAL TUBE DEFECTS

- Abnormalities of the neural tube that occur during _____ and _____ stages of development
- Developmental failure in proximal portion, anencephaly may result
- Abnormality in development in the distal end results in spina bifida

SPINA BIFIDA

- Spina bifida occulta is most benign form
- _____ occurs when the meninges protrude through spina bifida
- Spina bifida with myelomeningocele
- Treatment
  - Surgery

HYDROCEPHALUS

- Excessive _____ present in arachnoid and ventricular spaces of brain
- Occurs more commonly in infants and children
- Sometimes occurs in adults as result of tumors or trauma
- Treatment
  - Surgical insertion of a shunt

CEREBRAL PALSY

- Group of _____ disorders that result from CNS damage sustained during the prenatal, neonatal, or postnatal periods
- Impairment ranges from slight motor dysfunction to catastrophic physical and mental disabilities
- Treatment is supportive and rehabilitative
- Currently, no cure exists

TRAUMA

- Traumatic injuries are _____ of neurological disorders
- Trauma often occurs as result of preventable injuries
- To help prevent these injuries
  - Encourage parents to require helmets for their children
  - Bike riding
  - Skateboarding
  - Encourage all patients to wear seat belts in motor vehicles

TRAUMATIC BRAIN INJURIES

- _____ population is particularly at risk for head trauma
  - Head is large in proportion to rest of body
  - They often fall head first
  - Reflex systems are immature
- Traumatic injuries include
  - Concussions
  - Contusions
  - Intracranial hemorrhages

CONCUSSIONS

- Nonlethal brain injury that results from blunt trauma
- Patient may experience momentary _____ but returns to an awake and alert state promptly
- Treatment involves rest and observations for signs of more serious injury

CONTUSION

- Involves a _____ of cerebral circulation
- Hemorrhages and extravasation of blood and fluid can result
- Loss of consciousness
- Brain damage may occur
- Patient may become confused, lethargic, and have nausea and vomiting

INTRACRANIAL HEMORRHAGES

- Bleeding of a vessel _____ due to
  - Trauma
  - Congenital abnormalities
  - Aneurysms

INTRACRANIAL HEMORRHAGES
(continued)

- ■ Treatment for contusions and hemorrhages
  - • Surgery
  - • Drug therapy
  - • Supportive care
- ■ Prognosis for all brain injuries
  - • Depends on _____ of damage and _____ of injury

Answer

_____

_____

_____

_____

_____

SPINAL CORD INJURIES

- ■ _____ spinal cord injury
  - • Cord is transected
  - • No neurologic abilities remain below point of injury
- ■ _____ spinal cord injury
  - • Cord is injured or partially severed
  - • Minor to severe neurologic disabilities below point of injury

SPINAL CORD INJURIES *(continued)*

- ■ Treatment
  - • Initial consideration is to _____ _____
  - • Treatment in emergency department focuses on stabilization
- ■ Patients usually require extended hospitalization and rehabilitation

SPINAL CORD INJURIES *(continued)*

- ■ In physician's office, patients
  - • May receive follow-up treatment and evaluation
  - • Be monitored for changes in their _____
  - • Be evaluated for physical and occupation therapy

CHECKPOINT QUESTION 4

How does a complete spinal cord injury differ from an incomplete one?

BRAIN TUMORS

- ■ May be either malignant or benign, many occur as metastatic sites
- ■ Symptoms
  - • Vague complaints of headaches
  - • _____
  - • Personality changes
  - • Memory loss

BRAIN TUMORS *(continued)*

- ■ More advanced cases
  - • Seizures
  - • Blindness
  - • _____
- ■ Treatment
  - • Surgery
  - • Radiation therapy
  - • Chemotherapy

HEADACHES

- ■ 70% of population experiences _____ or headaches
  - • May have variety of origins including
    - • Trauma
    - • Bone pathology
    - • Infections
    - • Vascular disturbances
- ■ In many instances
  - • Etiology will never be known

MIGRAINE HEADACHES

- ■ One of the most common types of headaches
- ■ Symptoms
  - • Preceded by an _____
  - • Unilateral temporal headache

- Photophobia
- Diplopia
- Nausea

MIGRAINE HEADACHES *(continued)*

- Treatment
  - _____
  - Rest in a dark, quiet room
  - Medications to stop headache when migraine begins

OTHER COMMON HEADACHES

- _____ headaches
  - Contraction of muscles of neck and scalp due to stress
  - Treatment involves muscle relaxants, analgesics, and reversing precipitating factors
- _____ headaches
  - Similar to migraine headaches
  - Typically occur at night
  - Treatment requires muscle relaxants, analgesics, and stress relief techniques

COMMON DIAGNOSTIC TESTS FOR DISORDERS OF THE NERVOUS SYSTEM

- Physical examination
- Radiologic tests
- _____
- Lumbar puncture

PHYSICAL EXAMINATION

- Key component in diagnosing nervous system disorders
  - Mental status and orientation
  - _____ assessment
  - Sensory and motor functions
  - Reflex assessment

RADIOLOGIC TESTS

- Computed tomography (CT) scan
- Magnetic resonance imaging (MRI)
- CT or MRI with contrast medium or dye

- _____
- Cerebral angiogram
- Radiography of skull

ELECTRICAL TESTS

- _____
  (EEG)
  - Noninvasive test
  - Records electrical impulses in brain
  - Variety of electrodes placed on patient's scalp
  - Tracings of brain wave activity are recorded
  - Patient typically given mild sedative to induce quiet state
  - Used to assess hyperactive electrical responses in brain as seen in patients with seizure disorders

 CHECKPOINT QUESTION 5

What are the differences between a myelogram and an EEG?

Answer

_____

_____

_____

_____

_____

LUMBAR PUNCTURE

- Procedure used to diagnose infectious, inflammatory, or bleeding disorders affecting the

  _____

  or as a means of injecting medications for pain control into the spinal column

LUMBAR PUNCTURE *(continued)*

- Needle is inserted into _____ space at level of L-4 to L-5, below the level of the spinal cord

- CSF is removed and sent to laboratory to be tested for
  - Glucose
  - Protein
  - Bacteria
  - Cell counts
  - Presence of red blood cells indicating intracranial bleeding
  - Evaluate intracranial pressure

LUMBAR PUNCTURE (continued)

- _____ test
  - Used to determine presence of an obstruction in the CSF flow

- Medical assistant presses against patient's jugular veins in the neck while physician monitors pressure of CSF

LUMBAR PUNCTURE (continued)

- If lumbar puncture is performed in medical office, medical assistant will
  - Assist patient into a side-lying, curled position or a supported, forward-bending sitting position
  - Maintain sterility of items used during puncture
  - Help patient to relax by encouraging slow, _____

Chapter 36

Allergy and Immunology

THE LYMPHATIC AND IMMUNE SYSTEMS

- Environment contains many infectious agents
  - Viruses
  - Bacteria
  - Fungi
  - Parasites
- Agents can cause _____ damage
- Intact immune system
  - Most infections do not last long
  - Permanent damage is rare

THE LYMPHATIC SYSTEM

- Includes
  - Lymph fluid
  - Lymph vessels
  - Lymph nodes
- Organs function as filters
  - _____
  - _____
  - _____

THE IMMUNE SYSTEM

- Body is protected by two types of defense
  - Nonspecific defense
  - Specific defense
- Defenses work against any invading pathogen (_____ defense) or against only a particular pathogen (_____ defenses)

NONSPECIFIC DEFENSES

- Include _____ defenses
  - Intact skin
  - Respiratory barriers
  - Digestive enzymes
  - Acidity of the genitourinary tract
  - Tears
  - Protective reflexes

NONSPECIFIC DEFENSES (continued)

- Other nonspecific defenses include
  - _____
  - Fever
  - Inflammation
  - Production of interferon

SPECIFIC DEFENSES

- _____
  - Ability to fight off a microorganism once infection has occurred

- ■ B cells
  - • Produced in bone marrow
  - • Mature in the spleen and lymph nodes
- ■ T cells
  - • Produced in thymus gland
  - • Circulate between blood and lymph

ANTIGENS

- ■ Antigens
  - • _____ that identify cells
- ■ When antigens are foreign
  - • Body recognizes them as dangerous
  - • Attempts to destroy them

ANTIBODIES

- ■ In response to foreign antigens
  - • Body produces proteins called antibodies
- ■ Antibodies become attached to foreign antigens and label them for _____ by phagocytes

CHECKPOINT QUESTION 1

What are antigens? What does the body form in response to foreign antigens?

Answer

_____
_____
_____
_____
_____

TYPES OF IMMUNITY

- ■ _____
- ■ _____
  - • Natural or artificial
  - • Active or passive
- ■ _____
  - • Active acquired artificial immunity

CHECKPOINT QUESTION 2

What are the three types of vaccines?

Answer

_____
_____
_____
_____
_____

COMMON LYMPHATIC DISORDERS

- ■ _____
- ■ _____
- ■ _____

LYMPHADENITIS

- ■ Inflammatory condition that results from a bacterial or viral infection
- ■ Symptoms
  - • Enlarged, tender _____
- ■ Treatment
  - • Directed at eliminating primary infection

MONONUCLEOSIS

- ■ Caused by _____ virus and affects entire lymphatic system
- ■ Symptoms
  - • Fatigue
  - • Asthenia
  - • Sore throat
  - • Enlarged tender lymph nodes
- ■ Treatment
  - • Symptomatic and palliative
- ■ Recovery
  - • Usually takes 4 to 8 weeks

CHECKPOINT QUESTION 3

In lymphadenitis, why do the lymph nodes become enlarged and tender?

Answer

_____
_____
_____
_____
_____

HODGKIN'S DISEASE

- _____ of lymph nodes
- Symptoms
  - Lymphadenopathy
  - Splenomegaly
  - Fever
  - Weakness
  - Anorexia
  - Weight loss
- Treatment
  - Radiotherapy
  - Chemotherapy

COMMON IMMUNE DISORDERS

- _____
- _____
- _____

ALLERGIES

- _____ to particular allergen
- Allergens
  - Plant pollens
  - Foods
  - Chemicals
  - Antibiotics
  - Mold spores

ALLERGIES (continued)

- Mild reaction
  - Severe rhinitis or hay fever
- Severe reaction
  - _____
- Treatment
  - Antihistamine medications

AUTOIMMUNITY

- Body fails to recognize its own proteins and produces antibodies that will _____ its own cells and tissues
- Examples
  - Rheumatoid arthritis
  - Chronic thyroiditis
  - Lupus erythematosus
  - Pernicious anemia
- No cure for autoimmune diseases

HUMAN IMMUNODEFICIENCY VIRUS (HIV)

- Pathogen that causes AIDS by destroying _____ and suppressing body's cell-mediated immune response
- Most often transmitted through
  - Exchange of blood or body fluids
  - Sharing contaminated needles
  - Transfusions of contaminated blood
  - Accidental injury from sharp instruments

HIV (continued)

- Stages
  1. Acute infectious stage
  2. Latent period
  3. Complaints of weight loss, lymphadenopathy, fever, diarrhea, anorexia, fatigue, and skin rashes
  4. Onset of immunodeficiency disorders
- HIV positive patients
  - Treated _____

CHECKPOINT QUESTION 4

How is HIV spread?

Answer

_____

_____

_____

_____

_____

COMMON DIAGNOSTIC AND THERAPEUTIC PROCEDURES

- Allergy testing
- Laboratory testing for HIV

ALLERGY TESTING

- Medical assistant's responsibilities
  - Obtain careful history of _____ _____
  - Prepare allergens as ordered by physician

- Assist with or perform allergy testing
- Follow up with patient education

- Patch tests
- Laboratory blood tests

ALLERGY TESTING *(continued)*

- Because of potential for anaphylaxis
  - Emergency equipment and medications must be available
- Allergy testing methods
  - Scratch tests
  - _____

LABORATORY TESTING FOR HIV

- _____ used to screen blood for antibodies to the AIDS virus
- Western blot test used to confirm positive findings
- Medical assistant's responsibility
  - Collecting specimen by phlebotomy and routing to proper laboratory

Chapter 37

Urology

INTRODUCTION

- Metabolism creates _____ that must be eliminated from body
- Several body systems prevent build-up of end-products
  - Gastrointestinal system
  - Respiratory system
  - Integumentary system

INTRODUCTION *(continued)*

- Urinary system
  - Removes waste from _____
  - Regulates fluid volume, electrolytes, blood pressure, and pH balance

COMMON URINARY DISORDERS

- Renal failure
- _____
- Tumors
- Hydronephrosis
- Urinary system infections

RENAL FAILURE

- Acute or chronic disorder of _____ _____ manifested by inability

of kidney to excrete wastes, concentrate urine, and aid in homeostatic electrolyte conservation
- Symptoms
  - General weakness
  - Edema of lungs and tissues
  - Neurologic symptoms

RENAL FAILURE *(continued)*

- Treatment
  - _____ to remove nitrogenous waste products and excess fluid from body
  - Hemodialysis
  - Peritoneal dialysis
- Dialysis is not a cure for renal dysfunction

CALCULI

- _____ formations found anywhere in urinary system
- Symptoms vary
  - Hematuria
  - Flank pain
- Treatment
  - May not be needed if stones are small
  - Lithotripsy
  - Diet adjustment

 CHECKPOINT QUESTION I

What are calculi and when are they more likely to form?

Answer

_____

_____

_____

_____

_____

TUMORS

- Urinary system may be primary or secondary site for tumors
- Symptoms vary
  - _____
  - Unexplained abdominal mass
- Treatment
  - Based on extent and type of tumor
  - May include surgery, chemotherapy, radiation, or combination

HYDRONEPHROSIS

- Distention of the renal pelvis and calyces resulting from an obstruction in the kidney or ureter
- Symptoms
  - _____
  - Hematuria
  - Pyuria
  - Fever
  - Chills
- Treatment
  - Cystoscopy
  - Nephrostomy
  - Ureterostomy

URINARY SYSTEM INFECTIONS

- Glomerulonephritis
- Pyelonephritis
- Cystitis
- _____

GLOMERULONEPHRITIS

- Inflammation of the _____
- Symptoms
  - Very mild edema
  - Proteinuria

- Hematuria
- Oliguria
- Complete renal failure
- Treatment
  - Usually symptomatic
  - Antibiotics

PYELONEPHRITIS

- Inflammation of _____ and body of the kidney
  - Usually results from ascending infection from ureters
  - May be acute or chronic

CYSTITIS

- Inflammation of the _____
  - More common in women due to shorter length of urethra
- Symptoms
  - Urinary frequency
  - Dysuria
  - Chills
  - Fever
  - Nausea
  - Vomiting
  - Flank pain
- Treatment
  - Antibiotics

URETHRITIS

- Inflammation of the _____
- Treatment for cystitis is also effective for urethritis

CHECKPOINT QUESTION 2

Why are women more likely than men to experience cystitis?

Answer

_____

_____

_____

_____

_____

COMMON DISORDERS OF THE MALE REPRODUCTIVE SYSTEM

- ■ _____
  - ■ Carcinoma of prostate gland
  - ■ Testicular cancer

BENIGN PROSTATIC HYPERPLASIA

- ■ Nonmalignant _____ of the prostate gland
- ■ As prostate gland enlarges
- ■ Causes urinary symptoms such as frequency and nocturia
- ■ Condition not usually serious problem
- ■ Treatment
  - • Medications
  - • Surgery

PROSTATE CANCER

- ■ Malignancy in tissues of prostate
- ■ If prostate gland is enlarged
  - • Biopsy of prostate
  - • _____
- ■ Treatment
  - • Surgery
  - • Chemotherapy
  - • Radiation

 CHECKPOINT QUESTION 3

Would the patient with BPH have an elevated prostate-specific antigen? Why or why not?

Answer

_____

_____

_____

_____

_____

TESTICULAR CANCER

- ■ Accounts for only _____ of all malignancies
- ■ Seen in men between ages of 15 and 34

- ■ Symptoms are gradual and painless
  - • Vague feeling of scrotal heaviness
- ■ Treatment
  - • Orchiectomy
  - • Chemotherapy
  - • Radiation

HYDROCELE

- ■ Collection of _____ within the scrotum and around the testes
- ■ If condition is extremely uncomfortable
  - • Excess fluid aspirated
- ■ If condition persists
  - • Surgical intervention
- ■ In most cases, no treatment is necessary

CRYPTORCHIDISM

- ■ One or both _____ testes
- ■ Treatment
  - • Orchiopexy
  - • Usually performed before age of 4 years
- ■ If not surgically corrected
  - • Will result in sterility of undescended organ
  - • May increase risk of testicular malignancy

INGUINAL HERNIA

- ■ Protrusion of _____ through abdominal wall
- ■ Symptoms
  - • Often asymptomatic
  - • May result in noticeable bulge and pain
- ■ Treatment
  - • Depends on patient's physical condition
  - • Herniorrhaphy

INFECTIONS

- ■ Most common infections of male reproductive system
  - • _____
  - • Orchitis
  - • Prostatitis

EPIDIDYMITIS

- ■ Usually results from an _____ or other inflammation in the urinary tract

■ Treatment
  • Antibiotics
  • Bed rest
  • Fluids
  • Palliative measures for pain

ORCHITIS

■ Inflammation of the _____
■ May also result in development of a hydrocele
■ Treatment
  • Antibiotics
  • Bed rest
  • Fluids
  • Palliative measures for pain

CHRONIC PROSTATITIS

■ Common among the _____
  and may be confused with prostatic
  hypertrophy
■ Symptoms
  • Inguinal pain
  • Fever
  • Low back and joint pain
  • Burning
  • Dysuria
  • Urethral discharge
■ Treatment
  • Antibiotics

IMPOTENCE

■ Inability to either achieve or maintain an
  _____
  • Psychogenic impotence
  • Organic impotence
■ Treatment
  • Vacuum tube system
  • Vitamin E injections
  • Medications
  • Penile implants

CHECKPOINT QUESTION 4

What are some microorganisms responsible for causing
infections in the male reproductive system?

Answer

_____

_____

_____

_____

_____

COMMON DIAGNOSTIC AND THERAPEUTIC PROCEDURES

■ _____
■ Blood tests
■ Cystoscopy (cystourethroscopy)
■ Intravenous pyelogram (IVP) and retrograde
  pyelogram
■ Ultrasound
■ Rectal and scrotal examinations
■ Vasectomy

URINALYSIS

■ Most important step in diagnosing urinary
  system diseases
■ Use _____ urine specimen
  • Patient performs clean-catch midstream
    procedure
  • Catheterization
■ Urinalysis includes
  • Physical and chemical evaluation
  • Specific gravity
  • Microscopic examination
  • Urine culture

BLOOD TESTS

■ Serum levels of _____,
  blood urea nitrogen (BUN), or creatinine may
  be indicated
■ Medical assistant's responsibilities
  • Draw patient's blood specimen
  • Process it on site or direct it to proper testing
    facility

CYSTOSCOPY (CYSTOURETHROSCOPY)

■ Direct visualization of the bladder and urethra
  with a _____
■ Medical assistant's responsibility
  • Provide preoperative instructions to patient

CHECKPOINT QUESTION 5

What is the most commonly performed test for disorders of the urinary system in the medical office?

Answer

_____

_____

_____

_____

_____

INTRAVENOUS PYELOGRAM (IVP)

- X-ray examination of kidneys and urinary tract using a _____ injected into circulatory system
- Medical assistant's responsibilities
  - Schedule examination at appropriate facility
  - Instruct patient in procedure preparations
  - Question patient about iodine allergies

RETROGRADE PYELOGRAM

- X-ray examination dye is introduced through a catheter into the _____
- Medical assistant's responsibilities
  - Make arrangements with appropriate facility
  - Give patient necessary instructions

 CHECKPOINT QUESTION 6

How does a retrograde pyelogram differ from an intravenous pyelogram?

Answer

_____

_____

_____

_____

_____

ULTRASOUND

- Noninvasive use of sound waves that can show the presence of stones and _____ in the urinary system and tissues
  - No special preparation required other than explanation of procedure to patient

RECTAL AND SCROTAL EXAMINATIONS

- Medical assistant's responsibilities
  - Instruct patient to disrobe from waist down
  - Provide appropriate material
- Physician will
  - Inspect and palpate _____
  - Perform digital rectal examination

RECTAL AND SCROTAL EXAMINATIONS (*continued*)

- Patients should perform testicular _____ at home
- Medical assistant's responsibilities
  - Educate patient about self-exam
  - Best time is following a warm shower
  - Perform frequently
  - Notify physician immediately if lumps or thickened areas are found

VASECTOMY

- Surgical removal of all or a segment of the _____ to prevent the passage of sperm from the testes
- Medical assistant's responsibilities
  - Instructing patient on preoperative orders
  - Assist physician
  - Assist patient into lithotomy position with appropriate draping

Chapter 38

Obstetrics and Gynecology

INTRODUCTION

- Gynecology
  - Specialty that deals with development and disorders of _____
    _____
- Obstetrics
  - Branch of medicine that cares patients through _____, childbirth, and postpartum period

INTRODUCTION (continued)

- _____
  - Age at which girl begins menses
- Menstrual cycle
  - About 28 days in length
  - Involves series of complex events in internal organs
  - Medical assistant should remind patients to record their cycle

GYNECOLOGIC DISORDERS

- Dysfunctional uterine bleeding
- Premenstrual syndrome (PMS)
- _____
- Uterine prolapse and displacement
- _____
- Gynecologic cancers
- Infertility
- Sexually transmitted diseases

DYSFUNCTIONAL UTERINE BLEEDING

- Abnormal or irregular uterine bleeding caused by an _____ imbalance
  - Menorrhagia
  - Metrorrhagia
  - Polymenorrhea
  - Postmenopausal bleeding

- Treatment
  - Hormone therapy
  - Oral contraceptives
  - Curettage of uterine cavity
  - Hysterectomy

 CHECKPOINT QUESTION I

What is the difference between menorrhagia and metrorrhagia?

Answer

_____

_____

_____

_____

_____

PREMENSTRUAL SYNDROME (PMS)

- Characterized by variety of physical, psychological, and behavioral symptoms occurring on regular, cyclic basis
- Symptoms usually diminish a few hours after onset of menses
- Treatment
  - Regular exercise
  - Dietary _____
  - Adequate rest and avoid unnecessary stress

ENDOMETRIOSIS

- Condition which endometrial tissue grows outside the _____
- Found in
  - Fallopian tubes
  - Ovaries
  - Uterosacral ligaments
  - Other parts of abdominal cavity
- Symptoms
  - Infertility
  - Dysmenorrhea
  - Pelvic pain
  - Dyspareunia

ENDOMETRIOSIS (continued)

- Treatment
  - Hormone and drug therapy to _____
    _____ growth of tissue

- Laparoscopic excision of tissue using laser or cautery
- Severe cases, hysterectomy with possible bilateral salpingo-oophorectomy

CHECKPOINT QUESTION 2

What are some symptoms of endometriosis?

Answer

_____

_____

_____

_____

_____

UTERINE PROLAPSE

- Uterus droops or protrudes downward into
  _____
- Symptoms
  - Pelvic pressure
  - Dyspareunia
  - Urinary problems
  - Constipation

UTERINE PROLAPSE (continued)

- Treatment
  - Hysterectomy
  - _____
  - Colpocleisis
- Medical management
  - Hormone therapy
  - Use of pessary

UTERINE DISPLACEMENT

- Uterus is _____
  from natural position
- Symptoms
  - Pressure in rectal area or against bladder
  - Usually just troublesome to patient
- Treatment
  - Follows same protocol as required for uterine prolapse

LEIOMYOMAS

- _____ tumors of uterus, including fibroid tumors, myomas, and fibromyomas
- May be located in
  - Endometrium
  - Myometrium
  - Perimetrium
- Most patients are asymptomatic

LEIOMYOMAS (continued)

- Large tumors
  - Tend to distort uterus
  - More likely to be _____
  - Abnormal bleeding
  - Pelvic pressure and discomfort
  - Constipation
  - Urinary frequency
  - Infertility

LEIOMYOMAS (continued)

- Treatment depends on size of tumor
  - Small asymptomatic tumors monitored to detect excessive growth
  - _____ or hysterectomy for large tumors

CHECKPOINT QUESTION 3

How are uterine prolapse and uterine displacement different?

Answer

_____

_____

_____

_____

_____

OVARIAN CYSTS

- Numerous types of benign ovarian cysts
  - Functional cysts
  - _____ ovaries

FUNCTIONAL CYSTS

- Fairly common
- _____ that causes few, if any, problems
- Patient is most often asymptomatic unless cyst is large or ruptures
- Treatment
  - Puncture
  - Excision

POLYCYSTIC OVARY SYNDROME

- More troublesome and complex disorder
- Affects both ovaries
- Symptoms
  - _____
  - Irregular menses or amenorrhea
  - Hirsutism
- Treatment
  - Depends on patient's desire for future pregnancy
  - Management includes hormone therapy or oral contraceptives

GYNECOLOGIC CANCERS

- Cervical and breast cancers
  - Excellent prognosis when detected and treated early
  - If left untreated or diagnosed in later stages, these cancers are deadly
  - Instruct all female patients to perform _____ every month
  - Encourage yearly physical that includes breast exam and Pap smear

INFERTILITY

- Causes of female infertility may include
  - Uterine or cervical abnormalities
  - _____ or scarring
  - Hormonal imbalance
  - Psychological factors
- Treatment involves identifying and correcting problem

CHECKPOINT QUESTION 4

What two factors greatly affect the prognosis of all cancers?

Answer

_____

_____

_____

_____

_____

SEXUALLY TRANSMITTED DISEASES (STDS)

- STDs are easily transmitted
  - Must be reported to local _____ _____ by medical office
  - Patient should be encouraged to notify sexual partners so that they may also receive treatment

ACQUIRED IMMUNODEFICIENCY SYNDROME (AIDS)

- Infectious disease that overwhelms the body's _____
  - Caused by human immunodeficiency virus (HIV)
- Transmission of HIV occurs through exchange of blood or body fluids

AIDS (continued)

- Stages as infection progresses to AIDS
  1. Acute infectious state
  2. _____ period
  3. Weight loss, lymphadenopathy, fever, diarrhea, anorexia, fatigue, and skin rashes
  4. Onset of immunodeficiency disorders

CHLAMYDIA

- Infections by *Chlamydia trachomatis* cause
  - _____ in men
  - Cervicitis in women
  - Lymphogranuloma venereum in both
- Chlamydia is one of leading causes of pelvic inflammatory disease

CHLAMYDIA (continued)

- Symptoms
  - Women may be asymptomatic or present with vague, flu-like symptoms
  - Severe cases, extensive _____ involvement known as lymphogranuloma venereum
- Treatment
  - Antibiotics such as doxycycline, tetracycline, or sulfamethoxazole

CONDYLOMATA ACUMINATA

- _____ of genital area causing growth of soft, papillary warts
  - Vulva
  - Vagina
  - Cervical perineum
- Treatment
  - Cryotherapy
  - Laser ablation

GONORRHEA

- Second most common STD, caused by *N. gonorrhoeae*
- Symptoms
  - Appear in genitalia 2 to 8 days after exposure
  - In some women, Bartholin's and Skene's glands fill with pus and infection may spread
- Treatment
  - _____

SYPHILIS

- After AIDS, syphilis most serious STD, caused by *Treponema pallidum*
- Symptoms
  - First phase, _____ or ulcerated lesion
  - Second phase, rash that may appear anywhere on body
- Treatment
  - Penicillin

HERPES GENITALIS

- Virus caused by herpes simplex virus 2
- Symptoms
  - Painful _____ in genital area

- Rupture and leave equally painful ulcers
- Swollen and tender lymph nodes
- Flu-like symptoms

HERPES GENITALIS (continued)

- Patients should be advised to avoid sexual contact during episodes of _____ _____
- No cure
  - Somewhat controlled with antiviral agents such as acyclovir

VULVOVAGINITIS

- Inflammation of the vulva and vagina
- Symptoms
  - _____
  - Burning of the vulva or the vagina (or both)
  - Increased vaginal discharge
- Type of discharge often indicates cause of disorder
- Effective treatment depends on cause

SALPINGITIS/PID

- Bacterial infection of the _____ most often transmitted by sexual intercourse; sometimes called PID when surrounding structures are inflamed
  - Pelvic peritoneum
  - Uterus
  - Ovaries, and surrounding tissues

SALPINGITIS/PID (continued)

- Symptoms
  - Abdominal pain and tenderness, with or without fever
  - _____
- Treatment for mild infections
  - Antibiotic and analgesic therapy
  - Bed rest
  - Removal of source of infection

SALPINGITIS/PID (continued)

- Treatment for serious infections
  - _____ with bilateral salpingectomy-oophorectomy

- Incision and drainage for patients with pyosalpinx, tubal obstruction, abscess, serious inflammation and edema

CHECKPOINT QUESTION 5

Which sexually transmitted disease is associated with a female reproductive cancer?

Answer

_____

_____

_____

_____

_____

COMMON DIAGNOSTIC AND THERAPEUTIC PROCEDURES

- The gynecologic examination
- Colposcopy
- _____
- Dilatation and curettage (D&C)

THE GYNECOLOGIC EXAMINATION

- As physician
  - Examines breasts
  - Performs pelvic examination
  - Obtains _____ smear
- Medical assistant will instruct patient not to
  - Douche
  - Use vaginal medications
  - Have sexual intercourse for 24 hours before examination

THE GYNECOLOGIC EXAMINATION *(continued)*

- When preparing for pelvic examination
  - Ensure that vaginal speculum is correct size for patient
  - Warm speculum
  - Establish rapport with patient

CHECKPOINT QUESTION 6

What procedures does the physician perform as part of a complete gynecologic examination?

Answer

_____

_____

_____

_____

COLPOSCOPY

- Visual examination of vaginal and cervical surfaces using a _____
- Used to evaluate patients with atypical Pap smear results
- If biopsy is to be done
  - Obtain written consent
  - Label specimen containers and complete laboratory request forms

HYSTEROSALPINGOGRAPHY

- Uterus and fallopian tubes are radiographed after injection of _____ _____
- Determines
  - Configuration of uterus
  - Patency of fallopian tubes
- Medical assistant's responsibilities
  - Schedule procedure
  - Educate patient

DILATATION AND CURETTAGE (D&C)

- Surgical procedure performed to
  - Remove uterine tissue for diagnostic testing
  - Remove _____ tissue
  - Prevent or treat menorrhagia
  - Remove retained products of conception
- Procedure usually requires anesthesia

DILATATION AND CURETTAGE
(continued)

- Medical assistant's responsibilities
  - Obtain signed _____
  - Give preoperative and postoperative instructions

OBSTETRIC CARE

- Obstetricians frequently called to hospital to deliver infants during regular office hours
- In absence of physician
  - Medical assistant must use good judgment
  - Follow _____ listed in policy and procedure manual
  - Help ensure that safe procedures are followed for patients

DIAGNOSIS OF PREGNANCY

- _____ signs
  - Amenorrhea
  - Nausea
  - Vomiting
  - Breast enlargement and tenderness
  - Fatigue
  - Urinary frequency

DIAGNOSIS OF PREGNANCY
(continued)

- _____ signs
  - Presence of HCG in maternal urine or blood
  - Changes in uterus and cervix
  - Occurrence of Braxton-Hicks contractions
  - Enlargement of uterus

 CHECKPOINT QUESTION 7

Why are presumptive signs and symptoms of pregnancy not considered to be conclusive?

Answer

_____

_____

_____

_____

_____

FIRST PRENATAL VISIT

- First visit includes
  - Confirmation of pregnancy
  - Complete history and physical
  - Determination of _____ or
    _____
  - Assessment of gestational age
  - Identification of risk factors
  - Patient education

FIRST PRENATAL VISIT *(continued)*

- Physical exam and laboratory tests include
  - Pelvic examination with Pap smear
  - Pregnancy test
  - Clinical _____
  - Laboratory blood tests
- Medical assistant should
  - Reinforce physician's instructions
  - Encourage patient to call with questions

FIRST PRENATAL VISIT *(continued)*

- Patients notify physician if any of the following occur
  - Vaginal bleeding or spotting
  - Persistent vomiting
  - Fever or chills
  - Dysuria
  - Abdominal or uterine cramping
  - Leaking _____
  - Alteration in fetal development
  - Dizziness or blurred vision
  - Other problems

SUBSEQUENT PRENATAL VISITS

- If pregnancy is progressing without
  _____
  - Patient is seen at 12, 16, 20, 24, and 28 weeks
  - Seen every 2 weeks during last 2 months and weekly after 36th week

 CHECKPOINT QUESTION 8

The pregnant patient should be advised to contact the physician when what problems occur?

Answer

_____

_____

_____

_____

_____

ONSET OF LABOR

- Labor is the _____
  leading to expelling the fetus from the uterus
- Characterized by
  - Regular uterine contractions
  - Appearance of "bloody show"
  - Rupture of amniotic sac

POSTPARTUM CARE

- _____ is period
  from childbirth until reproductive structures
  return to normal
- Postpartum visit includes
  - Complete gynecologic and breast
    examination
  - Patient counseling
  - Weight and vital signs
  - Urinalysis
  - Hematocrit
  - Hemoglobin
  - Physician may assess lochia

CHECKPOINT QUESTION 9

What is lochia? Name and describe the three types.

Answer

_____

_____

_____

_____

_____

OBSTETRIC DISORDERS

- Ectopic pregnancy
- _____

- Abortion
- Preeclampsia and eclampsia
- Placenta previa and abruptio placentae

ECTOPIC PREGNANCY

- Gestation in which fertilized ovum implants
  somewhere other than uterine cavity
  - Usually, in fallopian tube
  - Referred to as _____
- Patient may present with signs of early
  pregnancy including
  - Breast enlargement or tenderness
  - Nausea
  - Absent or delayed menses

ECTOPIC PREGNANCY *(continued)*

- Present early in pregnancy
  - _____
  - Syncope
  - Abdominal symptoms
  - Painful sexual intercourse
  - Irregular bleeding

ECTOPIC PREGNANCY *(continued)*

- If not diagnosed early
  - Potential for _____
    of fallopian tube
- Treatment
  - Surgical excision of ectopic pregnancy
    through either laparoscopy or laparotomy

HYPEREMESIS GRAVIDARUM

- Nausea and vomiting, commonly called
  _____
  - Expected during early pregnancy
- Treatment
  - Small, frequent meals
  - Adequate hydration
  - Patient reassurance

HYPEREMESIS GRAVIDARUM
(continued)

- If vomiting becomes unrelenting, can lead to
  - _____
  - Electrolyte imbalance
  - Weight loss
- Occasionally, patient must be hospitalized

ABORTION

- Spontaneous abortion
  - More common in _____
  - Defined as loss of pregnancy before the fetus is viable
- First symptom—vaginal bleeding followed by uterine cramps and low back pain

PREECLAMPSIA AND ECLAMPSIA

- _____ that is directly related to pregnancy
  - Preeclampsia
  - Eclampsia

PREECLAMPSIA

- Hypertension occurring after _____ of gestation
  - Proteinuria
  - Edema of lower extremities
- As condition progresses
  - Blurred vision
  - Headaches
  - Edema
  - Vomiting

PREECLAMPSIA (continued)

- Management includes
  - Restricted activities
  - _____
  - Sexual abstinence
  - Antihypertensive therapy
  - Well-balanced meals
- Close monitoring of patient
- Risk of developing eclampsia increases with advancing pregnancy

ECLAMPSIA

- Almost always preceded by preeclampsia
- Sudden onset
- Clinical signs of preeclampsia become more severe
- Characterized by _____ that may be followed by coma, hypertensive crisis, shock
- Management
  - Stabilizing patient
  - Inducing delivery of baby

PLACENTA PREVIA

- Condition in which placenta is implanted either partially or completely over the internal _____
- Symptoms
  - May have painless vaginal bleeding during 2nd or 3rd trimester

PLACENTA PREVIA (continued)

- Easily diagnosed by _____
- Medical management includes
  - Bed rest
  - Drug therapy if patient is preterm
- If patient is near term and bleeding is severe
  - Delivery of baby is essential

ABRUPTION PLACENTAE

- Premature _____ of placenta from uterus
- Symptoms
  - Pain
  - Uterine tenderness
  - Bleeding
  - Signs of impending shock
  - Fetal distress or death
- If confirmed
  - Baby is usually delivered by cesarean section

CHECKPOINT QUESTION 10

What is placenta previa and how is it managed in a preterm patient?

Answer

_____

_____

_____

_____

_____

COMMON OBSTETRIC TESTS AND PROCEDURES

- Pregnancy test
- _____ (AFP)
- Fetal ultrasonography
- Contraction stress test and nonstress test

PREGNANCY TEST

- Many OTC pregnancy tests are available for patients to use at home

ALPHA FETOPROTEIN (AFP)

- Test performed at 16 to 18 weeks of gestation
- Levels of AFP are obtained to screen for possible defects in _____
- Positive results indicate need for further studies

AMNIOCENTESIS

- Involves insertion of needle through abdomen into gravid uterus to remove fluid from _____
- Fluid is analyzed for variety of disorders
- Medical assistant's responsibilities
  - Preparing patient
  - Assisting physician
  - Preparing specimen for transportation to laboratory
  - Giving patient postprocedure instructions

FETAL ULTRASONOGRAPHY

- Use of high-frequency sound waves to create an image of the fetus
- Performed to assess the size, _____ _____, position, number of fetuses, fetal structures, development

CONTRACTION STRESS TEST (CST)

- Performed to determine how fetus will tolerate uterine contractions in third trimester
  - Nipple-stimulating CST
  - Oxytocin-stimulated CST
- Fetal _____ and movement are monitored in relation to uterine contractions

NONSTRESS TEST

- _____ obstetric procedure used to evaluate fetal heart tones and movement in relation to spontaneous uterine contractions
  - Can be safely performed in medical office

CONTRACEPTION

- Many methods available
- Decision involves many factors
  - Patient's religious, cultural, and personal beliefs
  - Health history, financial situation, and motivation
- Help patient understand
  - Indications
  - Risk factors
  - Cost
  - _____

MENOPAUSE

- Developmental stage of life during which ovulation ceases
- Changes early in menopause
  - _____
  - Amenorrhea
  - Dysfunctional uterine bleeding
  - _____
  - Flushing
  - Perspiration

MENOPAUSE (continued)

- Decrease in circulating estrogen is risk factor for
  - _____
  - Coronary heart disease
  - Osteoporosis
- Supplemental estrogen
  - Protects cardiovascular and skeletal disorders
  - Decreases menopausal symptoms

MENOPAUSE (continued)

- To ease transition through menopause, recommend
  - _____
  - Healthy diet
  - Vitamin and mineral supplements
- Encourage
  - Regular pelvic examinations
  - Pap smears
  - Breast examinations
  - Mammograms

Chapter 39

Pediatrics

THE PEDIATRIC PRACTICE

- Pediatrics is the medical specialty devoted to the care of infants, children, and adolescents
- Medical assistants must understand the needs of _____

SAFETY

- Safety is a prime concern when choosing toys and equipment for a pediatric office
- Toys should be examined frequently and _____ when damaged or soiled

SAFETY *(continued)*

- Follow these tips
  - Place infant scales on sturdy table
  - Store disinfection solutions away from patient care areas
  - Dispose of all sharps in proper containers
  - Practice stringent _____ and standard precautions

 CHECKPOINT QUESTION 1

What are three safety precautions that should be used in a pediatric office?

Answer

_____

_____

_____

_____

_____

THE WELL-CHILD OFFICE VISIT

- Regularly scheduled office visits based on child's age with goal of maintaining child's optimum health

- Includes complete examination, evaluation of child's _____ and _____ development, and immunizations

IMMUNIZATIONS

- Hepatitis B (HBV)
- Diphtheria, tetanus, acellular pertussis (DTaP)
- Poliomyelitis (IPV)
- Mumps, measles, and rubella (_____)
- Haemophilus influenzae type B (HiB)
- Varicella zoster (VZV)
- Hepatitis A
- Pneumococcal vaccine

IMMUNIZATIONS *(continued)*

- Influenza vaccine
- Meningococcal vaccine
- If responsible for administering vaccines, you must read all package inserts and become familiar with the correct administration and

  _____
- In addition, give caregiver written information about each vaccine your are administering

THE SICK-CHILD OFFICE VISIT

- Diagnosis and treatment of the child's immediate _____
- After examining child, physician may pursue diagnostic tests and treatments
  - X-rays
  - Laboratory tests
  - Medication
  - Reassurance that illness will run predictable and manageable course

 CHECKPOINT QUESTION 2

What is the difference between well-child and sick-child visits?

Answer

_____

_____

_____

_____

_____

_____

CHILD DEVELOPMENT

- ■ _____ aspects of care
- ■ _____ aspects of care

PSYCHOLOGICAL ASPECTS OF CARE

- ■ During an office visit, pediatric patient may feel fearful and _____
- ■ Medical assistant should reassure pediatric patients and family members
- ■ Encourage parents to remain with children and assist in care

PSYCHOLOGICAL ASPECTS OF CARE *(continued)*

- ■ Many _____ patients prefer to be alone with physician to
  - • Demonstrate their independence
  - • Discuss matters without parents present
- ■ Depending on maturity ask patient if parent should be present during examination

CHECKPOINT QUESTION 3

What kinds of feelings might a pediatric patient experience during an office visit?

Answer

_____

_____

_____

_____

_____

PHYSIOLOGIC ASPECTS OF CARE

- ■ Medical assistant must have a broad knowledge of child growth and development patterns
- ■ _____ is complete, but immature at birth
- ■ Denver Developmental Screening Test (DDST) is a popular tool

THE PEDIATRIC PHYSICAL EXAMINATION

- ■ Medical assistant's responsibilities
  - • _____

- • Restrain patient as necessary
- • Document history and chief complaint
- • Collect specimens

THE PEDIATRIC PHYSICAL EXAMINATION *(continued)*

- ■ When approaching pediatric patient, you should
  - • Have calm and cheerful manner
  - • Use _____ but gentle touch
  - • Involve parents as much as possible

THE PEDIATRIC HISTORY

- ■ Starts with history of mother's pregnancy, labor, and delivery
- ■ As child grows, includes
  - • Childhood illnesses
  - • _____
  - • Immunizations
  - • Nutritional status

OBTAINING AND RECORDING MEASUREMENTS AND VITAL SIGNS

- ■ Before physical exam, obtain
  - • _____
  - • Head and chest circumference
  - • Weight
  - • Temperature
  - • Pulse and respiratory rate
  - • Blood pressure
  - • Graph on growth chart and determine percentiles

CHECKPOINT QUESTION 4

Why is it important to track a child's anthropometric measurements?

Answer

_____

_____

_____

_____

_____

PEDIATRIC VITAL SIGNS

- Temperature
- Pulse and respiration
- _____

TEMPERATURE

- May be measured by axillary, oral, rectal, or tympanic methods
- If child is compliant, axillary route is viable choice
- Tympanic method is gaining popularity
- Oral measurements may be used with older child
- Rectal route used for _____

PULSE AND RESPIRATION

- Pulse rate affected by
  - Activity
  - Body temperature
  - Emotions
  - Illness
- Children's heart rates are considerably _____ than adults
- Measure respiratory rate by observing rise and fall of child's chest

BLOOD PRESSURE

- Difficult measurement to obtain in an infant or child
- Not required for most pediatric patients
- Children have _____ blood pressures than adults

 CHECKPOINT QUESTION 5

How does a child's pulse and respiratory rate differ from an adult's?

Answer

_____

_____

_____

_____

_____

USING RESTRAINTS

- Restraining is sometimes necessary to protect child from injury and to help physician complete examination
- Many children resist examination or procedures because they are frightened
- Use calm and _____ restraint

ADMINISTERING MEDICATIONS

- Medication dosages for children are calculated by weight or _____
- To prevent errors, always check drug dosage calculations for an infant or child with another staff member

THE SEVEN "RIGHTS" OF DRUG ADMINISTRATION

- Right _____
- Right _____
- Right _____
- Right _____
- Right _____
- Right _____
- Right _____

ORAL MEDICATIONS

- Use caution to prevent aspiration
- Hold infants in semi-reclining position, place medication on either side of tongue
- Depending on age, use medication spoon, syringe, dropper, or medicine cup
- Administer small amounts, allowing child time to _____

INJECTIONS

- Children fear injections
- Approach child in calm and firm manner
- Never _____ to child or say that injection will not hurt
- After injection, praise and comfort child

 CHECKPOINT QUESTION 6

How is medication dosage calculated for children?

Answer

_____

_____

_____

_____

_____

COLLECTING A URINE SPECIMEN

- ■ For infants and small children, use pediatric
  _____
- ■ Once applied, device should be left in place until infant urinates in bag
- ■ Diaper may be placed on infant with collection device in place

UNDERSTANDING CHILD ABUSE

- ■ Federal Child Abuse Prevention and Treatment Act mandates that threats to a child's physical and mental welfare must be reported by anyone having contact with children in a professional or employment setting
- ■ Medical assistants are _____
  _____
- ■ Medical assistants must be aware of the signs of abuse

SIGNS OF ABUSE

- ■ Obvious implications
  - Reports of physical or sexual abuse by child
  - Previous reports of abuse
  - _____ stories about injury
  - Injuries inconsistent with history
  - Injuries blamed on
    _____
  - Repeated emergency room visits
  - Fractures, burns, or skeletal injuries of suspicious nature

SIGNS OF ABUSE *(continued)*

- ■ Hidden indications
  - _____
  - Nervous system trauma
  - Internal injuries

- ■ Behavioral indications
  - Children who are overly _____
  - Passive avoidance
  - Extremely aggressive behavior
  - Role reversal, "parenting" the parent
  - Developmental delays

SIGNS OF ABUSE *(continued)*

- ■ Warning signs
  - Malnutrition
  - _____
  - Poor hygiene
  - Gross dental disorders
  - Unattended medical needs

PEDIATRIC ILLNESSES AND DISORDERS

- ■ Because children do not have well-developed
  _____
  - More susceptible to viruses and bacterial infections
  - Sick-child visits occur frequently during early childhood
  - Some children experience febrile seizures

PEDIATRIC ILLNESS AND DISORDERS *(continued)*

- ■ Parents should be instructed
  - How to obtain child's temperature and be encouraged to call office for any evidence of fever
  - To never give _____ to young children with viral fevers

IMPETIGO

- ■ Patches of _____
  vesicles that produce honey-colored crusts
- ■ Common integumentary disorder
- ■ Contagious
- ■ Treatment
  - Wash area 2 to 3 times a day
  - Apply topical antibiotic
  - Oral antibiotics
  - Discourage scratching
  - Advise parents to separate and wash towels, washcloths, and bed linens

MENINGITIS

- Inflammation of meninges covering spinal cord and brain
- Viral meningitis is usually not life-threatening and is short lived
- _____ meningitis is often severe and may be fatal

MENINGITIS *(continued)*

- Signs and symptoms
  - _____
  - Vomiting
  - Fever
  - Headaches
  - _____
  - Rash with small, reddish purple dots
  - May become comatose and develop seizures

MENINGITIS *(continued)*

- Treatment is based on microorganism
- Viral meningitis
  - Treated with oral fluids and bed rest
- Bacterial meningitis
  - Treated with antibiotics
  - Generally requires _____

 CHECKPOINT QUESTION 7

How does the treatment of viral meningitis differ from that of bacterial meningitis?

Answer

_____

_____

_____

_____

_____

ENCEPHALITIS

- Inflammation of the _____
- Symptoms
  - Drowsiness
  - Headaches
  - Fever in early stages
  - Seizures and coma may occur in later stages

- Treatment
  - Requires hospitalization for intravenous therapy and supportive care

TETANUS

- Infection of nervous tissue caused by *Clostridium tetani*
- Bacilli enter body through _____ or open areas in skin
- All deep, dirty wounds should be treated as high risk for tetanus

 CHECKPOINT QUESTION 8

What is the best way to prevent polio?

Answer

_____

_____

_____

_____

_____

CEREBRAL PALSY

- Group of _____ that result from CNS damage during prenatal, neonatal, or postnatal development
- Impairments may range from slight to catastrophic
- Treatment
  - Supportive and rehabilitative

CROUP

- _____ primarily seen in children 3 months to 3 years of age
- Symptoms
  - High-pitched crowing wheeze on inspiration
  - Sharp barking cough
- Treatment
  - Hospitalization
  - Cool mist vaporizers
  - Medications to decrease swelling

EPIGLOTTITIS

- _____ of epiglottis, may present similarly to croup
- Usually more serious and may be life threatening
- Child must be transported immediately to the hospital

CYSTIC FIBROSIS

- Inherited disease that causes _____ to be extremely thick and sticky
- Most serious complications are usually respiratory
- Treatment
  - Medications to reduce thickness of secretions
  - Frequent breathing treatments to maintain open airways

CHECKPOINT QUESTION 9

Why is epiglottitis considered a medical emergency?

Answer

_____

_____

_____

_____

_____

ASTHMA

- Reversible inflammatory process involving bronchi and _____
- Attacks triggered by
  - Exposure to allergens
  - Inhaled irritants
  - Upper respiratory infections
- Treatment
  - Bronchodilators through inhaler
  - Pulse rate should be monitored

OTITIS MEDIA

- Inflammation or infection of the

  _____

- Symptoms
  - Severe pain
  - Fever
  - Mild to moderate hearing loss
  - Infants may be fussy

- Treatment
  - Antibiotics and analgesics
  - Decongestants
  - Surgery

TONSILLITIS

- Inflammation of the throat and/or the tonsils
- Signs and symptoms
  - Tissue of throat _____
  - Pustules on tonsils or in throat
- Throat culture to rule out streptococcus
- Treatment
  - Antibiotics
  - Tonsillectomy

CHECKPOINT QUESTION 10

Why is otitis media more common in children rather than adults?

Answer

_____

_____

_____

_____

_____

OBESITY

- Obesity in children has become an epidemic
- Prevention of obesity is important
- Ask parents about
  - Eating patterns
  - Nutrition status
  - _____ of child
- Educate parents about eating in moderation and increasing physical activity

ATTENTION DEFICIT HYPERACTIVITY DISORDER (ADHD)

- Condition of the brain that causes difficulty in

  _____

- Problematic behavior in school
  - Daydreaming
  - Easily distracted
  - Inability to complete tasks
  - Forgetfulness

- Reluctance in performing tasks that require mental effort
- Low grades in school

ADHD *(continued)*

- ■ Hyperactivity often seen as
  - • _____
  - • Inability to sit quietly

- • Breaking rules regarding running or jumping
- ■ Treatment
  - • Behavior therapy
  - • Psychological counseling
  - • Education about ADHD
  - • Coordination plan with family and teachers
  - • Stimulant medications

Chapter 40

Geriatrics

CONCEPTS OF AGING

- ■ Established concepts about the aging process have changed
- ■ _____
  - • Specialists who study aging process
- ■ Geriatrics
  - • Branch of medicine that deals with the elderly population

REINFORCING MEDICAL COMPLIANCE IN THE ELDERLY

- ■ Establish good rapport with elderly clients to ensure compliance
  - • Write instructions in easy-to-understand terms
  - • Use _____
  - • Have patient repeat instructions
  - • Ask patient to perform a procedure
  - • Give patient appointment calendar

REINFORCING MEDICAL COMPLIANCE IN THE ELDERLY (CONTINUED)

- ■ At every visit, take complete account of all medications
  - • Prescribed
  - • _____
  - • Herbal supplements or vitamins
- ■ Have patients bring all medications to office

 CHECKPOINT QUESTION 1

What are some reasons that a patient may not be compliant with a prescribed treatment plan?

Answer

_____

_____

_____

_____

_____

REINFORCING MENTAL HEALTH IN THE ELDERLY

- ■ _____ between mental and physical health
- ■ Be aware of mental health status in patients with physical conditions

REINFORCING MENTAL HEALTH IN THE ELDERLY *(continued)*

- ■ Maintain open communication
- ■ Help patient express feelings of guilt or _____
- ■ Encourage positive self-image
- ■ Assist family in positive support system
- ■ Don't be discouraging or offer false hope
- ■ Direct to support groups

 CHECKPOINT QUESTION 2

How can you help promote good mental health in your elderly patients?

Answer

_____

_____

_____

_____

_____

COPING WITH AGING

- Most elderly people are generally _____
  _____
- But some feel overwhelming stress and grief
- Stress
  - Compromises immune system
  - Raises blood pressure and blood sugar levels
  - Strains heart and lungs

COPING WITH AGING *(continued)*

- Help patients cope with stress by
  - Listening to their fears
  - _____
    their right to have these feelings
  - Helping them reduce the stressors in their lives

ALCOHOL

- Alcohol abuse may be mistaken for
  - _____
  - TIAs
  - CNS impairment
- Medications may react badly with alcohol
- Identifying these patients can be difficult
- Refer to mental health professional or
  community resource

SUICIDE

- With ill health, multiple losses, deep
  depression, suicide may seem preferable to life
- Generally well planned and successful
- Often involve white men over 65, who have
  recently lost a _____

SUICIDE *(continued)*

- Watch for
  - Deepening _____

- Increasing anger
- Increase in alcoholism
- Loss of interest in health
- _____ behavior
- Sharp mood swings
- Giving away favored objects
- Take seriously those who express intent to
  commit suicide

CHECKPOINT QUESTION 3

What are some signs of suicidal intent?

Answer

_____

_____

_____

_____

_____

LONG-TERM CARE

- Three types
  1. Group homes or assisted living facilities
  2. Long-term care facilities
  3. _____ facilities

CHECKPOINT QUESTION 4

How are long-term facilities and skill nursing facilities
different?

Answer

_____

_____

_____

_____

_____

ELDER ABUSE

- As prevalent as child abuse
- Common risk factors
  - Multiple, chronic illnesses that stress
    family's resources

- Senile dementia
- _____
- Sleep disturbances
- Dependence on caretaker for daily living

ELDER ABUSE (continued)

- Several forms
  - _____
  - Active neglect
  - Psychological abuse
  - Financial abuse
  - Physical abuse
- If you suspect abuse or neglect, bring to attention of physician

SIGNS OF ABUSE

- Wounds of suspicious origin
- Signs of _____
- Neglected pressure ulcers
- Poor hygiene or nutrition
- Dehydration
- Untreated injuries or medical conditions
- Excessive agitation or apathetic resignation

CHECKPOINT QUESTION 5

What are the different types of elder abuse?

Answer

_____

_____

_____

_____

_____

MEDICATIONS AND THE ELDERLY

- Body's systems slow down
  - GI system has _____ in peristalsis
  - Circulatory system does not absorb or deliver medications quickly
  - Liver does not biotransform as well
  - Kidneys don't filter as well

MEDICATIONS AND ELDERLY
(continued)

- Guidelines
  1. Explain side effects, precautions, interactions, expected actions
  2. Explain proper dosage and how to measure it.
  3. Write out _____ and suggest methods to help patient remember

MEDICATIONS AND ELDERLY
(continued)

  4. Tell patient to take most important medication _____
  5. Encourage patient not to rush
  6. Tell them to ask pharmacist for large print on label

CHECKPOINT QUESTION 6

How can you help your elderly patients follow the medication regimen prescribed by the physician?

Answer

_____

_____

_____

_____

_____

SYSTEMIC CHANGES IN THE ELDERLY

- Longevity is largely

  _____
- When cells have reached a specific reproduction level, they either will not replace themselves or they will replicate more slowly or ineffectively

DISEASES OF THE ELDERLY

- _____ disease
- _____ disease

PARKINSON'S DISEASE

- Slow, progressive _____
  _____ that affects specific cells
  of the brain
- Affects men more than women
- Cause unknown

PARKINSON'S DISEASE *(continued)*

- Signs and symptoms
  - _____
  - Bradykinesia
  - Difficulty walking
  - Forward bending posture
  - Laryngeal rigidity
  - Pharyngeal rigidity
  - Facial muscle rigidity
  - Small tremors in fingers

PARKINSON'S DISEASE *(continued)*

- Parkinson's has no cure
- Treatment is symptomatic, supportive, and
  _____
  - Medications
  - Deep brain stimulation

PARKINSON'S DISEASE *(continued)*

- Patients retain _____
  functions
- They require psychological support
  - Encourage participation in all activities of
    daily living
  - Promote independence
  - Suggest increased fluid intake and balanced
    diet

PARKINSON'S DISEASE *(continued)*

- Encourage patient to use eating aids, raised
  toilet seats, handrails
- Listen to patient
- Educate patient about
  _____
- Enlist help of support groups

CHECKPOINT QUESTION 7

How can you assist a patient with Parkinson's disease?

Answer

_____
_____
_____
_____
_____

ALZHEIMER'S DISEASE

- Roughly half the cases of _____
  can be traced to Alzheimer's disease
- Symptoms may be similar to
  - TIAs
  - Cerebral tumors
  - Dementias
- Symptoms may begin as early as age 40

ALZHEIMER'S DISEASE *(continued)*

- When caring for Alzheimer's patients
  - Remember that anger and hostility are
    _____ of the disease
  - Respond with patience and compassion
  - Speak calmly and without condescension

ALZHEIMER'S DISEASE *(continued)*

- Never argue with patient
- _____ yourself at
  each visit
- Explain common procedures
- Approach quietly and professionally
- Speak in short, simple sentences
- Keep list of support contacts for family
  members

MAINTAINING OPTIMUM HEALTH

- It is possible to maintain a good level of health
  after age 70
  - _____ with physician's
    approval
  - Good nutrition

EXERCISE

- Guidelines for starting an exercise program
  1. Always warm up cold muscles for at least 10
     minutes
  2. Begin by exercising for brief time periods

3. Stop if you feel _____,
shortness of breath, or dizziness

EXERCISE (continued)

4. Breathe deeply and evenly
5. Rest when _____
6. Keep record of progress
7. Exercise with a friend, group, or to music
8. Make exercise part of daily routine

DIET

- Elderly patients often have difficulty maintaining good nutrition
- Smaller, more frequent meals may be easier to _____
- Water should be encouraged to maintain hydration
- Consider a service such as Meals on Wheels

SAFETY

- Alert patient and caregivers to hazards in the home
  - Remove scatter rugs
  - Never allow electrical cords to cross passageways
  - Remove or reduce
  - _____
  - Strengthen handrails

SAFETY (continued)

- Install _____ by bedside and favorite chair
- Install and maintain smoke alarms and carbon monoxide detectors
- Establish system to call and check on patient every day
- Use community programs

Chapter 41

Introduction to the Clinical Laboratory

INTRODUCTION

- Medical laboratory provides physician with powerful _____ tools
- Laboratory staff analyze blood, urine, and other body samples to facilitate identification of diseases and disorders

INTRODUCTION (continued)

- Laboratory testing used for
  - Detecting/diagnosing disease
  - Following progress of disease
  - Meeting _____ requirements
  - Monitoring medication and treatment
  - Determining levels of essential substances in body
  - Identifying cause of infection
  - Determining baseline value
  - Disease prevention

INTRODUCTION (continued)

- Medical assistant's responsibilities
  - Educate patients before obtaining laboratory specimens
  - Obtain quality specimens
  - Arrange for appropriate transport
  - Perform common laboratory tests
  - Document and maintain quality assurance program
  - _____ laboratory instrument and equipment

TYPES OF LABORATORIES

- Three types
  - _____
  - _____
  - Physician's office laboratories (_____)

REFERENCE LABORATORY

- Large facility, where thousands of tests of different types are performed each day
  - Receives specimens from satellite procurement stations, physicians offices, hospitals, clinics
- Tests are performed in

_____

REFERENCE LABORATORY *(continued)*

- Staff includes
  - _____
  - Medical technologists
  - Medical laboratory technicians
  - Laboratory assistants
  - Customer services personnel
- Medical assistant may work in specimen processing, client services, or in testing

HOSPITAL LABORATORY

- Hospital laboratory serves inpatients and outpatients
- Staff includes
  - _____
  - Laboratory assistants
  - Medical laboratory technicians and medical technologists
  - Receptionists or secretaries

HOSPITAL LABORATORY *(continued)*

- Medical assistants work as
  - Laboratory secretaries
  - Receptionists
  - Phlebotomists
  - _____

PHYSICIAN'S OFFICE LABORATORY

- Perform limited number of _____ to moderate-complexity tests
- Most common tests
  - Urinalysis
  - Blood cell counts
  - Hemoglobin and hematocrit
  - Blood glucose or cholesterol levels
  - Pregnancy tests
  - Quick screening tests

PHYSICIAN'S OFFICE LABORATORY *(continued)*

- Medical assistants may
  - _____
  - Perform tests

- Manage quality control
- Maintain instruments
- Keep accurate records
- Report results

 CHECKPOINT QUESTION I

What is a reference laboratory and how does it differ from a physician's office laboratory? Name and describe the kinds of positions that a medical assistant may hold in a reference laboratory.

Answer

_____

_____

_____

_____

_____

LABORATORY DEPARTMENTS

- Large laboratories are divided into departments to divide workload and to group similar kinds of tests together
- Small laboratories, such as _____ may have only one department

HEMATOLOGY

- Performs tests that detect abnormalities of blood and blood-forming tissues
- Common tests
  - _____
  - White blood cell count
  - Red blood cell count
  - Platelet count
  - Hemoglobin

HEMATOLOGY *(continued)*

- Common tests *(continued)*
  - Hematocrit
  - Differential
  - Erythrocyte sedimentation rate
  - _____

COAGULATION

- Evaluates how well the body reacts when blood vessels are _____
- Most common tests
  - Prothrombin times
  - Partial prothrombin times
  - Fibrinogens
  - Bleeding times

CLINICAL CHEMISTRY

- Measures _____ in blood or serum
- Substances include
  - Hormones
  - Enzymes
  - Electrolytes
  - Gases
  - Medicines and drugs
  - Sugars
  - Proteins
  - Fats
  - Waste products

CLINICAL CHEMISTRY (continued)

- Chemistry profiles often contain 20 or more chemical analyses
- Most common tests in small laboratories
  - Glucose
  - _____
  - Blood urea nitrogen
  - Electrolytes

TOXICOLOGY

- Measures blood levels of _____ drugs and drugs of _____

URINALYSIS

- Performs complete urinalysis to evaluate the physical, chemical, and _____ properties of urine

IMMUNOHEMATOLOGY

- _____ performs blood typing and compatibility testing of

patient's blood with blood products for transfusion purposes
- Prepares, stores, and dispenses blood products
- Other services
  - Autologous donation
  - Tissue typing
  - Paternity testing

IMMUNOLOGY

- Tests the reactions of _____ formed against certain diseases in the presence of antigens
- Produces quick and accurate tests for diagnosing
  - Syphilis
  - HIV
  - Mononucleosis
  - Streptococcus A and B

MICROBIOLOGY

- Identifies various microorganisms that cause disease
- Includes
  - Bacteriology
  - Virology
  - _____
  - Parasitology

ANATOMIC AND SURGICAL PATHOLOGY

- Studies tissue and _____ specimens from aspirations, autopsies, biopsies, organ removal, and other procedures to identify presence of or evaluate the effects of cancer and other diseases

HISTOLOGY

- Studies the microscopic structure of _____
- Samples of tissue are prepared, stained, and evaluated under a microscope
- Types of specimens examined
  - Tissue obtained through biopsy
  - Surgical frozen sections

CYTOLOGY AND CYTOGENETICS

- Cytology is the study of the microscopic structure of cells

- Cytogenetics studies the genetic structure of cells to test for presence of _____

CHECKPOINT QUESTION 2

What departments may be found in a large laboratory? Summarize the testing done in each one.

Answer

_____

_____

_____

_____

_____

LABORATORY PERSONNEL

- Specially trained professionals oversee laboratory operations and
  _____
- Each position requires a particular level of education and training

PHYSICIAN'S OFFICE LABORATORY TESTING (POL)

- Many tests can be performed in POL
- Must meet standards of 1988 Clinical Laboratory Improvement Amendments (CLIA)
- Two categories
  - Performed on _____ machine
  - Conducted using self-contained kit

LABORATORY EQUIPMENT

- Basic pieces of equipment
  - Automated cell counter
  - Microscope
  - Chemistry analyzer
  - _____
  - Incubator
  - Refrigerator or freezer
  - Glassware

CELL COUNTER

- Automated analyzer used to perform _____ testing on blood specimens

- Medical assistants may use cell counter if they have received documented training from a CLIA-qualified person

CHECKPOINT QUESTION 3

Why are package inserts crucial for safe and accurate testing?

Answer

_____

_____

_____

_____

_____

MICROSCOPE

- Used to identify and count cells and microorganisms in blood and other specimens
- Proper use requires time and repeated practice
- _____ microscope commonly used in medical office

MICROSCOPE *(continued)*

- Consists of
  - Frame
  - _____
  - Binocular microscopes
  - Coarse adjustment knob
  - Fine adjustment knob
  - Nosepiece
  - Stage
  - Diaphragm
  - Light source

CHECKPOINT QUESTION 4

How do the three objective lenses of the microscope differ?

Answer

_____

_____

_____

_____

_____

CHEMISTRY ANALYZERS

- Vary from simple to complex
- Portable testing devices designed for _____ testing
- For higher volume testing and a larger variety of tests, use bench top analyzers

CENTRIFUGES

- Uses centrifugal force to separate liquids into component parts
- Tubes must always be balanced
- NEVER open centrifuge until all motion has _____
- NEVER stop the spin with your hand

INCUBATOR

- Culture media are stored in an incubator for 24 hours to allow microbes to reproduce to be identified
- Incubator set at about body temperature
- Maintain _____ to record temperature

REFRIGERATORS AND FREEZERS

- Used to store reagents, kits, patient specimens
- _____ is critical
  - Must be measured and recorded daily
- Food should never be stored in these refrigerators

GLASSWARE

- Term also includes disposable plastic supplies
  - _____
  - Flasks
  - Glass slides and coverslips
  - Graduated cylinders
  - Petri dishes or plates
  - _____
  - Pipettes marked TC (To Contain)
  - Pipettes marked TD (To Deliver)

LABORATORY SAFETY

- All specimens should be considered potentially _____

- Three basic types of hazards
  - Physical hazards (fire, broken glass, liquid spills)
  - Chemical hazards (acids, alkalis, chemical fumes)
  - Biologic hazards (diseases such as HIV, hepatitis, and tuberculosis)

PHYSICAL HAZARDS

- Fires
  - Staff must operate fire extinguishers and identify fire escape routes
- Maintain and use electrical equipment properly
- Avoid using _____
- Unplug instruments before servicing

CHEMICAL HAZARDS

- Minimize by labeling all chemicals with the _____
  _____ (MSDS)
- Facility's Chemical Hygiene Plan includes
  - Up-to-date MSDSs for all chemicals used
  - Chemical safety protocols

HAZARDOUS CHEMICALS

- NFPA classification system
  - _____ section—health hazards
  - _____ section—fire hazards
  - _____ section—reactive hazards
  - _____ section—specific hazard
  - Numbered from 0 (no hazard) to 4 (dangerous hazard)

BIOLOGIC HAZARDS

- Specimens capable of transmitting _____
- Wear personal protective equipment per OSHA requirements
- Methods for handling hazards must be outlined in your facility's policy and procedure manuals

OCCUPATIONAL SAFETY AND HEALTH ADMINISTRATION (OSHA)

- OSHA is a federal agency within U.S. Department of Labor
- OSHA standards are federal laws that protect workers
- OSHA standards _____ all other regulatory agency requirements

OSHA *(continued)*

- Two standards of particular importance to medical laboratories
  - Occupational Exposure to Bloodborne Pathogens Standards
  - Hazardous Communication (_____) Standard

BLOODBORNE PATHOGENS STANDARD

- Requires all medical employers to provide training for employees to protect them from occupational exposure to _____
- Safety manuals must be available

BLOODBORNE PATHOGENS STANDARD *(continued)*

- OSHA standards require that all workers at risk wear _____ supplied by employer
  - Gloves
  - Gowns
  - Aprons
  - Face shields
  - Goggles
  - Glasses with side shields
  - Masks
  - Lab coats

HAZCOM STANDARD

- Requires all _____ materials be labeled by manufacturers
- Hazardous chemicals must be labeled with a warning
- Manufacturer's must supply MSDS for products
- Employers must develop protocol for each hazardous agent

 CHECKPOINT QUESTION 5

What are three types of hazards found in the laboratory? Give examples of and suggestions to prevent each.

Answer

_____

_____

_____

_____

_____

SAFETY GUIDELINES

- Important safety factors required in all laboratories
  1. Never eat, drink, or _____ in laboratory areas
  2. Never touch your face, mouth or eyes with your gloves or with items such as pens or pencils

SAFETY GUIDELINES *(continued)*

  3. Do not apply makeup or insert contact lenses
  4. Wear _____ and appropriate protective barriers whenever in contact with body fluids
  5. Label all specimen containers with biohazard labels

SAFETY GUIDELINES *(continued)*

  6. Store all chemicals according to manufacturer's recommendations
  7. _____ frequently
  8. Clean reusable glassware with recommended disinfectant and dry thoroughly

SAFETY GUIDELINES *(continued)*

  9. Avoid inhaling fumes of any chemicals or wearing contacts
  10. Know location and operation of all _____ equipment
  11. Use safe practices when operating laboratory equipment

SAFETY GUIDELINES *(continued)*

  12. _____ all laboratory surfaces at end of day
  13. Dispose of needles and broken glass in sharps containers
  14. Use mechanical pipettes to apply suction

SAFETY GUIDELINES *(continued)*

  15. Use proper procedure for removing chemical or biologic spills
  16. Avoid _____
  17. Use splatter guards or splash shields
  18. When removing stoppers, hold the opening away

SAFETY GUIDELINES *(continued)*

19. Report all work-related injuries or biohazard exposure to supervisor immediately
20. Follow all guidelines for Standard Precautions
21. When opening tubes or containers, open them _____ from you

CHECKPOINT QUESTION 6

How would you clean up a biologic spill?

Answer

_____

_____

_____

_____

_____

INCIDENT REPORTS

- Complete when
  - _____ could be considered
  - Patient, employee, or visitor is injured
  - Employee is stuck with contaminated needle
  - Medication errors occur
  - Blood is drawn from wrong patient

INCIDENT REPORTS *(continued)*

- Information includes
  - Injured person's name, address, telephone number and date of birth
  - Date, time, and location of incident
  - Brief _____
  - Witness's account and information
  - Signature of person completing form and supervisor

CLINICAL LABORATORY IMPROVEMENT AMENDMENTS

- Congress passed CLIA in 1988 to establish regulations governing facilities that perform testing
- Centers for Medicare and Medicaid Services (CMS) regulate all _____ testing

CLIA *(continued)*

- CLIA regulations set standards for
  - Laboratory operations
  - Application and user fees
  - Procedures for enforcement of the amendment
  - Approval of programs for _____

LEVELS OF TESTING

- CLIA regulations established three levels of testing based on complexity
  1. Waived tests
  2. _____ tests
  3. High-complexity tests

LABORATORY STANDARDS

- Laboratories that perform moderate- or high-complexity testing may be inspected in an _____ visit every year by representatives from CMS or the Centers for Disease Control and Prevention (CDC)

PATIENT TEST MANAGEMENT

- Policies must be written for standards of patient care and employee conduct
- Each test performed will be evaluated for safety, _____, and diagnostic indication for its performance

PATIENT TEST MANAGEMENT *(continued)*

- Policy and procedure manuals will clearly outline
  - Patient _____
  - Specimen handling
  - How tests are to be performed
  - Alternatives to usual testing methods
  - What to do in event of questionable test results

QUALITY CONTROL (QC)

- Comprehensive QC program
  - _____ each phase of laboratory process

- Monitors reagents, instrumentations and personnel
- Each laboratory must have written policies to ensure QC

CONTROL SAMPLE

- Specimens with known reference ranges provided by manufacturers for testing equipment
  - _____ performances of controls in QC log book
  - If controls fail, patient testing cannot be conducted

MANAGEMENT OF REAGENTS

- Reagents are chemicals used to produce a _____ in a testing situation
  - Record lot number and expiration date in QC log book
  - If reagent performs inappropriately, lot number will help manufacturer identify defects

INSTRUMENT CALIBRATION

- Laboratory equipment is sensitive and requires strict compliance with operation and maintenance standards

- Maintenance must be _____ in QC log book

QUALITY ASSURANCE

- Laboratory's policy and procedure manual should cover
  - Recommendations for continuing _____
  - Evaluation methods for ensuring worker competence
- Qualifications and responsibilities of laboratory workers are specified by CLIA

PROFICIENCY TESTING

- All laboratories must participate in three proficiency tests a year and must be available for at least one

  _____

QUALITY CONTROL LOG BOOK

- To comply with CLIA measures
  - Keep record of each

    _____ and standard test
  - Log date and time of test, results expected, results obtained, action taken for correction

Chapter 42

Microbiology

INTRODUCTION

- Microbiology is the study of small life such as bacteria, parasites, fungi
- Microorganisms likely to present problems in the health care field
- _____ are nonpathogenic
- Pathogens capable of producing disease

INTRODUCTION (continued)

- Microorganisms require five elements for survival

- _____
- Warmth
- Moisture
- Darkness
- Oxygen
- Human body provides all five elements

INTRODUCTION (continued)

- Specimens taken from wounds or other areas
  - Throat
  - Vagina
  - Urethra
  - Skin
- Specimens may be drawn from body by
  - _____
  - Venipuncture

- Specimens also excreted from body as
  - Sputum
  - Stool
  - Urine

MICROBIOLOGIC LIFE FORMS

- Bacteria
- Rickettsias and chlamydias
- _____
- Viruses
- Protozoa
- Metazoa

BACTERIA

- Unicellular simple organisms, each with its own specific characteristics
- _____ is science and study of bacteria
- Organisms named with a genus and species name

BACTERIA *(continued)*

- Organisms identified by distinct shape
  - Cocci
  - _____
  - Spirochetes
  - Vibrios

BACTERIAL SPORE FORMATION

- Some microorganisms produce spores to protect themselves under adverse conditions
- Examples
  - *Clostridium botulinum*–food poisoning
  - *Clostridium tetani*–tetanus
- Spores are destroyed _____

CHECKPOINT QUESTION 1

What are the four main categories of bacteria?

Answer

_____

_____

_____

_____

_____

RICKETTSIAS AND CHLAMYDIAS

- Specialized forms of bacteria
  - _____ than bacteria
  - Larger than _____
- Obligate intracellular parasites
- Rickettsias
  - Cause Rocky Mountain spotted fever
- Chlamydias
  - Cause trachoma and lymphogranuloma venereum

FUNGI

- Small organisms that resemble plants
- _____ is science and study of fungi
- Opportunistic, usually becoming pathogenic when normal flora can no longer counterbalance colony's growth

FUNGI *(continued)*

- Fungal diseases called mycoses or mycotic infections
- _____
  - Aspergillus
  - Blastomycosis
  - Coccidiomycosis
  - Histoplasmosis
  - Tinea
- _____
  - Candidiasis: thrush, vaginitis, endocarditis
  - May be spread by contact

VIRUSES

- Smallest form of microorganisms
- Virology is science and study of viruses
- Viruses cause
  - _____
  - Infectious hepatitis
  - Rabies
  - Polio
  - AIDS
- Require living host for survival and replication

VIRUSES *(continued)*

- Because viruses are not susceptible to _____, most are extremely difficult to treat

- Antiviral therapy
  - Now being developed
  - Work continues on cures for viral diseases

PROTOZOA

- Single-celled parasitic animals
- Protozoas cause
  - Entamoeba
  - Giardia
  - _____
  - Plasmodium
  - Toxoplasma

METAZOA

- Includes
  - _____
  - Nematodes
  - Arthropods

HELMINTH FAMILY

- Includes
  - Round worms
  - Flat worms
  - Flukes
- Most will survive almost anywhere in
  _____

NEMATODES

- Cause
  - Roundworm infestation
  - Gastrointestinal obstruction
  - Bronchial damage
  - _____ infestation
  - Trichinosis

ARTHROPODS

- Include
  - Mites
  - Lice
  - Ticks
  - Fleas
  - Bees
  - Spiders
  - Wasps
  - Mosquitoes
  - Scorpions
- All cause injury by their
  _____

MICROBIOLOGIC TESTING: THE MEDICAL ASSISTANT'S ROLE

- Role in microbiologic testing may be extensive
- Includes both administrative and
  _____ responsibilities

ADMINISTRATIVE DUTIES

- Routing specimens
- Handling and filing reports
- Ensuring patient safety and education
- Billing and _____
  filing

CLINICAL SKILLS

- Collecting and processing _____
- Assisting physician and patient
- Maintaining standard precautions and safety
- Performing terminal cleaning procedures after testing is complete

SPECIMEN COLLECTING AND HANDLING

- Laboratory tests most often performed on specimens that are easily obtained from body
  - Blood
  - Urine
  - Feces
  - _____
  - Other body secretions and fluids

TYPES OF SPECIMENS

- Cultures are media that will support the growth of microorganisms
  - Primary cultures
  - Secondary cultures
  - _____ cultures

TYPES OF SPECIMENS (continued)

- Blood frequently examined for microbiological organisms
- _____ must be done carefully
- Specimen must remain uncontaminated

TYPES OF SPECIMENS *(continued)*

- Sputum often tested for diagnosis of respiratory disease
- Wound specimens
- Other commonly obtained specimens
  - _____ cultures
  - Urine cultures
  - Stool specimens

CHECKPOINT QUESTION 2

What are the differences between mixed cultures, secondary cultures, and pure cultures?

Answer

_____

_____

_____

_____

_____

TYPES OF CULTURE MEDIA

- _____ (liquid, solid or semisolid preparations) support the growth of microorganisms
- Selective media contain additives to support the growth of specific organisms
- Nonselective media will grow almost any microorganism

CARING FOR THE MEDIA

- Commercially prepared culture media
  - Must be stored in refrigerator media side up
  - Discard plates that are past _____
  - Check and record temperature of refrigerator

CARING FOR CULTURE MEDIA
(continued)

- Culture media prepared in medical office
  - Follow manufacturer's _____
  - Use strict sterile technique

CARING FOR CULTURE MEDIA
(continued)

- Culture medium effective for 72 hours

- _____ medium
  - Must be refrigerated until needed, then warmed to room temperature before use
- Check and record incubator temperature

CHECKPOINT QUESTION 3

Why is it important to store the Petri plates with the media side uppermost?

Answer

_____

_____

_____

_____

_____

TRANSPORTING THE SPECIMEN

- Transport or process specimens

  _____

  - Place in transport media
  - Fill out identification slips and information carefully

MICROSCOPIC EXAMINATION OF MICROORGANISMS

- Smears and slides
- Identification by staining
- Microbiologic _____
- Sensitivity testing
- Streptococcal testing

SMEARS AND SLIDES

- Specimens grown on a culture are spread onto glass slide and inspected with a microscope
- Sometimes stains or _____ will be applied to aid in identification

IDENTIFICATION BY STAINING

- Staining
  - May help physician determine possible pathogens and initiate treatment before culture has been incubated
  - Most bacteria are _____ and hard to see without staining

MICROBIOLOGIC INOCULATION

- The practice of introducing a microorganism into culture medium placed in a hospitable environment.
  - Medical assistant will inoculate specimen
  - Culture plates are then _____

CHECKPOINT QUESTION 4

Why are bacteria stained?

Answer

_____

_____

_____

_____

_____

SENSITIVITY TESTING

- Suspected pathogen is inoculated in a broth medium and incubated
  - Then impregnated with various antibiotic disks
  - Inspected for _____ around each disk

Chapter 43

Urinalysis

INTRODUCTION

- Urinalysis
  - Physical and chemical examination of urine to assess renal function and other possible problems
- Some disorders diagnosed or assessed by examination of urine
  - _____
  - Shock
  - Malnutrition

SENSITIVITY TRAINING *(continued)*

- Those with a margin with _____ indicate pathogen is sensitive or susceptible to medication
- If no zone around disk, organism is resistant to antibiotic

STREPTOCOCCAL TESTING

- Streptococcal _____ most common infection in medical office
- Kits available to test quickly for the pathogen
- Results read in a few minutes while patient waits
- Treatment begins at once

CHECKPOINT QUESTION 5

What is the purpose of sensitivity testing?

Answer

_____

_____

_____

_____

_____

- _____
- Blood transfusion reactions

SPECIMEN COLLECTION METHODS

- Proper collection varies depending on test to be performed
- _____ specimen is fine unless otherwise specified by physician
- Random urine
  - Patient voids into clean dry container

SPECIMEN COLLECTION METHODS *(continued)*

- All cultures require the specimen not be _____

- Once collected, many urine elements deteriorate if not tested within 1 hour
- If testing cannot be performed, specimen is refrigerated at 4°C–8°C for up to 4 hours

SPECIMEN COLLECTION METHODS
(continued)

- Timing of collection
- First-morning specimens are the most _____
- Useful for many tests

CLEAN CATCH MIDSTREAM URINE SPECIMEN

- Most commonly ordered random specimen
  - Used for culture if not contaminated
  - Urinary meatus and surrounding skin are

  _____
  - Urine voided in sterile container

BLADDER CATHETERIZATION

- Thin sterile catheter is placed into bladder through _____
  - Usually performed by physician or nurse
  - Medical assistants may be trained to perform catheterizations

SUPRAPUBIC ASPIRATION

- Needle is inserted into bladder through skin of

  _____
  - Urine is aspirated
  - Performed by physician

24-HOUR URINE COLLECTION

- Better indicator of values than a random specimen
  - Creatinine
  - Electrolytes
- Medical assistant provides written instructions
- Patient collects all voided urine within

  _____

CHECKPOINT QUESTION 1

What is the time frame for testing urine that is not refrigerated? Why is this important?

Answer

_____

_____

_____

_____

_____

PHYSICAL PROPERTIES OF URINE

- Color
- Appearance
- _____
- Odor

COLOR

- Urine color affected by
  - Diet
  - Drugs
  - Diseases
  - Concentration
- Normal color is pale straw to _____

CLARITY

- Normal, freshly voided urine is usually

  _____
- Haziness or turbidity indicates presence of particulate matter
- Three terms used to describe clarity
  - Clear
  - Hazy
  - Cloudy

SPECIFIC GRAVITY

- The concentration of the specimen
- Weight of urine is compared with weight of water
- Low specific gravity indicates more

  _____ urine
- High specific gravity indicates concentrated urine

CHECKPOINT QUESTION 2

What are the three physical properties of urine and which two are assessed visually?

Answer

_____

_____

_____

_____

_____

CHEMICAL PROPERTIES OF URINE

- Urine contains chemicals produced in body and ingested from _____
- Ten chemical measurements are performed in UA test
- Reagent strips dipped into urine and react with chemicals in the urine

pH

- Because body produces more acids than bases, pH of urine is more _____
- Expected values range from 5.0 (acidic) to 8.0 (slightly acidic)

pH *(continued)*

- Typical value for freshly voided urine
  - Slightly acidic at 6.0
- Acidic urine also occurs with
  - High-protein diets
  - Uncontrolled _____

pH *(continued)*

- Alkaline urine (above 7.0)
  - Occurs after meals
  - Vegetarian diets
  - Certain renal diseases
  - _____

GLUCOSE

- Filtered and reabsorbed in the kidneys
- Amount in urine corresponds to _____ levels
- Normal urine does not contain glucose

KETONES

- A group of chemicals that result from fat metabolism
- In normal urine, ketones are typically too low to be measurable
- Positive ketone test indicates that body is burning more _____ than normal

PROTEINS

- Normal urine has small quantities
- _____ is indicator of renal disease
- Other conditions that can cause protein in urine
  - Strenuous physical exercise
  - Pregnancy
  - Infections
  - Hematuria
  - Pyuria
  - Multiple myeloma

BLOOD

- Small numbers of red blood cells occasionally in urine
- _____ indicates bleeding in the urinary tract
  - Renal disorders
  - Certain neoplasms
  - UTI
  - Trauma
  - Intact capillaries in glomerulus usually do not allow passage of cells into Bowman's capsule

BILIRUBIN

- Bilirubin formed from breakdown of _____
- Urine contains very low levels of bilirubin
- Bilirubinuria can occur with
  - Certain liver diseases
  - Biliary tract obstruction
  - Hemolytic states

UROBILINOGEN

- Small amounts of urobilinogen normally found in urine
- Increased levels of urobilinogen found in conditions with a high rate of red cell destruction
  - _____
  - Liver impairment

CHECKPOINT QUESTION 3

What does a positive bilirubin test indicate?

Answer

_____

_____

_____

_____

_____

NITRITE

- Some types of bacteria enzyme that can reduce nitrate to nitrite
- Positive nitrite test indicates _____
  - Urinary tract infection

LEUKOCYTE ESTERASE

- Normal urine may contain few white cells
- _____ in urine indicate urinary tract infection

CHECKPOINT QUESTION 4

Which two indicators on a dipstick would suggest a urinary tract infection?

Answer

_____

_____

_____

_____

_____

URINE SEDIMENT

- _____ examination of urine
  - Can corroborate findings of the UA
  - May produce new data of diagnostic value
  - Cells and other structures are noted and counted

URINE SEDIMENT *(continued)*

- Prepared by _____ urine and saving particulate matter that collects in bottom of tube
- Button is resuspended, placed on slide, and viewed with microscope

STRUCTURES FOUND IN URINE SEDIMENT

- Red blood cells
- White blood cells
- Bacteria
- _____
- Crystals
- Casts
- Others

CHECKPOINT QUESTION 5

What are three of the most common crystals found in urine?

Answer

_____

_____

_____

_____

_____

URINE PREGNANCY TESTING

- Human chorionic gonadotropin is secreted by developing _____ shortly after conception
- Its appearance and rapid rise in urine make an excellent marker for pregnancy confirmation
- First morning urine specimens are best

URINE DRUG TESTING

- Several techniques screen for five drug classes
  - _____ tests required for positive drug result
  - Initial test eliminates negative urine specimens
  - Gas chromatography/mass spectrometry technology used for confirmation testing

Chapter 44

Phlebotomy

INTRODUCTION

- Blood collection methods
  - Arterial puncture
  - Skin puncture
  - Venipuncture
- Blood is _____ material
  - Needle stick injuries
  - May expose workers to bloodborne pathogens

GENERAL BLOOD DRAWING EQUIPMENT

- Blood drawing station
- Gloves
- _____
- Spill kit supplies and instructions
- Gauze pads
- Bandages
- Needle and sharps disposal containers

BLOOD DRAWING STATION

- Includes
  - _____
  - Chair or bed for patient

GLOVES

- New pair must be used for each patient and removed when the procedure is finished
- Standard precautions
  - _____ after glove removal
  - Good glove fit
  - Do not use powder in latex gloves

ANTISEPTICS

- Inhibit growth of _____
- Used to clean skin before skin puncture or venipuncture
- Most commonly used is 70% isopropyl alcohol

SPILL KIT SUPPLIES AND INSTRUCTIONS

- Spill kit should include
  - Copy of instructions
  - Nitrile disposable gloves
  - Lab coat
  - _____
  - All-purpose disinfectant
  - Bucket
  - Dustpan and hand broom
  - Sharps container
  - Biohazard waste bags

CLEANING UP BLOOD/BODY FLUIDS

1. _____ spill area
2. Locate clean-up kit
3. Wear gloves
4. Pour or place absorbent material over spill

CLEANING UP BLOOD/BODY FLUIDS (continued)

5. Use scoop or dustpan to pick up material
6. Wipe blood up with absorbent towel
7. Apply disinfectant to area
8. _____ all cleanup materials

CLEANING UP GLASS AND BLOOD/BODY FLUIDS

- Wear double gloves
- Pick up glass with _____
- Place broken glass into a sharps container
- Follow steps for cleaning up blood/body fluid spills

GAUZE PADS

- Clean 2 × 2 gauze pads folded in fourths
  - Used to hold _____ over puncture site
- Cotton or rayon balls not recommended

BANDAGES

- Used to cover site once bleeding has stopped

- If patient is _____ to adhesive bandages
  - Use paper, cloth, or knitted tape over folded gauze square

NEEDLE AND SHARPS DISPOSAL CONTAINERS

- Immediately dispose of used needles in puncture-resistant, leakproof sharps container

CHECKPOINT QUESTION 1

What are disinfectants and antiseptics used for?

Answer

_____

_____

_____

_____

_____

VENIPUNCTURE EQUIPMENT

- _____
- _____

TOURNIQUETS

- Constricts venous blood flow and makes _____ more prominent
  - Soft, pliable rubber strip
  - Can easily be released with one hand
  - Does not cut into patient's arm
  - Use new one for each patient

NEEDLES

- Sterile, disposable, single-use needles are used for venipuncture
- _____
  - Long, cylindrical portion
- _____
  - End that connects to blood-drawing apparatus
- _____
  - Indicates size based on lumen
  - Selected for size and condition of vein

BLOOD COLLECTION SYSTEMS

- Two systems commonly used for venipuncture
  - _____ or evacuated tube system
  - _____ system

EVACUATED TUBE SYSTEM

- Consists of a tube holder and evacuated tube needle
- Three components:
  - Multisample needle
  - Plastic needle holder
  - Various _____ tubes

TUBE ADDITIVES

- Any substance (other than tube coating) that is placed in a tube
- Most common additives
  - Anticoagulant
  - _____
  - Thixotropic gel separator

SYRINGE SYSTEM

- Syringes made of glass or disposable plastic
- Choose syringe volume to accommodate total specimen collection
- _____ the syringe to fill with blood
- Transfer blood to collection tube

WINGED INFUSION SET

- _____ collection system has stainless steel beveled needle with plastic extensions
- Essential tool for collecting blood from difficult or small veins

CHECKPOINT QUESTION 2

What are three chemical substances that may be added to collection tubes? Explain the function of each.

Answer

_____

_____

_____

_____

_____

ORDER OF DRAW

- Designated "order of draw" is recommended to avoid _____
  - Of nonadditive tubes by additive tubes
  - Between different types of additive tubes
  - With tissue thromboplastin and microbial contamination

 CHECKPOINT QUESTION 3

What is the proper order of draw when using the evacuated tube system? Why is this important?

Answer

_____

_____

_____

_____

_____

SKIN PUNCTURE (MICROCOLLECTION) EQUIPMENT

- _____ puncture requires penetration of capillary bed in the dermis
- Small specimen volumes required by point-of-care instruments
- Equipment used to collect specimen depends on test being performed

LANCETS

- Sterile, disposable lancets
  - Used to pierce skin to obtain drops of blood
  - Designed to control _____ of puncture
  - Have safety features to reduce accidental sharps injuries
  - Available in range of lengths and depths

MICROHEMATOCRIT TUBES

- Narrow-bore glass or plastic disposable tubes used for hematocrit determinations
  - Plain tubes have _____ band on one end
  - Ammonium heparin-coated tubes have _____ band

MICROCOLLECTION CONTAINERS

- Microtainers consist of
  - Nonsterile, small, round-bottomed plastic tubes
  - Color-coded stoppers that indicate presence or absence of _____
- Used for filling, measuring, stoppering, centrifuging, and storing blood all in one container

FILTER PAPER TEST REQUISITIONS

- Blood collection on filter paper
- Used to test newborns for _____ defects
- Lateral surface of heel is punctured
- Specimen should air dry in horizontal position

WARMING DEVICES

- Increase _____ before skin is punctured
- Provide a temperature not exceeding 42°C

PATIENT PREPARATION

- Gain patient's trust and confidence
- Identify patient and explain procedure
- Verify that patient has followed dietary instructions
- Always believe patients who say they might _____

PERFORMING A VENIPUNCTURE

- _____ veins commonly used for venipuncture
  - Cephalic
  - Median cubital (primary vein for venipuncture)
  - Basilic

PERFORMING A VENIPUNCTURE
(continued)

- Procedure
  1. Wash hands and put on _____
  2. Place tourniquet 3 to 4 inches above planned venipuncture site
  3. Secure tourniquet by using half-bow

PERFORMING A VENIPUNCTURE
(continued)

4. Apply tourniquet tightly enough to slow venous blood flow
5. Ask patient to make fist so that veins in arm become more _____
6. Do not allow patient to open and close fist

SELECTION OF THE VENIPUNCTURE SITE

■ Locate by _____
■ If no suitable vein is found
   • Release tourniquet and repeat procedure on other arm

SELECTION OF THE VENIPUNCTURE SITE *(continued)*

■ If suitable vein is not found in either arm
   • Check hand veins and wrist veins
   • _____ arm from wrist to elbow increases blood flow
   • Warming site with warm towel can produce same effect

SELECTION OF THE VENIPUNCTURE SITE *(continued)*

■ If blood sample cannot be obtained
   • May need to change _____ of needle
   • Rotate needle half a turn
   • Slowly advance needle further into vein or pull back a little

SELECTION OF THE VENIPUNCTURE SITE *(continued)*

■ Never attempt a venipuncture more than _____
■ Have another person attempt the draw or do a microcollection

COMPLICATIONS OF VENIPUNCTURE

■ _____
■ Accidental puncture of an artery
■ Infection of venipuncture site
■ Permanent nerve damage

PERFORMING A SKIN PUNCTURE

■ Adult
   • Performed when no veins are _____
   • Saves veins for other procedures
■ Infants and children
   • Preferred method

 CHECKPOINT QUESTION 4

How should you label the patient's blood sample?

Answer

_____

_____

_____

_____

_____

Chapter 45

Hematology

INTRODUCTION

■ Hematology laboratory analyzes blood cells, their quantities, and their characteristics
■ Hematology includes the study of _____

FORMATION OF BLOOD CELLS

■ Blood is made of
   • Plasma
   • _____ (red blood cells)
   • _____ (white blood cells)
   • _____ (platelets)
■ Blood cells form in bone marrow
   • Alternative sites include liver, spleen

CHECKPOINT QUESTION 1

What is hematopoiesis and how is it influenced?

Answer

_____

_____

_____

_____

_____

HEMATOLOGIC TESTING

- Used to diagnose and manage disease of blood cells and of nonhematologic disease
- Common tests include
  - Complete blood count (_____)
  - Erythrocyte sedimentation rate (_____)
  - Coagulation tests

COMPLETE BLOOD COUNT (CBC)

- Parameters
  - White blood cell count and differential
  - Red blood cell count
  - _____
    determination
  - Hematocrit determination
  - Mean cell volume
  - Mean corpuscular hemoglobin
  - Mean corpuscular hemoglobin concentration
  - _____ count

COMPLETE BLOOD COUNT (CBC)
(continued)

- Dilution of whole blood is prepared
- Blood cells counted using a _____ or hemocytometer

WHITE BLOOD CELL (WBC) COUNT

- Leukocytes provide main line of defense against foreign invaders
- Normal range is _____ to _____/mm^3

WBC COUNT (continued)

- _____ results from
  - Chemical toxicity
  - Nutritional deficiencies
  - Chronic or overwhelming infections
  - Certain malignancies

WBC COUNT (continued)

- Leukocytosis results from
  - Infections
  - _____
  - Certain drugs
  - Injuries to tissues
  - Certain malignancies

WBC DIFFERENTIAL

- Performed to determine amounts of various WBC types present in peripheral blood
  - _____
  - Lymphocytes
  - Monocytes
  - _____
  - Basophils

CHECKPOINT QUESTION 2

What is leukopenia and what are four conditions that may cause it?

Answer

_____

_____

_____

_____

_____

NEUTROPHILS

- Defend against _____ by phagocytizing them
- Normal percentage is 50% to 70%
- Number increases with bacterial infections

CHECKPOINT QUESTION 3

What is the function of neutrophils?

Answer

_____

_____

_____

_____

_____

Answer

_____

_____

_____

_____

_____

LYMPHOCYTES

- Recognize that a particle is foreign to the body and make antibodies specific to its destruction
- Normal percentage is _____ to
  _____
- Higher numbers signal a viral infection

MONOCYTES

- Capable of phagocytizing foreign material
- Normal percentage is _____ to
  _____
- Monocytosis occurs with inflammatory responses and bacterial infections
- Monocytopenia occurs after administration of certain drugs or an overwhelming infection

EOSINOPHILS

- Function is not completely understood
- Normal percentage is _____ to
  _____
- Higher in allergic reactions and some infections

BASOPHILS

- Appear to be involved in _____, in contact allergies, and in hypothyroidism and chronic myeloid leukemia
- Represent less than 1% of circulating WBCs

CHECKPOINT QUESTION 4

Elevated eosinophils and basophils are both seen with what condition?

RED BLOOD CELL (RBC) COUNT

- Erythrocytes transport _____ (mainly oxygen and carbon dioxide) between lungs and tissue
- Normal range
  - For men, 4.6 to 6.2 million/mm^3
  - For women, 4.2 to 5.4 million/mm^3

HEMOGLOBIN

- Functioning unit of the red blood cell
- Each hemoglobin molecule contains four _____ called globins
- Each globin contains a heme unit with one iron molecule each

HEMOGLOBIN *(continued)*

- Millions of hemoglobin molecules in each RBC
  - Normal range for men, _____ to 18 g/dL
  - Normal range for women, _____ to 16 g/dL
- Anemia
  - Detected with hemoglobin measurement

HEMATOCRIT

- _____ of red blood cells contained in whole blood
- Purpose for measuring hematocrit is to detect anemia
  - Normal range for men, 45% to 50%
  - Normal range for women, 37% to 48%

CHECKPOINT QUESTION 5

A patient has a hematocrit of 20%. What does this percentage signify?

Answer

_____

_____

_____

_____

_____

MEAN CELL VOLUME

- Measures average size of red blood cells
- Used as an indicator for _____
- Normal range is 80 to 95 fL
- Microcytosis commonly caused by iron deficiency
- Macrocytosis may be caused by deficiency of vitamin B_{12} or folic acid

MEAN CELL HEMOGLOBIN AND MEAN CELL HEMOGLOBIN CONCENTRATION

- Indicate relative hemoglobin concentration in blood
- Normal range for MCG, 27 to _____ picograms
  - Increase seen in macrocytic anemias
- Normal range for MCHC, 32 to _____ g/dL
  - Reduced in true hypochromic anemia

PLATELET COUNT

- Essential to hemostasis
- Normal range is 200,000 to 400,000/mm^3
- _____ caused by many conditions
- Treatment requires specific diagnosis of cause
- Thrombocytosis most often benign

ERYTHROCYTE SEDIMENTATION RATE (ESR OR SED RATE)

- Measures rate at which RBCs settle out in a tube
- Normal ranges
  - For men, 0 to _____ mm/h
  - For women, 0 to _____ mm/h
- Elevations not specific for any disorder

COAGULATION TESTS

- Measure ability of whole blood to form a ____
- When vascular damage occurs, sequence of events occurs

1. Vasoconstriction
2. Platelet plug formation
3. Fibrin clot formation
4. Clot lysis and vascular repair

PROTHROMBIN TIME (PT)

- Test in which calcium and thromboplastin are added to plasma then, clotting time is observed
- Normal range is _____ to _____ seconds
- Prolonged when a deficiency exists or due to coumarin therapy

PARTIAL THROMBOPLASTIN TIME (PTT)

- Two-stage test in which partially activated thromboplastin is incubated with plasma, calcium is added, and clotting time is determined
- Normal range is 32 to 51
- May be prolonged in certain _____

BLEEDING TIME

- Performed to determine time required for blood to stop flowing from a very small wound
- Normal range is from _____ to _____ minutes

BLEEDING TIME *(continued)*

- Prolonged times can occur from
  - Decreased or impaired _____
  - Use of medications
  - Disease states
  - Ingestion antiinflammatory medications

CHECKPOINT QUESTION 6

What are the two most common tests used to determine how well a fibrin clot will form?

Answer

_____

_____

_____

_____

_____

Chapter 46

Serology and Immunohematology

- Gently rock reagent and sample back and forth
- Observe for agglutination

INTRODUCTION

- Serology is the study of _____ and _____
- Immunohematology refers to testing done in blood banks on red blood cells
- All testing requires the use of Standard Precautions

AGGLUTINATION TEST (continued)

- If specific antigen is in reagent, then serum can be tested for the specific antibody
  - Infectious mononucleosis
  - _____
  - Syphilis
  - Rubella.
- If reagent has antibody attached, then specimen can be tested for specific antigen
  - Streptococci

ANTIGENS AND ANTIBODIES

- Antigens are substances recognized as _____ by the body
- Antibodies are _____ produced by the body in response to specific antigens

ENZYME LINKED IMMUNOSORBENT ASSAYS

- _____ tests come with necessary reagents packaged in a kit
- Be sure to follow manufacturer's instructions
- Results are easy-to-read color change

 CHECKPOINT QUESTION 1

How would you describe a test that is both specific and sensitive?

Answer

_____

_____

_____

_____

_____

 CHECKPOINT QUESTION 2

What are two serology test methods and how do they indicate the presence of the test substance?

Answer

_____

_____

_____

_____

SEROLOGY TEST METHODS AND PRINCIPLES

- _____ of visible particles
- Enzyme linked immunosorbent assays (ELISA)
- Other methods
  - Agglutination inhibition
  - Competitive binding assays

REAGENT AND KIT STORAGE AND HANDLING

- Kits must be stored at _____ recommended on box
  - Room temperature
  - Refrigerator
- Reagents should never be used past expiration date
- Follow specific specimen collection guidelines for each kit

AGGLUTINATION TEST

- Mix together _____ and sample on paper card or glass plate

© Lippincott Williams & Wilkins, 2005, West-Stack, Study Guide, Lippincott Williams & Wilkins' Comprehensive Medical Assisting

CHECKPOINT QUESTION 3

Why is it important to store reagent kits at specified temperatures?

Answer

_____

_____

_____

_____

_____

FOLLOWING TEST PROCEDURES

- Test principle and clinical use of test
- Reagents and materials needed to do test
- _____
- Specimen collection and handling
- Controls to be run and how often

FOLLOWING TEST PROCEDURES
(continued)

- Step-by-step procedure to follow
- _____ and reporting of results
- Normal or expected values
- Test limitations

QUALITY ASSURANCE AND QUALITY CONTROL

- Kits should be tested periodically for continued _____ of all reagents
- Quality control (QC) test needs to be performed each time the reagents are used

EXTERNAL CONTROLS

- Solution similar to a patient sample is tested as patient sample
- Its value or expected result is _____
- If controls do not give the expected result, patient results should not be reported

INTERNAL CONTROLS

- _____ are built into the test packs

- Monitor that test procedure is followed correctly and reagents are working properly
- Do not report patient results if controls do not give proper reactions

SEROLOGY TESTS

- Many serological tests exist
- Some common tests are performed in medical office

RHEUMATOID FACTOR/RHEUMATOID ARTHRITIS

- Autoimmune _____ inflammatory disease of the joints
- Test for agglutination
- False-negative result
  - Negative result when patient does have disease
- False-positive result
  - Positive result when patient does not have disease

CHECKPOINT QUESTION 4

What is the difference between a false-negative and a false-positive test result, and why do these sometimes occur?

Answer

_____

_____

_____

_____

_____

INFECTIOUS MONONUCLEOSIS

- Caused by Epstein-Barr virus
- Testing
  - Agglutination of RBCs or latex particles
  - ELISAs
- Results
  - _____ early in the disease
  - _____ results by waiting too long to read agglutination tests

RAPID PLASMA REAGIN TEST FOR SYPHILIS

- Sexually transmitted disease caused by *Treponema pallidum*
- RPR is agglutination test
- Physician and _____ must be notified of reactive results for syphilis

PREGNANCY TEST

- Based on detection of human chorionic gonadotropin (_____)
- Testing
  - Agglutination
  - ELISA
- Urine or serum is added to test pack
- Internal positive and negative control areas must react appropriately for valid results

GROUP A STREPTOCOCCUS

- One of most common bacterial causes of sore throat and upper respiratory tract infections
- Testing
  - _____
  - Agglutination
  - ELISA

CHECKPOINT QUESTION 5

What are the benefits and drawbacks of using serology tests versus cultures for group A streptococcus?

Answer

_____

_____

_____

_____

_____

IMMUNOHEMATOLOGY

- Determines if _____ blood is compatible for transfusion
- If compatible, RBCs circulate in recipient's body for longer time
- If incompatible, recipient's body will begin destroying donor blood
  - Rapidly leads to death

BLOOD GROUP ANTIGENS

- Transfusion compatibility determined by testing antigens present on donor and recipient RBCs and antibodies present in recipient's serum
  - ABO group
  - _____
  - Other blood groups

ABO GROUP

- Four blood groups: A, B, O, or AB
- Almost all serum contains antibodies to ABO antigens it lacks
- Antibodies are crucial to safe _____

Rh TYPE

- Rh group includes antigens D, E, C, e, c
- Presence of D antigen is Rh _____
- Absence is Rh negative
- Antibodies to D do not occur naturally

Rh TYPE *(continued)*

- Those lacking D antigen must be exposed to D antigen of foreign RBCs to produce antibodies
  - Rh-negative patient is transfused with Rh-_____ blood
  - Rh-negative mother is exposed to Rh-positive cells of her baby before or during childbirth

OTHER BLOOD GROUPS

- Other RBC antigens
  - Duffy, Lewis, MNS, Kidd, Kell
- White blood cells and _____ also have antigens
  - Human leukocyte antigens

BLOOD GROUP TESTING

- ABO Testing
  - Direct or _____ typing
  - Indirect or _____ typing
- Rh Testing
  - Anti-D reagent is used to determine the Rh of RBCs

CHECKPOINT QUESTION 6

Which ABO blood group is the universal donor? What does this mean?

Answer

_____

_____

_____

_____

_____

BLOOD SUPPLY

- American Red Cross and other agencies collect donor blood
- Shortage of donor blood

- Donor blood divided into three products
  1. Packed RBCs
  2. _____
  3. Platelet concentrates

CHECKPOINT QUESTION 7

What are three products that can be obtained from 1 U whole blood and how are they used?

Answer

_____

_____

_____

_____

_____

Chapter 47

Clinical Chemistry

INTRODUCTION

- Clinical chemistry involves testing for chemical components found in
  - Serum
  - Plasma
  - Whole blood
  - Other body fluids
- Chemical components can be
  - Electrically charged atoms called _____
  - Metabolic by-products
  - Proteins
  - Hormones

INTRODUCTION *(continued)*

- Quantifying the amount of these chemicals can help physician to
  - Assess _____ function
  - Gain better understanding of patient's overall health status

INSTRUMENTATION AND METHODOLOGY

- Much of chemistry analysis is performed in reference laboratories on _____ that mechanically sample, dilute, or add reagents to patient's blood for quantifying components
- Automation
  - Allows more rapid analyses
  - Reduces occurrence of operator error
  - Helps control costs

CHECKPOINT QUESTION 1

How does the physician utilize chemistry test results?

Answer

_____

_____

_____

_____

_____

RENAL FUNCTION

- Kidneys
  - Rid body of waste products
  - Help maintain fluid and _____ balance
- When kidneys fail, waste products build up in blood
  - Patient becomes edematous
  - Delicate acid-base balance is upset

RENAL FUNCTION (continued)

- To assess renal function, physician may order tests for serum measurements of
  - Electrolytes
  - _____
  - Creatinine
  - Other components

ELECTROLYTES

- Conduct electric impulses across cell membranes to maintain fluid and acid-base balance and aid in function of nerve cells and muscle tissue
  - Sodium
  - Potassium
  - Chloride
  - _____
  - _____
  - Phosphorus
  - Bicarbonate

 CHECKPOINT QUESTION 2

What is hyperkalemia? Name three possible causes.

Answer

_____

_____

_____

_____

_____

NONPROTEIN NITROGENOUS COMPOUNDS

- Three compounds can be increased as a consequence of impaired renal function

- Urea
- _____
- Uric acid
- Diseases can affect concentrations
  - Makes this relatively nonspecific indicator

LIVER FUNCTION

- Liver
  - Largest gland of body
  - One of most complex
- Among its major functions are
  - Production of bile
  - Metabolism of many compounds
  - Processing of _____
  - Detoxifying dangerous substances

LIVER FUNCTION (continued)

- Commonly tested chemistries that help determine liver function
  - Bilirubin
  - _____
  - Alanine aminotransferase
  - Aspartate aminotransferase

BILIRUBIN

- _____ product from worn out RBCs
- If excess amounts settle into skin and sclera, its presence will make patient appear yellow (jaundiced)

 CHECKPOINT QUESTION 3

Name the nonprotein nitrogenous compounds important for assessing renal function.

Answer

_____

_____

_____

_____

ENZYMES

- Proteins produced by living cells that speed up chemical reactions

■ Liver has many to speed up its processes
- Alkaline phosphatase
- Alanine aminotransferase
- _____

? CHECKPOINT QUESTION 4

Name four common tests that evaluate liver function.

Answer

_____

_____

_____

_____

_____

THYROID FUNCTION

■ Thyroid gland regulates _____
by secreting triiodothyronine (T_3) and
thyroxine (T_4)

■ Thyroid gland controlled by TSH

THYROID-STIMULATING HORMONE (TSH)

■ Many situations can cause an imbalance in
delicate _____ system

■ If thyroid gland is malfunctioning, it cannot be
stimulated, regardless of amount of TSH
secreted

CARDIAC FUNCTION

■ When myocardial infarction occurs, specific
_____ are released in
large quantities by damaged heart muscle into
bloodstream

CREATINE KINASE-MB

■ Creatine kinase (CK) has three isoenzymes
- MM (muscle)
- MB (heart)
- BB (brain)

■ Within 2 to 8 hours of MI, CK levels will
increase

■ High _____ suggests heart
muscle is damaged

TROPONIN

■ Protein specific to _____

■ Troponin blood levels begin to rise within 4
hours of onset of myocardial damage

PANCREATIC FUNCTION

■ Pancreas functions in both _____
and _____ systems

■ Exocrine system products
- Amylase and lipase

■ Endocrine system products
- Insulin and glucagon

AMYLASE AND LIPASE

■ Amylase markedly increased in
_____

■ Lipase levels also rise with pancreatitis

PANCREATIC HORMONES AND CARBOHYDRATE METABOLISM

■ Glucose is primary _____
for body

■ Two hormones regulate process of bringing
glucose into cells
- Insulin
- Glucagon

GLUCOSE-REGULATING HORMONES

■ _____ brings the glucose
used for energy into cells for immediate use or
for storage

■ _____ causes glucose
stored in the form of glycogen to be released
into the bloodstream

? CHECKPOINT QUESTION 5

Which enzymes can assist the physician to diagnose an
MI within 3 hours of onset? Why?

Answer

_____

_____

_____

_____

_____

COMMON GLUCOSE TESTS

- Fasting blood glucose (sugar)
- Random blood glucose
- 2-Hour postprandial glucose
- Glucose tolerance test
- _____ glucose testing
- Obstetric glucose testing

CHECKPOINT QUESTION 6

What is hypoglycemia? List the symptoms associated with this disorder.

Answer

_____

_____

_____

_____

_____

LIPIDS AND LIPOPROTEINS

- Cholesterol, associated lipids, and lipoproteins are part of important building blocks of our bodies

- Testing for these aids physicians in assessing risk of _____

CHOLESTEROL

- Is considered a health hazard only in proportions not necessary for cell maintenance
- Ideal range is less than _____ mg/dL
- Anyone over 200 mg/dL is at increased risk of developing atherosclerosis

LOW-DENSITY LIPOPROTEIN

- Plasma protein that transports cholesterol from liver and deposits it on walls of large and medium-sized arteries
  - _____ plaques form, vessel thickens, circulation is reduced

HIGH-DENSITY LIPOPROTEIN

- Protein molecule that carries _____ deposited on arterial walls back to liver
- Higher levels correlate with decreased risk of heart disease
- Decreased levels correlate with increased risk of heart disease

TRIGLYCERIDES

- Triglycerides store energy
- _____ tissue composed almost entirely of triglycerides
- Normal range is less than 150 mg/dL
- Identified as risk factor in heart disease

Chapter 48

Making the Transition: Student to Employee

EXTERNSHIPS

An externship is a training program that gives you the experience of working in a _____ _____ under the supervision of a preceptor or supervisor who will help you apply the theories and procedures you learned during classroom training.

TYPES OF FACILITIES

As a medical assisting student, you will experience an extensive scope of procedures during an externship in a general or family practice clinic or office.

Family practices

General practice facilities

Specialty practices

EXTERN SITES

An ideal site should provide a variety of experiences, both in administrative (front office) and clinical (back office) procedures.

A _____ works with externship students

 CHECKPOINT QUESTION 1

What is the role of the preceptor?

Answer

_____

_____

_____

BENEFITS OF EXTERNSHIP

To the student

To the medical assisting program

To the externship site

BENEFITS TO THE STUDENT

_____

_____

_____

_____

BENEFITS TO THE MEDICAL ASSISTING PROGRAM

Medical assisting programs also rely on the medical profession to aid in updating and revising the curriculum and course content to ensure that the methods and procedures presented to the students from year to year are current.

BENEFITS TO THE EXTERNSHIP SITE

Gain information

Review or add policies

RESPONSIBILITIES OF EXTERNSHIP

Student's responsibilities

Program's responsibilities

Externship site's responsibilities

RESPONSIBILITIES OF THE STUDENT

You must be _____ .

You must act in a _____ manner.

You must be well groomed and meet the program's dress code.

CHECKPOINT QUESTION 2

List three responsibilities that you have during your externship.

Answer

You must be:

- ■ _____
- ■ _____
- ■ _____

RESPONSIBILITIES OF THE MEDICAL ASSISTING PROGRAM

Arrange for best clinical experiences possible

Externship coordinator:

- ■ Matches students to appropriate sites
- ■ Visits frequently
- ■ Evaluates progress

RESPONSIBILITIES OF THE EXTERNSHIP SITE

Provide opportunities for training

Orient students to the office

Provide opportunities to observe and ask questions

GUIDELINES FOR A SUCCESSFUL EXTERNSHIP

_____

_____

_____

_____

PROCEDURAL PERFORMANCE

You will be judged on your ability to measure up to the standard of care for an entry-level medical assistant.

Arrive prepared

Ask questions

Perform procedures only when preceptor is present

PREPAREDNESS

Arrange to have:

- ■ Reliable transportation
- ■ Day care
- ■ Financial coverage if necessary

ATTENDANCE

If at any time you will be late or will not be able to attend the site for any reason, you must notify both the clinical coordinator and the site preceptor.

APPEARANCE

Clean, laundered uniform

Conservatively styled hair

Minimal makeup

No perfume or cologne

Short fingernails

Minimal, tasteful jewelry

 CHECKPOINT QUESTION 3

Describe the proper attire for your externship.

Answer

_____

_____

_____

ATTITUDE

Much attitude is determined by how well you handle change and direction and how adaptable and flexible you are during difficult assignments.

EXTERNSHIP DOCUMENTATION

Time records

Site evaluation

Self-evaluation

TIME RECORDS

Most programs use a time sheet or record of some sort to document your hours in the externship.

Used to validate your time

Requirement for completion

SITE EVALUATION

Used to gather impressions of the site and the experience

Be objective and honest

- Positive or negative experience?
- Opportunities for learning?
- Staff open to questions?
- Availability of preceptor

SELF-EVALUATION

Used to help you determine additional skills or experience you need

Encourages introspection and honesty

 CHECKPOINT QUESTION 4

What three types of documentation are often required in externship programs?

Answer

Documentation includes:

- _____
- _____
- _____

ESTABLISH THE JOB FOR YOU

Setting employment goals

Self-analysis

SETTING EMPLOYMENT GOALS

Employment goal: decide what you want and need from a job

Describe the best job for yourself

- Specialty
- Duties
- Type of employer
- Atmosphere
- Hours

To win the job you want, you have to learn to _____.

SELF-ANALYSIS

Know your _____ and _____.

Use strengths to _____ and your value

_____ and _____ weaknesses

 CHECKPOINT QUESTION 5

What is the purpose of self-analysis?

Answer

_____

_____

_____

_____

FINDING THE RIGHT JOB

Many studies show that most positions are never advertised in the media.

Sources of information:

- _____
- _____
- _____
- _____
- _____

CHECKPOINT QUESTION 6

List four resources that you may use to identify potential job opportunities.

Answer

_____

_____

_____

_____

APPLYING FOR THE JOB

Answering newspaper advertisements

Preparing your _____

Preparing your _____

Completing an employment application

ANSWERING NEWSPAPER ADVERTISEMENTS

Do exactly what the ad asks

Make your response distinctive

PREPARING YOUR RÉSUMÉ

Consult resources

- Books
- Websites
- Templates

Neat, professional flash picture of yourself

PREPARING YOUR RÉSUMÉ *(continued)*

Guidelines

- List your skills and goals
- Keep it to one page
- Include key information:
  - Contact information
  - Education
  - Affiliations

- Experience
- References

When you have chosen the people you want to use as references, be sure to ask their permission.

PREPARING YOUR RÉSUMÉ *(continued)*

Use action words

Use regular type, black ink

Proofread

Use letter-quality printer

Be honest.

 CHECKPOINT QUESTION 7

What is the difference between a functional and a chronological résumé?

Answer

A functional résumé _____ .

A chronological résumé _____

_____ .

PREPARING YOUR COVER LETTER

Must be included with résumé

Keep it _____ **and**

_____

Address the correct person

Format:

- First paragraph: _____
- Second paragraph: _____
- Third paragraph: _____

COMPLETING AN EMPLOYMENT APPLICATION

Read completely

Follow instructions

Answer all questions

Enter "negotiable" in wage line

Make reason for leaving previous position positive

Write neatly with blue or black pen

INTERVIEWING

A skill that must be developed and practiced

Role-play with family or friends

Practice answering tricky questions

Crucial for obtaining a job

PREPARING FOR THE INTERVIEW

_____

- Reputation
- Employee turnover
- Procedures performed

_____

_____

_____

_____

_____

_____

CRUCIAL INTERVIEW QUESTIONS

Do you have _____**?**

Do you have _____**?**

Do you _____**?**

Ask the interviewer questions:

- Job responsibilities
- Advancement opportunities
- Continuing education
- Performance evaluation process
- Benefits

Thank interviewer and offer handshake

 WHAT IF?

_____

You become tongue-tied during an interview. What should you do?

FOLLOW-UP

_____

_____

WHY SOME APPLICANTS FAIL TO GET THE JOB

Lack of necessary skills

- Technical skills
- Confidentiality
- Human relations
- Communication

Lack of professionalism

KEEP THE JOB OR MOVE ON?

Considerations for seeking other employment:

- Salary
- Sense of achievement
- Recognition
- Status
- Job security

Leave with positive feelings

EMPLOYMENT LAWS

Federal and state laws regulate employment

- Americans with Disabilities Act (ADA)
- Age Discrimination in Employment Act (ADEA)
- Discrimination is illegal
  - Race
  - National origin
  - Religion
  - Sex
  - Age
  - Marital status
- Equal Pay Act

COMPETENCY EVALUATION FORMS: SKILL SHEETS

Introduction to Competency Evaluation Forms

These competency evaluation forms (skill sheets) are designed to help you practice and then test your proficiency in many of the skills you will be responsible for knowing as a medical assistant. On each form, you will find a procedure, broken down step-by-step, and the specific equipment you will need to complete the procedure. Before you begin, your instructor will tell you how long you have to complete the procedure and what the passing score will be. These procedures can also be found in your textbook (Procedures 17-1 and 18-1 are from Box 17-4 and Chapter 18, respectively).

How to Calculate Your Score

Each form has three columns. The first is for self-evaluation, the second is for your partner's evaluation, and the third is for your instructor's evaluation. You will find that having two chances to practice the skills on your own will not only help you retain the information but also build your confidence when you have to complete the procedure for your instructor during a test.

You can earn one of three possible scores for each step in the procedure: 4, satisfactory; 0, unsatisfactory; NA, not counted. Each procedure has a total number of points that can be earned. To get this number, add the number of steps (do not include steps with NA) and multiply that number by 4. Then, to calculate your score, add the total number of points you earned and multiply that number by 100. Divide this number by the total possible points, and you will get your final percentage.

List of Procedures

Name_____ Date _____ Time_____

PROCEDURE 5-1: Handling Incoming Calls

Equipment/Supplies: Telephone, message pad, pen or pencil, headset (if applicable)

Standards: Given the needed equipment and a place to work the student will perform this skill with _____% accuracy in a total of _____ minutes. *(Your instructor will tell you what the percentage and time limits will be before you begin.)*

Key: 4 = Satisfactory   0 = Unsatisfactory   NA = this step is not counted

Procedure Steps	Self	Partner	Instructor
1. Answer the phone within two rings.	☐	☐	☐
2. Greet the caller with your name and name of the office.	☐	☐	☐
3. Determine the nature of or reason for the call.	☐	☐	☐
4. Triage the call according to office policy.	☐	☐	☐
5. Record the message correctly on a message pad. Include name of the caller, date and time, telephone number where the caller can be reached, description of the caller's concerns, and the person to whom the message is routed. Clarify information as needed.	☐	☐	☐
6. Give the caller an approximate time frame for a return call.	☐	☐	☐
7. Ask the caller whether he or she has any additional questions or if they need any other help. Allow the caller to disconnect first.	☐	☐	☐
8. Place the message in an appropriate place or note any follow-up action necessary.	☐	☐	☐

Calculation

Total Possible Points: _____
Total Points Earned: _____ Multiplied by 100 = _____ Divided by Total Possible Points = _____%

Pass   Fail

☐   ☐

Comments:

Student signature_____ Date_____
Partner signature_____ Date_____
Instructor's signature_____ Date_____

Name_____ Date _____ Time_____

SKILL

PROCEDURE 5-2: Calling Emergency Medical Services

Equipment/Supplies: Telephone, patient information, pen or pencil

Standards: Given the needed equipment and a place to work the student will perform this skill with _____% accuracy in a total of _____ minutes. *(Your instructor will tell you what the percentage and time limits will be before you begin.)*

Key: 4 = Satisfactory   0 = Unsatisfactory   NA = this step is not counted

Procedure Steps	Self	Partner	Instructor
1. Obtain the following information before dialing EMS: patient's name, age, sex, nature of medical condition, type of service the physician is requesting, any special instructions or requests by the physician, your location, and any special information for access.	❑	❑	❑
2. Dial 911 or other EMS number.	❑	❑	❑
3. Calmly provide the dispatcher with the information.	❑	❑	❑
4. Answer the dispatcher's questions calmly and professionally. Follow the dispatcher's instructions if applicable.	❑	❑	❑
5. End the call per the dispatcher's instructions.	❑	❑	❑

Calculation

Total Possible Points: _____
Total Points Earned: _____ Multiplied by 100 = _____ Divided by Total Possible Points = _____%

Pass   Fail   Comments:
❑   ❑

Student signature_____ Date_____
Partner signature_____ Date_____
Instructor's signature_____ Date_____

SKILL

PROCEDURE 6-1: Making an Appointment for a New Patient

Equipment/Supplies: Appointment book, telephone, pen or pencil

Standards: Given the needed equipment and a place to work the student will perform this skill with _____% accuracy in a total of _____ minutes. *(Your instructor will tell you what the percentage and time limits will be before you begin.)*

Key: 4 = Satisfactory   0 = Unsatisfactory   NA = this step is not counted

Procedure Steps

	Self	Partner	Instructor
1. Obtain as much information as possible from the patient: full name with correct spelling, mailing address, day and evening telephone numbers, reason for the visit, name of the referring physician or individual.	☐	☐	☐
2. Explain the payment policy of the practice. Most offices require full or partial payment at the time of an initial visit. Instruct patients to bring all pertinent insurance information.	☐	☐	☐
3. Ensure that the patient knows how to get to the office; if needed, give concise directions.	☐	☐	☐
4. Tell the patient approximately how long the office visit will be.	☐	☐	☐
5. To avoid violating confidentiality, ask the patient whether it is permissible to call at home or at work.	☐	☐	☐
6. Before ending the call, confirm the time and date of the appointment.	☐	☐	☐
7. Always check your appointment book to be sure that you have placed the appointment on the correct day in the right time slot.	☐	☐	☐

Calculation

Total Possible Points: _____
Total Points Earned: _____   Multiplied by 100 = _____   Divided by Total Possible Points = _____%

Pass   Fail
☐   ☐

Student signature_____   Date_____
Partner signature_____   Date_____
Instructor's signature_____   Date_____

SKILL

PROCEDURE 6-2: Making an Appointment for an Established Patient

Equipment/Supplies: Appointment book, telephone, pen or pencil, appointment cards

Standards: Given the needed equipment and a place to work the student will perform this skill with _____% accuracy in a total of _____ minutes. *(Your instructor will tell you what the percentage and time limits will be before you begin.)*

Key: 4 = Satisfactory   0 = Unsatisfactory   NA = this step is not counted

Procedure Steps	Self	Partner	Instructor
1. Review the patient's chart to determine what will be done at the return visit. Carefully check your appointment book or computer system before offering an appointment.	❑	❑	❑
2. Offer the patient a specific time and date. Give the patient a choice and, if neither time is convenient, offer another specific time and date.	❑	❑	❑
3. Write the patient's name and telephone number in the appointment book.	❑	❑	❑
4. Transfer the pertinent information to an appointment card and give it to the patient.	❑	❑	❑
5. Repeat aloud the appointment day, date, and time to the patient as you hand over the card.	❑	❑	❑
6. Double-check your book to be sure you have not made an error.	❑	❑	❑
7. End your conversation with a pleasant word and a smile.	❑	❑	❑

Calculation

Total Possible Points: _____
Total Points Earned: _____   Multiplied by 100 = _____   Divided by Total Possible Points = _____%

Pass   Fail   Comments:
❑   ❑

Student signature_____ Date_____
Partner signature_____ Date_____
Instructor's signature_____ Date_____

Name_____ Date _____ Time_____

PROCEDURE 6-3: Making an Appointment for a Referral to Another Provider

Equipment/Supplies: Chart, preferred provider list, telephone, pen or pencil

Standards: Given the needed equipment and a place to work the student will perform this skill with _____% accuracy in a total of _____ minutes. *(Your instructor will tell you what the percentage and time limits will be before you begin.)*

Key: 4 = Satisfactory   0 = Unsatisfactory   NA = this step is not counted

Procedure Steps	Self	Partner	Instructor
1. Review the patient's chart to determine what kind of appointment is needed. Make certain the requirements of any third-party payers are met.	☐	☐	☐
2. Refer to the preferred provider list for the patient's insurance company. Allow the patient to choose a provider from the list.	☐	☐	☐
3. Call the provider to schedule the appointment. Have the following information available when you make the call: ■ Physician's name and telephone number ■ Patient's name, address, and telephone number ■ Reason for the call ■ Degree of urgency ■ Whether the patient is being sent for consultation or referral	☐	☐	☐
4. Record in the patient's chart the time, date of the call, and person who received your call.	☐	☐	☐
5. Tell the person you are calling that you wish to be notified if your patient does not keep the appointment. If this occurs, be sure to tell your physician and enter this information in the patient's record.	☐	☐	☐
6. Write down the name, address, and telephone number of the doctor you are referring your patient to and include the date and time of the appointment. Give or mail this information to your patient.	☐	☐	☐

Calculation

Total Possible Points: _____
Total Points Earned: _____   Multiplied by 100 = _____   Divided by Total Possible Points = _____%

Pass   Fail
☐   ☐

Comments:

Student signature_____ Date_____
Partner signature_____ Date_____
Instructor's signature_____ Date_____

508

SKILL

PROCEDURE 7-1: How to Fold a Letter for a No. 10 Envelope

Equipment/Supplies: Letter, 8.5 × 11; envelope, no. 10

Standards: Given the needed equipment and a place to work the student will perform this skill with _____% accuracy in a total of _____ minutes. *(Your instructor will tell you what the percentage and time limits will be before you begin.)*

Key: 4 = Satisfactory 0 = Unsatisfactory NA = this step is not counted

Procedure Steps

	Self	Partner	Instructor
1. Place the letter right side up and flat on a table.	☐	☐	☐
2. Bring the bottom third of the letter up. Make a solid crease.	☐	☐	☐
3. Fold the top third of the letter down to within three eighths of an inch of the first fold. Make a solid crease.	☐	☐	☐
4. Place the letter in the envelope with the last fold at the top of the envelope.	☐	☐	☐

Calculation

Total Possible Points: _____
Total Points Earned: _____ Multiplied by 100 = _____ Divided by Total Possible Points = _____%

Pass Fail
☐ ☐

Comments:

Student signature_____ Date_____
Partner signature_____ Date_____
Instructor's signature_____ Date_____

SKILL

PROCEDURE 7-2: How to Fold a Letter for an Envelope With a Window

Equipment/Supplies: Letter, 8.5 × 11; envelope, no. 10 with a window

Standards: Given the needed equipment and a place to work the student will perform this skill with _____% accuracy in a total of _____ minutes. *(Your instructor will tell you what the percentage and time limits will be before you begin.)*

Key: 4 = Satisfactory   0 = Unsatisfactory   NA = this step is not counted

Procedure Steps

	Self	Partner	Instructor
1. Place the letter face down on a flat surface.	☐	☐	☐
2. Bring the bottom third of the letter up. Make a solid crease line.	☐	☐	☐
3. Fold the top third of the letter down to within three eighths of an inch of the first fold. Make a solid crease.	☐	☐	☐
4. Place the letter in the envelope.	☐	☐	☐
5. Turn the envelope over and look at the window; verify that the address is visible in the center of the window.	☐	☐	☐

Calculation

Total Possible Points: _____
Total Points Earned: _____   Multiplied by 100 = _____   Divided by Total Possible Points = _____%

Pass   Fail
☐   ☐

Comments:

Student signature_____ Date_____
Partner signature_____ Date_____
Instructor's signature_____ Date_____

SKILL

PROCEDURE 8-1: Preparing a Medical File

Equipment/Supplies: File folder, title, year, alphabetic or numeric labels

Standards: Given the needed equipment and a place to work the student will perform this skill with _____% accuracy in a total of _____ minutes. *(Your instructor will tell you what the percentage and time limits will be before you begin.)*

Key: 4 = Satisfactory   0 = Unsatisfactory   NA = this step is not counted

Procedure Steps	Self	Partner	Instructor
1. Decide the name of the file (a patient's name, company name, or the name of the type of information to be stored within the record).	☐	☐	☐
2. Type a label with the selected title on it *in unit order*.	☐	☐	☐
3. Place the label along the tabbed edge of the folder so that the title extends out farther than the file folder itself. (Tabs can either be the length of the folder or tabbed in various positions, such as left, center, and right, based on the type of filing system used.)	☐	☐	☐
4. Place a year label along the top edge of the tab before the label with the title. This will be changed each year that the patient has been seen.	☐	☐	☐
5. Place the appropriate alphabetic or numeric labels below the title.	☐	☐	☐
6. Apply any additional labels that your office may decide to use	☐	☐	☐

Calculation

Total Possible Points: _____
Total Points Earned: _____   Multiplied by 100 = _____   Divided by Total Possible Points = _____%

Pass   Fail   Comments:
☐   ☐

Student signature_____   Date_____
Partner signature_____   Date_____
Instructor's signature_____   Date_____

SKILL

PROCEDURE 9-1: Transcribing a Medical Document

Equipment/Supplies: Transcribing machine, headphones, transcription (dictation) tapes, computer or typewriter, paper, letterhead, envelopes

Standards: Given the needed equipment and a place to work the student will perform this skill with _____% accuracy in a total of _____ minutes. *(Your instructor will tell you what the percentage and time limits will be before you begin.)*

Key: 4 = Satisfactory   0 = Unsatisfactory   NA = this step is not counted

Procedure Steps

	Self	Partner	Instructor
1. Assemble the equipment.	☐	☐	☐
2. Select a transcription tape with the oldest date unless there are special requests for priority reports.	☐	☐	☐
3. Turn on the transcriber and insert and rewind the tape.	☐	☐	☐
4. Put on the headset and position the foot pedal in a comfortable location.	☐	☐	☐
5. Play a sample of the tape. Adjust the volume, speed, and tone to your comfort.	☐	☐	☐
6. Select the appropriate format and enter proper patient identification on the page.	☐	☐	☐
7. By pressing the foot pedal, play a short segment of the tape, stop the tape, and type the passage.	☐	☐	☐
8. If you come across an unfamiliar term, leave enough blank space in the document for the provider to write it in and continue transcribing.	☐	☐	☐
9. When you are finished, enter the initials of the provider, followed by a slash and your initials, on the bottom of the page. The date that each was done should be included.	☐	☐	☐
10. Spell-check the document by using medical spell check software.	☐	☐	☐
11. Print and proofread the document.	☐	☐	☐
12. Leave the document, along with the tape, in a designated area for review.	☐	☐	☐
13. Ensure that the provider has reviewed the document.	☐	☐	☐
14. Make any necessary corrections to the document and obtain approval from the provider.	☐	☐	☐
15. Copy the document for the patient's chart.	☐	☐	☐
16. Send the document to the recipient.	☐	☐	☐
17. Erase the tape and return it to the dictation area.	☐	☐	☐

Calculation

Total Possible Points: _____
Total Points Earned: _____ Multiplied by 100 = _____ Divided by Total Possible Points = _____%

Pass   Fail

☐   ☐

Comments:

Student signature_____ Date_____
Partner signature_____ Date_____
Instructor's signature_____ Date_____

SKILL

PROCEDURE 10-1: Searching on the Internet

Equipment/Supplies: Computer with Web browser, modem, active Internet connection account

Standards: Given the needed equipment and a place to work the student will perform this skill with _____% accuracy in a total of _____ minutes. *(Your instructor will tell you what the percentage and time limits will be before you begin.)*

Key: 4 = Satisfactory   0 = Unsatisfactory   NA = this step is not counted

Procedure Steps

	Self	Partner	Instructor
1. Connect your computer to the Internet.	☐	☐	☐
2. Locate a search engine.	☐	☐	☐
3. Select two or three key words. Then type the key words at the appropriate place on the Web page.	☐	☐	☐
4. View the number of search results. If no sites were found, check spelling and retype or choose new key words.	☐	☐	☐
5. If the search results showed an extensive list, do an advanced search and refine your key words.	☐	☐	☐
6. Select an appropriate site and open its home page.	☐	☐	☐
7. If you are satisfied with the site's information, download the material or bookmark the page.	☐	☐	☐
8. If you are unsatisfied with its information, either visit a site listed on the results page or return to the search engine.	☐	☐	☐

Calculation

Total Possible Points: _____

Total Points Earned: _____   Multiplied by 100 = _____   Divided by Total Possible Points = _____%

Pass   **Fail**

☐   ☐

Comments:

Student signature_____ Date_____

Partner signature_____ Date_____

Instructor's signature_____ Date_____

Name_____   Date_____   Time_____

PROCEDURE 12-1: Creating a Procedures Manual

Equipment/Supplies: Word processor, three-ring binder, paper

Standards: Given the needed equipment and a place to work the student will perform this skill with _____%
accuracy in a total of _____ minutes. *(Your instructor will tell you what the percentage and time limits will be
before you begin.)*

Key: 4 = Satisfactory   0 = Unsatisfactory   NA = this step is not counted

Procedure Steps

	Self	Partner	Instructor
1. Gather the information and resources needed to write the procedure.	☐	☐	☐
2. Title the procedure.	☐	☐	☐
3. Number the procedure, using a numbering system.	☐	☐	☐
4. Provide a purpose. This should be a sentence or two at most explaining the intent of the procedure.	☐	☐	☐
5. List all of the items needed to complete the procedure. If the procedure does not require any special equipment, note this on the manual page.	☐	☐	☐
6. List each step in the procedure.	☐	☐	☐
7. Include a rationale for each step if applicable.	☐	☐	☐
8. State the policy for not following a procedure as indicated in the manual.	☐	☐	☐
9. Provide spaces for the appropriate signatures.	☐	☐	☐
10. Record the date that the procedure was written.	☐	☐	☐

Calculation

Total Possible Points: _____
Total Points Earned: _____   Multiplied by 100 = _____   Divided by Total Possible Points = _____%

Pass   Fail
☐   ☐

Comments:

Student signature_____   Date_____
Partner signature_____   Date_____
Instructor's signature_____   Date_____

SKILL

PROCEDURE 14-1: Balancing the Day Sheet

Equipment/Supplies: Calculator, current day sheet with yesterday's balance total, carbon paper, all ledger cards with transactions on the day sheet, pencil, pen

Standards: Given the needed equipment and a place to work the student will perform this skill with _____% accuracy in a total of _____ minutes. *(Your instructor will tell you what the percentage and time limits will be before you begin.)*

Key: 4 = Satisfactory   0 = Unsatisfactory   NA = this step is not counted

Procedure Steps

	Self	Partner	Instructor
1. Determine whether all entries are complete.	☐	☐	☐
2. Add each column with a calculator and place the total in pencil in the appropriate column.	☐	☐	☐
3. Add the totals from the current day to the totals from the previous day sheet.	☐	☐	☐
4. To verify the accuracy of the entries, add the total of the previous balance column and the total of the current balance column.	☐	☐	☐
5. From this total, subtract the totals of the payment and adjustment columns. This amount will equal the current balance column total.	☐	☐	☐
6. When the totals are verified, go back over them in pen.	☐	☐	☐

Calculation

Total Possible Points: _____
Total Points Earned: _____   Multiplied by 100 = _____   Divided by Total Possible Points = _____%

Pass   **Fail**
☐   ☐

Comments:

Student signature_____ Date_____

Partner signature_____ Date_____

Instructor's signature_____ _____ Date_____

SKILL

PROCEDURE 14-2: Posting Charges to the Patient's Account

Equipment/Supplies: Day sheet, carbon paper, pegboard, ledger card, charge slip and/or encounter form, calculator, form, pen

Standards: Given the needed equipment and a place to work the student will perform this skill with _____% accuracy in a total of _____ minutes. *(Your instructor will tell you what the percentage and time limits will be before you begin.)*

Key: 4 = Satisfactory   0 = Unsatisfactory   NA = this step is not counted

Procedure Steps

	Self	Partner	Instructor
1. Align the patient's ledger card on the day sheet.	☐	☐	☐
2. Take the charge slip from the patient and check to be sure it is complete, including the proper procedures and diagnosis made by the physician.	☐	☐	☐
3. Make sure the provider has signed the charge slip.	☐	☐	☐
4. Verify that the charge slip belongs to the patient whose ledger card or account is in hand.	☐	☐	☐
5. Post the total amount of today's charges in the charge column on the ledger card. Each service can be listed in the description column by using abbreviations.	☐	☐	☐
6. If using a computer, post each charge separately on the charge screen.	☐	☐	☐

Calculation

Total Possible Points: _____
Total Points Earned: _____ Multiplied by 100 = _____ Divided by Total Possible Points = _____%

Pass   **Fail**
☐   ☐

Comments:

Student signature_____ Date_____
Partner signature_____ Date_____
Instructor's signature_____ Date_____

SKILL

PROCEDURE 14-3: Posting Payments to the Patient's Account

Equipment/Supplies: Day sheet, carbon paper, pegboard, ledger card, charge slip and/or encounter form, calculator, form, pen

Standards: Given the needed equipment and a place to work the student will perform this skill with _____% accuracy in a total of _____ minutes. *(Your instructor will tell you what the percentage and time limits will be before you begin.)*

Key: 4 = Satisfactory 0 = Unsatisfactory NA = this step is not counted

Procedure Steps	Self	Partner	Instructor
1. Align the patient's ledger card on the day sheet. If the patient is paying for services received by the physician today, the charge slip that shows today's charges should also be placed on the day sheet.	☐	☐	☐
2. Enter the patient's name and previous balance in the appropriate columns. If using a charge slip, make sure you enter the charge slip number in the receipt number column.	☐	☐	☐
3. Enter the posting date in the date column.	☐	☐	☐
4. Enter the type of payment in the description column, whether personal check (pers. ck.), money order (m. o.), credit card (MC, VISA), or insurance check (ins. ck.).	☐	☐	☐
5. Enter the amount of payment in the payment column.	☐	☐	☐
6. Enter the amount of payment on the deposit section of the day sheet in the cash or checks column.	☐	☐	☐
7. Subtract the payment amount from the previous balance and record the new balance in the new balance column.	☐	☐	☐

Calculation

Total Possible Points: _____
Total Points Earned: _____ Multiplied by 100 = _____ Divided by Total Possible Points = _____%

Pass ☐ Fail ☐

Comments:

Student signature_____ Date_____
Partner signature_____ Date_____
Instructor's signature_____ Date_____

SKILL

PROCEDURE 14-4: Posting a Credit Adjustment

Equipment/Supplies: Day sheet, carbon, pegboard, ledger card, calculator, pen

Standards: Given the needed equipment and a place to work the student will perform this skill with _____%
accuracy in a total of _____ minutes. *(Your instructor will tell you what the percentage and time limits will be
before you begin.)*

Key: 4 = Satisfactory   0 = Unsatisfactory   NA = this step is not counted

Procedure Steps

	Self	Partner	Instructor
1. Align the patient's ledger card on the day sheet.	☐	☐	☐
2. Record the patient's name, previous balance, and the date in the appropriate columns.	☐	☐	☐
3. Record [in brackets] the amount of the adjustment in the adjustment column of the ledger card. Brackets indicate that the amount is subtracted.	☐	☐	☐
4. Enter a description of the adjustment in the professional service column (insurance adjustment or correction adjustment).	☐	☐	☐
5. Subtract the amount of the adjustment from the previous balance and record the new balance in the balance column.	☐	☐	☐

Calculation

Total Possible Points: _____
Total Points Earned: _____   Multiplied by 100 = _____   Divided by Total Possible Points = _____%

Pass   Fail
☐   ☐

Comments:

Student signature_____ Date_____
Partner signature_____ Date_____
Instructor's signature_____ Date_____

SKILL

PROCEDURE 14-5: Reconciling a Bank Statement

Equipment/Supplies: Monthly bank statement, check register, calculator, pen

Standards: Given the needed equipment and a place to work the student will perform this skill with _____% accuracy in a total of _____ minutes. *(Your instructor will tell you what the percentage and time limits will be before you begin.)*

Key: 4 = Satisfactory   0 = Unsatisfactory   NA = this step is not counted

Procedure Steps	Self	Partner	Instructor
1. Determine which portion (dates and/or check numbers) of the checkbook is covered on this bank statement.	☐	☐	☐
2. Locate the ending balance and the list of checks and deposits on the bank statement.	☐	☐	☐
3. Check your check register or record of disbursements against the bank statement and check off each check and deposit on your record that has been recorded on the bank statement.	☐	☐	☐
4. Total all outstanding checks that are not listed on the bank statement. Write this total in the space provided on the worksheet on the back of the bank statement.	☐	☐	☐
5. Total all outstanding deposits that do no appear on the bank statement and write this total in the space provided on the worksheet.	☐	☐	☐
6. Note any additional charges, such as service charges, automatic teller machine charges, or charges for returned checks, that do not appear on the bank statement.	☐	☐	☐
7. Calculate the balance, using the worksheet provided on the back of the statement.	☐	☐	☐
8. Starting with the ending balance, add the total of outstanding deposits.	☐	☐	☐
9. Subtract the total of checks or withdrawals.	☐	☐	☐
10. Verify that the figure is the same as the ending balance on the bank statement.	☐	☐	☐
11. If the figures do not match, recheck your work. If the two numbers still do not match, contact the bank to check for possible bank errors.	☐	☐	☐

Calculation

Total Possible Points: _____

Total Points Earned: _____   Multiplied by 100 = _____   Divided by Total Possible Points = _____%

Pass ☐   Fail ☐

Comments.

Student signature_____ Date_____

Partner signature_____ Date_____

Instructor's signature_____ Date_____

SKILL

PROCEDURE 15-1: Issuing a Payroll Check Using the Pegboard System

Equipment/Supplies: Pegboard with checks, carbon paper, payroll register, tax tables, calculator, time card

Standards: Given the needed equipment and a place to work the student will perform this skill with _____% accuracy in a total of _____ minutes. *(Your instructor will tell you what the percentage and time limits will be before you begin.)*

Key: 4 = Satisfactory   0 = Unsatisfactory   NA = this step is not counted

Procedure Steps

	Self	Partner	Instructor
1. Align the carbon or transfer strip at the top of the check on the employee's payroll record, then align both the transfer strip or carbon and the employee's payroll record on the payroll journal.	☐	☐	☐
2. Enter the employee's name first, followed by the check number, payroll period, and gross income plus any additional earnings.	☐	☐	☐
3. From the gross income, subtract federal, state, local, and social security taxes.	☐	☐	☐
4. Enter the net pay on the detachable payroll slip. Fold this slip behind the check.	☐	☐	☐
5. Total the payroll journal as each page is completed.	☐	☐	☐

Calculation

Total Possible Points: _____
Total Points Earned: _____ Multiplied by 100 = _____ Divided by Total Possible Points = _____%

Pass **Fail**
☐   ☐

Comments:

Student signature_____ Date_____
Partner signature_____ Date_____
Instructor's signature_____ Date_____

SKILL

PROCEDURE 15-2: Calculating the Amount of an Employee's Payroll Check

Equipment/Supplies: Calculator, W-4 form, tax tables

Standards: Given the needed equipment and a place to work the student will perform this skill with _____% accuracy in a total of _____ minutes. *(Your instructor will tell you what the percentage and time limits will be before you begin.)*

Key: 4 = Satisfactory   0 = Unsatisfactory   NA = this step is not counted

Procedure Steps

	Self	Partner	Instructor
1. Calculate the number of hours worked from the employee's time card or record.	☐	☐	☐
2. Calculate the employee's annual gross wage using the following formula: Hourly wage × number of hours worked per week × 52 (number of weeks in a year) = gross annual wage	☐	☐	☐
3. If the pay period for your facility is biweekly or monthly, divide this sum by 26 or 12, respectively, to calculate this pay period's gross wages.	☐	☐	☐
4. Divide by 52 weeks in a year and then by 5 workdays in a week to get the amount of a day's pay.	☐	☐	☐
5. Deduct this amount from the gross wage to get the adjusted gross wage from which you will withhold taxes.	☐	☐	☐
6. Refer to the appropriate tax tables (e.g., federal, FICA, Medicare, state taxes) for the deductions for taxes.	☐	☐	☐
7. Subtract the taxes from the gross or adjusted gross wages to obtain net pay.	☐	☐	☐
8. Write the payroll check for this amount.	☐	☐	☐

Calculation

Total Possible Points: _____
Total Points Earned: _____   Multiplied by 100 = _____   Divided by Total Possible Points = _____%

Pass   Fail   Comments:
☐   ☐

Student signature_____ Date_____
Partner signature_____ Date_____
Instructor's signature_____ Date_____

SKILL

PROCEDURE 17-1: Locating a Diagnostic Code

Equipment/Supplies: Current code book, patient's medical record

Standards: Given the needed equipment and a place to work the student will perform this skill with _____%
accuracy in a total of _____ minutes. *(Your instructor will tell you what the percentage and time limits will be
before you begin.)*

Key: 4 = Satisfactory   0 = Unsatisfactory   NA = this step is not counted

Procedure Steps

	Self	Partner	Instructor
1. Choose the main term within the diagnostic statement.	☐	☐	☐
2. Locate the main term in Volume 2.	☐	☐	☐
3. Refer to all notes and conventions under the main term.	☐	☐	☐
4. Find the appropriate indented subordinate term.	☐	☐	☐
5. Follow any relevant instructional terms, such as "see also."	☐	☐	☐
6. Confirm the selected code by cross-referencing Volume 1. Make sure you have added any necessary fourth or fifth digits.	☐	☐	☐
7. Assign the code.	☐	☐	☐

Calculation

Total Possible Points: _____
Total Points Earned: _____   Multiplied by 100 = _____   Divided by Total Possible Points = _____%

Pass   Fail   Comments:
☐   ☐

Student signature_____ Date_____
Partner signature_____ Date_____
Instructor's signature_____ Date_____

Name_____ Date _____ _____ Time_____

PROCEDURE 18-1: Locating a CPT code

Equipment/Supplies: Current CPT code book, patient's medical record

Standards: Given the needed equipment and a place to work the student will perform this skill with _____% accuracy in a total of _____ minutes. *(Your instructor will tell you what the percentage and time limits will be before you begin.)*

Key: 4 = Satisfactory   0 = Unsatisfactory   NA = this step is not counted

Procedure Steps	Self	Partner	Instructor
1. Identify the type of procedure, service, or medical supplies provided to the patient.	❑	❑	❑
2. Select one of these sections and open the book to that section: ■ Evaluation and management (E/M) ■ Anesthesia ■ Surgery ■ Radiology ■ Pathology and laboratory ■ Medicine	❑	❑	❑
3. Review the section guidelines for any specific issues.	❑	❑	❑
4. If you are selecting an E/M code, check the medical record for documentation of the key components. Two of the three are required for established patients; three of three are required for new patients.	❑	❑	❑
5. Select the appropriate code based on the level of history, examination, and medical decision making.	❑	❑	❑
6. Attach the CPT modifier if the procedure or service requires additional clarification.	❑	❑	❑
7. Assign the CPT code.	❑	❑	❑

Calculation

Total Possible Points: _____
Total Points Earned: _____ Multiplied by 100 = _____ Divided by Total Possible Points = _____%

Pass   Fail   Comments:
❑   ❑

Student signature_____ Date_____
Partner signature_____ Date_____
Instructor's signature_____ Date_____

SKILL

PROCEDURE 19-1: Handwashing for Medical Asepsis

Equipment/Supplies: Liquid soap, disposable paper towels, an orangewood manicure stick, a waste can

Standards: Given the needed equipment and a place to work, the student will perform this skill with _____% accuracy in a total of _____ minutes. *(Your instructor will tell you what the percentage and time limits will be before you begin practicing.)*

Key: 4 = Satisfactory   0 = Unsatisfactory   NA = This step is not counted

Procedure Steps

	Self	Partner	Instructor
1. Remove all rings and wristwatch.	❑	❑	❑
2. Stand close to the sink without touching it.	❑	❑	❑
3. Turn on the faucet and adjust the temperature of the water to warm.	❑	❑	❑
4. Wet hands and wrists, apply soap, and work into a lather.	❑	❑	❑
5. Rub palms together and rub soap between your fingers at least 10 times.	❑	❑	❑
6. Scrub one palm with fingertips, work soap under nails, and then reverse hands.	❑	❑	❑
7. Rinse hands and wrists under warm running water.	❑	❑	❑
8. Hold hands lower than elbows and avoid touching the inside of the sink.	❑	❑	❑
9. Using the orangewood stick, clean under each nail on both hands.	❑	❑	❑
10. Reapply liquid soap and rewash hands and wrists.	❑	❑	❑
11. Rinse hands again while holding hands lower than the wrists and elbows.	❑	❑	❑
12. Use a dry paper towel to dry your hands and wrists gently.	❑	❑	❑
13. Use a dry paper towel to turn off the faucets and discard the paper towel.	❑	❑	❑

Calculation

Total Possible Points: _____
Total Points Earned: _____   Multiplied by 100 = _____   Divided by Total Possible Points = _____%

Pass   Fail   Comments:
❑   ❑

Student signature_____ Date_____

Partner signature_____ Date_____

Instructor's signature_____ Date_____

SKILL

PROCEDURE 19-2: Removing Contaminated Gloves

Equipment/Supplies: Clean examination gloves; biohazard waste container

Standards: Given the needed equipment and a place to work, the student will perform this skill with _____% accuracy in a total of _____ minutes. *(Your instructor will tell you what the percentage and time limits will be before you begin practicing.)*

Key: 4 = Satisfactory   0 = Unsatisfactory   NA = This step is not counted

Procedure Steps

	Self	Partner	Instructor
1. Choose the appropriate size gloves and apply one glove to each hand.	☐	☐	☐
2. After "contaminating" gloves, grasp the glove palm of the nondominant hand with fingers of the dominant hand.	☐	☐	☐
3. Pull the glove away from the nondominant hand.	☐	☐	☐
4. Slide the nondominant hand out of the contaminated glove while rolling the contaminated glove into the palm of the gloved dominant hand.	☐	☐	☐

5. Hold the soiled glove in the palm of your gloved hand.
  a. Slip ungloved fingers under the cuff of the gloved hand.
  b. Stretch the glove of the dominant hand up and away from your hand while
  c. Turning it inside out with the nondominant hand glove balled up inside.
	☐	☐	☐

6. Discard both gloves as one unit into a biohazard waste receptacle.	☐	☐	☐
7. Wash your hands.	☐	☐	☐

Calculation

Total Possible Points: _____
Total Points Earned: _____   Multiplied by 100 = _____   Divided by Total Possible Points = _____%

Pass   Fail

☐   ☐

Comments:

Student signature_____   Date_____

Partner signature_____   Date_____

Instructor's signature_____   Date_____

Name_____ Date _____ Time_____

PROCEDURE 19-3: Cleaning Biohazardous Spills

Equipment/Supplies: Commercially prepared germicide OR 1:10 bleach solution, gloves, disposable towels, chemical absorbent, biohazardous waste bag, protective eyewear (goggles or mask and face shield), disposable shoe coverings, disposable gown or apron made of plastic or other material that is impervious to soaking up contaminated fluids

Standards: Given the needed equipment and a place to work, the student will perform this skill with _____% accuracy in a total of _____ minutes. *(Your instructor will tell you what the percentage and time limits will be before you begin practicing.)*

Key: 4 = Satisfactory   0 = Unsatisfactory   NA = This step is not counted

Procedure Steps	Self	Partner	Instructor
1. Put on gloves.	☐	☐	☐
2. Wear protective eyewear, gown or apron, and shoe covers if splashing is anticipated.	☐	☐	☐
3. Apply chemical absorbent to the spill.	☐	☐	☐
4. Clean up the spill using disposable paper towels.	☐	☐	☐
5. Dispose of paper towels and absorbent material in a biohazard waste bag.	☐	☐	☐
6. Further decontaminate using a commercial germicide or bleach solution. a. Wipe with disposable paper towels. b. Discard the towels used for decontamination in a biohazard bag.	☐	☐	☐
7. With gloves on, remove the protective eyewear and discard or disinfect.	☐	☐	☐
8. Remove the gown/apron and shoe coverings and place in biohazard bag.	☐	☐	☐
9. Place the biohazard bag in an appropriate waste receptacle.	☐	☐	☐
10. Remove contaminated gloves and wash hands thoroughly.	☐	☐	☐

Calculation

Total Possible Points: _____
Total Points Earned: _____   Multiplied by 100 = _____   Divided by Total Possible Points = _____%

Pass   Fail
☐   ☐

Comments:

Student signature_____ Date_____
Partner signature_____ Date_____
Instructor's signature_____ Date_____

SKILL

PROCEDURE 20-1: Interviewing the Patient to Obtain a Medical History

Equipment/Supplies: Medical history form or questionnaire, black or blue pen

Standards: Given the needed equipment and a place to work, the student will perform this skill with _____% accuracy in a total of _____ minutes. *(Your instructor will tell you what the percentage and time limits will be before you begin practicing.)*

Key: 4 = Satisfactory   0 = Unsatisfactory   NA = This step is not counted

Procedure Steps	Self	Partner	Instructor
1. Gather the supplies.	☐	☐	☐
2. Review the medical history form.	☐	☐	☐
3. Take the patient to a private and comfortable area of the office.	☐	☐	☐
4. Sit across from the patient at eye level and maintain frequent eye contact.	☐	☐	☐
5. Introduce yourself and explain the purpose of the interview.	☐	☐	☐
6. Ask the appropriate questions clearly and distinctly.	☐	☐	☐
7. Document the patient's responses.	☐	☐	☐
8. Determine the patient's CC and PI.	☐	☐	☐
9. Listen actively.	☐	☐	☐
10. Avoid projecting a judgmental attitude with your words or your actions.	☐	☐	☐
11. Explain to the patient what to expect during any examinations or procedures.	☐	☐	☐
12. Thank the patient for cooperating and ask if there are further questions.	☐	☐	☐

Calculation

Total Possible Points: _____
Total Points Earned: _____   Multiplied by 100 = _____   Divided by Total Possible Points = _____%

Pass   Fail
☐   ☐

Comments:

Student signature_____ Date_____
Partner signature_____ Date_____
Instructor's signature_____ Date_____

PROCEDURE 20-2: Document a Chief Complaint (CC) and Present Illness (PI)

Equipment/Supplies: A cumulative problem list or progress notes form, black or blue ink pen

Standards: Given the needed equipment and a place to work, the student will perform this skill with _____% accuracy in a total of _____ minutes. *(Your instructor will tell you what the percentage and time limits will be before you begin practicing.)*

Key: 4 = Satisfactory   0 = Unsatisfactory   NA = This step is not counted

Procedure Steps	Self	Partner	Instructor
1. Gather the supplies: medical record, cumulative problem list or progress note.	❑	❑	❑
2. Review the new and established patient's medical history form.	❑	❑	❑
3. Greet and identify the patient and lead to the examination room.	❑	❑	❑
4. Using open-ended questions, elicit information from the patient about the reason for the visit.	❑	❑	❑
5. Determine the PI.	❑	❑	❑
6. Document the CC and PI correctly.	❑	❑	❑
7. Thank the patient for cooperating.	❑	❑	❑
8. Reassure the patient that the doctor will be in soon.	❑	❑	❑

Calculation

Total Possible Points: _____
Total Points Earned: _____ Multiplied by 100 = _____ Divided by Total Possible Points = _____%

Pass   Fail   Comments:
❑   ❑

Student signature_____ Date_____
Partner signature_____ Date_____
Instructor's signature_____ Date_____

SKILL

PROCEDURE 21-1: Measuring Weight

Equipment/Supplies: Calibrated balance beam scale, digital scale, or dial scale; paper towel

Standards: Given the needed equipment and a place to work, the student will perform this skill with _____% accuracy in a total of _____ minutes. *(Your instructor will tell you what the percentage and time limits will be before you begin practicing.)*

Key: 4 = Satisfactory   0 = Unsatisfactory   NA = This step is not counted

Procedure Steps	Self	Partner	Instructor
1. Wash your hands.	☐	☐	☐
2. Ensure that the scale is properly balanced at zero.	☐	☐	☐
3. Escort the patient to the scale and place a paper towel on the scale.	☐	☐	☐
4. Have the patient remove shoes, heavy coats, or jackets.	☐	☐	☐
5. Assist the patient onto the scale facing forward.	☐	☐	☐
6. Ask patient to stand still, without touching or holding on to anything if possible.	☐	☐	☐
7. Weigh the patient.	☐	☐	☐
8. Return the bars on the top and bottom to zero.	☐	☐	☐
9. Assist the patient from the scale if necessary and discard the paper towel.	☐	☐	☐
10. Record the patient's weight.	☐	☐	☐

Calculation

Total Possible Points: _____
Total Points Earned: _____   Multiplied by 100 = _____   Divided by Total Possible Points = _____%

Pass   **Fail**   Comments:
☐   ☐

Student signature_____   Date_____
Partner signature_____   Date_____
Instructor's signature_____   _____   Date_____

SKILL

PROCEDURE 21-2: Measuring Height

Equipment/Supplies: A scale with a ruler

Standards: Given the needed equipment and a place to work, the student will perform this skill with _____% accuracy in a total of _____ minutes. *(Your instructor will tell you what the percentage and time limits will be before you begin practicing.)*

Key: 4 = Satisfactory   0 = Unsatisfactory   NA = This step is not counted

Procedure Steps

	Self	Partner	Instructor
1. Wash your hands.	☐	☐	☐
2. Have the patient remove the shoes and stand straight and erect on the scale, heels together, and eyes straight ahead.	☐	☐	☐
3. With the measuring bar perpendicular to the ruler, slowly lower until it firmly touches patient's head.	☐	☐	☐
4. Read the measurement at the point of movement on the ruler.	☐	☐	☐
5. Assist the patient from the scale.	☐	☐	☐
6. Record the weight and height measurements in the medical record.	☐	☐	☐

Calculation

Total Possible Points: _____
Total Points Earned: _____   Multiplied by 100 = _____   Divided by Total Possible Points = _____%

Pass   Fail   Comments:
☐   ☐

Student signature_____   Date_____
Partner signature_____   Date_____
Instructor's signature_____   Date_____

SKILL

PROCEDURE 21-3: Measuring Oral Temperature Using a Glass Mercury Thermometer

Equipment/Supplies: Glass mercury oral thermometer, tissues or cotton balls, disposable plastic sheath, gloves, biohazard waste container, cool soapy water, disinfectant solution

Standards: Given the needed equipment and a place to work, the student will perform this skill with _____% accuracy in a total of _____ minutes. *(Your instructor will tell you what the percentage and time limits will be before you begin practicing.)*

Key: 4 = Satisfactory   0 = Unsatisfactory   NA = This step is not counted

Procedure Steps	Self	Partner	Instructor
1. Wash your hands and assemble the necessary supplies.	☐	☐	☐
2. Dry the thermometer if it has been stored in disinfectant.	☐	☐	☐
3. Carefully check the thermometer for chips or cracks.	☐	☐	☐
4. Check the level of the mercury in the thermometer.	☐	☐	☐
5. If the mercury level is above 94°F, carefully shake down.	☐	☐	☐
6. Insert the thermometer into the plastic sheath.	☐	☐	☐
7. Greet and identify the patient.	☐	☐	☐
8. Explain the procedure and ask about any eating, drinking hot or cold fluids, gum chewing, or smoking.	☐	☐	☐
9. Place the thermometer under the patient's tongue.	☐	☐	☐
10. Tell the patient to keep the mouth and lips closed but caution against biting down on the glass stem.	☐	☐	☐
11. Leave the thermometer in place for 3 to 5 minutes.	☐	☐	☐
12. At the appropriate time, remove the thermometer from the patient's mouth while wearing gloves.	☐	☐	☐
13. Remove the sheath by holding the very edge of the sheath with your thumb and forefinger.	☐	☐	☐
14. Discard the sheath into a biohazard waste container.	☐	☐	☐
15. Hold the thermometer horizontal at eye level and note the level of mercury in the column.	☐	☐	☐
16. Record the patient's temperature.	☐	☐	☐

Calculation

Total Possible Points: _____
Total Points Earned: _____   Multiplied by 100 = _____   Divided by Total Possible Points = _____%

Pass   Fail   Comments:
☐   ☐

Student signature_____ Date_____
Partner signature_____ Date_____
Instructor's signature_____ Date_____

SKILL

PROCEDURE 21-4: Measuring a Rectal Temperature

Equipment/Supplies: Glass mercury rectal thermometer, tissues or cotton balls, disposable plastic sheaths, surgical lubricant, biohazard waste container, cool soapy water, disinfectant solution, gloves

Standards: Given the needed equipment and a place to work, the student will perform this skill with _____% accuracy in a total of _____ minutes. *(Your instructor will tell you what the percentage and time limits will be before you begin practicing.)*

Key: 4 = Satisfactory   0 = Unsatisfactory   NA = This step is not counted

Procedure Steps

	Self	Partner	Instructor
1. Wash your hands and assemble the necessary supplies.	☐	☐	☐
2. Dry the thermometer if it has been stored in disinfectant.	☐	☐	☐
3. Carefully check the thermometer for chips or cracks.	☐	☐	☐
4. Check the level of the mercury in the thermometer.	☐	☐	☐
5. If the mercury level is above 94°F, carefully shake down.	☐	☐	☐
6. Insert the thermometer into the plastic sheath.	☐	☐	☐
7. Spread lubricant onto a tissue and then from the tissue onto the sheath of the thermometer.	☐	☐	☐
8. Greet and identify the patient and explain the procedure.	☐	☐	☐
9. Ensure patient privacy by placing the patient in a side-lying position facing the examination room door. Drape appropriately.	☐	☐	☐
10. Apply gloves and visualize the anus by lifting the top buttock with your nondominant hand.	☐	☐	☐
11. Gently insert thermometer past the sphincter muscle.	☐	☐	☐
12. Release the upper buttock and hold the thermometer in place with your dominant hand for 3 minutes.	☐	☐	☐
13. After 3 minutes, remove the thermometer and the sheath.	☐	☐	☐
14. Discard the sheath into a biohazard waste container.	☐	☐	☐
15. Note the reading with the thermometer horizontal at eye level.	☐	☐	☐
16. Give the patient a tissue to wipe away excess lubricant.	☐	☐	☐
17. Assist with dressing if necessary.	☐	☐	☐
18. Record the procedure and mark the letter R next to the reading.	☐	☐	☐

Calculation

Total Possible Points: _____
Total Points Earned: _____   Multiplied by 100 = _____   Divided by Total Possible Points = _____%

Pass ☐   Fail ☐

Comments:

Student signature_____ Date_____
Partner signature_____ Date_____
Instructor's signature_____ Date_____

Name_____   Date _____   Time_____

SKILL

PROCEDURE 21-5: Measuring an Axillary Temperature

Equipment/Supplies: Glass mercury (oral or rectal) thermometer, tissues or cotton balls, disposable plastic sheaths, biohazard waste container, cool soapy water, disinfectant solution

Standards: Given the needed equipment and a place to work, the student will perform this skill with _____% accuracy in a total of _____ minutes. *(Your instructor will tell you what the percentage and time limits will be before you begin practicing.)*

Key: 4 = Satisfactory   0 = Unsatisfactory   NA = This step is not counted

Procedure Steps	Self	Partner	Instructor
1. Wash your hands and assemble the necessary supplies.	☐	☐	☐
2. Dry the thermometer if it has been stored in disinfectant.	☐	☐	☐
3. Carefully check the thermometer for chips or cracks.	☐	☐	☐
4. Check the level of the mercury in the thermometer.	☐	☐	☐
5. If the mercury level is above 94°F, carefully shake down.	☐	☐	☐
6. Insert the thermometer into the plastic sheath.	☐	☐	☐
7. Expose the patient's axilla, exposing as little of upper body as possible.	☐	☐	☐
8. Place the bulb of the thermometer well into the axilla.	☐	☐	☐
9. Bring the patient's arm down, crossing the forearm over the chest.	☐	☐	☐
10. Leave the thermometer in place for 10 minutes.	☐	☐	☐
11. After 10 minutes, remove the thermometer from the patient's axilla.	☐	☐	☐
12. Remove the sheath and discard the sheath into a biohazard waste container.	☐	☐	☐
13. Hold the thermometer horizontal at eye level and note the level of mercury.	☐	☐	☐
14. Record the procedure and mark a letter A next to the reading, indicating an axillary temperature.	☐	☐	☐

Calculation

Total Possible Points: _____
Total Points Earned: _____   Multiplied by 100 = _____   Divided by Total Possible Points = _____%

Pass   Fail   Comments:

☐   ☐

Student signature_____   Date_____

Partner signature_____   Date_____

Instructor's signature_____   Date_____

SKILL

PROCEDURE 21-6: Measuring Temperature Using an Electronic Thermometer

Equipment/Supplies: Electronic thermometer with oral or rectal probe, lubricant and gloves for rectal temperatures, disposable probe covers, biohazard waste container

Standards: Given the needed equipment and a place to work, the student will perform this skill with _____% accuracy in a total of _____ minutes. *(Your instructor will tell you what the percentage and time limits will be before you begin practicing.)*

Key: 4 = Satisfactory   0 = Unsatisfactory   NA = This step is not counted

Procedure Steps	Self	Partner	Instructor
1. Wash your hands and assemble the necessary supplies.	☐	☐	☐
2. Greet and identify the patient and explain the procedure.	☐	☐	☐
3. Choose the method (oral, axillary, or rectal) most appropriate for the patient.	☐	☐	☐
4. Insert the probe into a probe cover.	☐	☐	☐
5. Position the thermometer.	☐	☐	☐
6. Wait for the electronic thermometer unit to "beep."	☐	☐	☐
7. Remove the probe and note the reading on the digital display screen on the unit.	☐	☐	☐
8. Discard the probe cover into a biohazard waste container.	☐	☐	☐
9. Record the procedure result.	☐	☐	☐
10. Return the unit and probe to the charging base.	☐	☐	☐

Calculation

Total Possible Points: _____
Total Points Earned: _____   Multiplied by 100 = _____   Divided by Total Possible Points = _____%

Pass   Fail   Comments:
☐   ☐

Student signature_____ Date_____
Partner signature_____ Date_____
Instructor's signature_____ Date_____

SKILL

PROCEDURE 21-7: Measuring Temperature Using a Tympanic Thermometer

Equipment/Supplies: Tympanic thermometer, disposable probe covers, biohazard waste container

Standards: Given the needed equipment and a place to work, the student will perform this skill with _____% accuracy in a total of _____ minutes. *(Your instructor will tell you what the percentage and time limits will be before you begin practicing.)*

Key: 4 = Satisfactory   0 = Unsatisfactory   NA = This step is not counted

Procedure Steps

	Self	Partner	Instructor
1. Wash your hands and assemble the necessary supplies.	☐	☐	☐
2. Greet and identify the patient and explain the procedure.	☐	☐	☐
3. Insert the ear probe into a probe cover.	☐	☐	☐
4. Place the end of the ear probe into the patient's ear.	☐	☐	☐
5. Press the button on the thermometer. Watch the digital display.	☐	☐	☐
6. Remove the probe at "beep" or other thermometer signal.	☐	☐	☐
7. Discard the probe cover into a biohazard waste container.	☐	☐	☐
8. Record the procedure result.	☐	☐	☐
9. Return the unit and probe to the charging base.	☐	☐	☐

Calculation

Total Possible Points: _____
Total Points Earned: _____   Multiplied by 100 = _____   Divided by Total Possible Points = _____%

Pass Fail   Comments:
☐   ☐

Student signature_____ Date_____

Partner signature_____ Date_____

Instructor's signature_____ Date_____

Name **SKILL**_____ Date _____ Time_____

PROCEDURE 21-8: Measuring the Radial Pulse

Equipment/Supplies: A watch with a sweeping second hand.

Standards: Given the needed equipment and a place to work, the student will perform this skill with _____%
accuracy in a total of _____ minutes. *(Your instructor will tell you what the percentage and time limits will be
before you begin practicing.)*

Key: 4 = Satisfactory   0 = Unsatisfactory   NA = This step is not counted

Procedure Steps	Self	Partner	Instructor
1. Wash your hands.	☐	☐	☐
2. Greet and identify the patient and explain the procedure.	☐	☐	☐
3. Position the patient with the arm relaxed and supported.	☐	☐	☐
4. Locate the radial artery.	☐	☐	☐
5. If the pulse is regular, count the pulse for 30 seconds (irregular, count 60 seconds).	☐	☐	☐
6. Multiply the number of pulsations in 30 seconds by 2 (record pulses in 60 seconds as is).	☐	☐	☐
7. Record the rate in the patient's medical record with the other vital signs.	☐	☐	☐
8. Also, note the rhythm if irregular and the volume if thready or bounding.	☐	☐	☐

Calculation

Total Possible Points: _____
Total Points Earned: _____   Multiplied by 100 = _____   Divided by Total Possible Points = _____%

Pass   Fail

☐   ☐

Comments:

Student signature_____ Date_____
Partner signature_____ Date_____
Instructor's signature_____ Date_____

SKILL

PROCEDURE 21-9: Measuring Respirations

Equipment/Supplies: A watch with a sweeping second hand

Standards: Given the needed equipment and a place to work, the student will perform this skill with _____% accuracy in a total of _____ minutes. *(Your instructor will tell you what the percentage and time limits will be before you begin practicing.)*

Key: 4 = Satisfactory   0 = Unsatisfactory   NA = This step is not counted

Procedure Steps	Self	Partner	Instructor
1. Wash your hands.	☐	☐	☐
2. Greet and identify the patient and explain the procedure.	☐	☐	☐
3. Observe watch second hand and count a rise and fall of the chest as one respiration.	☐	☐	☐
4. For a regular breathing pattern count for 30 seconds and multiply by 3 (irregular for 60 seconds).	☐	☐	☐
5. Record the respiratory rate.	☐	☐	☐
6. Note the rhythm if irregular and any unusual or abnormal sounds such as wheezing.	☐	☐	☐

Calculation

Total Possible Points: _____
Total Points Earned: _____   Multiplied by 100 = _____   Divided by Total Possible Points = _____%

Pass   Fail   Comments:
☐   ☐

Student signature_____ Date_____
Partner signature_____ Date_____
Instructor's signature_____ Date_____

SKILL

PROCEDURE 21-10: Measuring Blood Pressure

Equipment/Supplies: Sphygmomanometer, stethoscope

Standards: Given the needed equipment and a place to work, the student will perform this skill with _____% accuracy in a total of _____ minutes. *(Your instructor will tell you what the percentage and time limits will be before you begin practicing.)*

Key: 4 = Satisfactory   0 = Unsatisfactory   NA = This step is not counted

Procedure Steps

	Self	Partner	Instructor
1. Wash your hands and assemble your equipment.	☐	☐	☐
2. Greet and identify the patient and explain the procedure.	☐	☐	☐
3. Position the patient with upper arm supported and level with the patient's heart.	☐	☐	☐
4. Expose the patient's arm.	☐	☐	☐
5. Palpate the brachial pulse in the antecubital area.	☐	☐	☐
6. Center the deflated cuff directly over the brachial artery.	☐	☐	☐
7. Lower edge of the cuff should be 1 to 2 inches above the antecubital area.	☐	☐	☐
8. Wrap the cuff smoothly and snugly around the arm, secure with the Velcro edges.	☐	☐	☐
9. Turn the screw clockwise to tighten. Do not tighten it too tightly for easy release.	☐	☐	☐
10. Palpate the brachial pulse. Inflate the cuff.	☐	☐	☐
11. Note the point or number on the dial or mercury column at which the brachial pulse disappears.	☐	☐	☐
12. Deflate the cuff by turning the valve counterclockwise.	☐	☐	☐
13. Wait at least 30 seconds before reinflating the cuff.	☐	☐	☐
14. Place the stethoscope earpieces into your ear canals with the openings pointed slightly forward.	☐	☐	☐
15. Stand about 3 feet from the manometer with the gauge at eye level.	☐	☐	☐
16. Place the diaphragm of the stethoscope against the brachial artery and hold in place.	☐	☐	☐
17. Close the valve and inflate the cuff.	☐	☐	☐
18. Pump the valve bulb to about 30 mm Hg above the number noted during step 8.	☐	☐	☐
19. Once the cuff is inflated to proper level, release air at a rate of about 2–4 mm Hg per second.	☐	☐	☐
20. Note the point on the gauge at which you hear the first clear tapping sound.	☐	☐	☐

21. Maintaining control of the valve screw, continue to deflate the cuff. ❏ ❏ ❏

22. When you hear the last sound, note the reading and quickly deflate the cuff. ❏ ❏ ❏

23. Remove the cuff and press the air from the bladder of the cuff. ❏ ❏ ❏

24. If this is the first recording or the first time the patient has been into the office, the physician may also want a reading in the other arm or in a position other than sitting. ❏ ❏ ❏

25. Record the reading with the systolic over the diastolic pressure (note which arm was used or any position other than sitting). ❏ ❏ ❏

Calculation

Total Possible Points: _____
Total Points Earned: _____ Multiplied by 100 = _____ Divided by Total Possible Points = _____%

Pass   Fail   Comments:
❏   ❏

Student signature_____ Date_____
Partner signature_____ Date_____
Instructor's signature_____ Date_____

SKILL

PROCEDURE 22-1: Assisting with the Adult Physical Examination

Equipment/Supplies: A variety of basic instruments and supplies including a stethoscope, ophthalmoscope, otoscope, penlight, tuning fork, nasal speculum, tongue blade, percussion hammer, gloves, and patient gowning and draping supplies

Standards: Given the needed equipment and a place to work, the student will perform this skill with _____% accuracy in a total of _____ minutes. *(Your instructor will tell you what the percentage and time limits will be before you begin practicing.)*

Key: 4 = Satisfactory   0 = Unsatisfactory   NA = This step is not counted

Procedure Steps

	Self	Partner	Instructor
1. Wash your hands.	☐	☐	☐
2. Prepare the examination room and assemble the equipment.	☐	☐	☐
3. Greet the patient by name and escort him or her to the examining room.	☐	☐	☐
4. Explain the procedure.	☐	☐	☐
5. Obtain and record the medical history and chief complaint.	☐	☐	☐
6. Take and record the vital signs, height, weight, and visual acuity.	☐	☐	☐
7. Instruct the patient to obtain a urine specimen and escort him or her to the bathroom.	☐	☐	☐
8. When patient has returned, instruct him or her in disrobing. Leave the room unless the patient needs assistance.	☐	☐	☐
9. Assist patient into a sitting position on the edge of the examination table. Cover the lap and legs with a drape.	☐	☐	☐
10. Place the patient's medical record outside the examination room door. Notify the physician that the patient is ready.	☐	☐	☐
11. Assist the physician during the examination by a. handing him or her the instruments needed for the examination. b. positioning the patient appropriately.	☐	☐	☐
12. Help the patient return to a sitting position.	☐	☐	☐
13. Perform any follow-up procedures or treatments	☐	☐	☐
14. Leave the room while the patient dresses unless assistance is needed.	☐	☐	☐
15. Return to the examination room after the patient has dressed to a. answer questions. b. reinforce instructions. c. provide patient education.	☐	☐	☐
16. Escort the patient to the front desk.	☐	☐	☐
17. Properly clean or dispose of all used equipment and supplies.	☐	☐	☐
18. Clean the room with a disinfectant and prepare for the next patient.	☐	☐	☐

19. Wash your hands. ❏ ❏ ❏
    a. Record any instructions that were ordered for the patient.
    b. Note if any specimens were obtained.
    c. Indicate the results of the test or note the laboratory where the specimens are being sent for testing.

Calculation

Total Possible Points: _____
Total Points Earned: _____   Multiplied by 100 = _____   Divided by Total Possible Points = _____%

Pass   Fail   Comments:
❏   ❏

Student signature_____ Date_____
Partner signature_____ Date_____
Instructor's signature_____ Date_____

Name_____ Date _____ Time_____

PROCEDURE 23-1: Sanitizing Equipment for Disinfection or Sterilization

Equipment/Supplies: Instruments or equipment to be sanitized, gloves, eye protection, impervious gown, soap and water, small hand-held scrub brush

Standards: Given the needed equipment and a place to work, the student will perform this skill with _____ % accuracy in a total of _____ minutes. *(Your instructor will tell you what the percentage and time limits will be before you begin practicing.)*

Key: 4 = Satisfactory   0 = Unsatisfactory   NA = This step is not counted

Procedure Steps

	Self	Partner	Instructor
1. Put on gloves, gown, and eye protection.	☐	☐	☐
2. For equipment that requires assembly, take removable sections apart.	☐	☐	☐
3. Check the operation and integrity of the equipment.	☐	☐	☐
4. Rinse the instrument with cool water.	☐	☐	☐
5. Force streams of soapy water through any tubular or grooved instruments.	☐	☐	☐
6. Use a hot, soapy solution to dissolve fats or lubricants left on the surface.	☐	☐	☐

7. Soak 5 to 10 minutes.
   a. Use friction (brush or gauze) to wipe down the instruments.
   b. Check jaws of scissors/forceps to ensure that all debris has been removed.
	☐	☐	☐

8. Rinse well.	☐	☐	☐
9. Dry well before autoclaving if sterilizing or soaking in disinfecting solution.	☐	☐	☐
10. Items (brushes, gauze, solution) used in sanitation process must be disinfected or discarded.	☐	☐	☐

Calculation

Total Possible Points: _____
Total Points Earned: _____   Multiplied by 100 = _____   Divided by Total Possible Points = _____ %

Pass   Fail   Comments:
☐   ☐

Student signature_____ Date_____
Partner signature_____ _____ Date_____
Instructor's signature_____ Date_____

SKILL

PROCEDURE 23-2: Wrapping Instruments for Sterilization in an Autoclave

Equipment/Supplies: Sanitized and wrapped instruments or equipment, distilled water, autoclave operating manual

Standards: Given the needed equipment and a place to work, the student will perform this skill with _____% accuracy in a total of _____ minutes. *(Your instructor will tell you what the percentage and time limits will be before you begin practicing.)*

Key: 4 = Satisfactory   0 = Unsatisfactory   NA = This step is not counted

Procedure Steps	Self	Partner	Instructor
1. Assemble the equipment and supplies.	☐	☐	☐
2. Check the instruments being wrapped for working order.	☐	☐	☐
3. Obtain correct material for wrapping instruments to be autoclaved.	☐	☐	☐
4. Tear off 1 to 2 pieces of autoclave tape. On one piece, label the contents of the pack, the date, and your initials.	☐	☐	☐

5. Lay the wrap on a flat, clean, dry surface diagonally.
  a. Place instrument in the center, with ratchets or handles in open position.
  b. Include a sterilization indicator.
	☐	☐	☐

6. Fold the first flap at the bottom of the diagonal wrap up. Fold back the corner to make a tab.	☐	☐	☐
7. Fold left corner of the wrap toward the center. Fold back the corner to make a tab.	☐	☐	☐
8. Fold right corner of the wrap toward the center. Fold back the corner to make a tab.	☐	☐	☐
9. Fold the top corner down, making the tab tucked under the material.	☐	☐	☐
10. Secure the package with labeled autoclave tape.	☐	☐	☐

Calculation

Total Possible Points: _____
Total Points Earned: _____   Multiplied by 100 = _____   Divided by Total Possible Points = _____%

Pass   Fail
☐   ☐

Comments:

Student signature_____   Date_____
Partner signature_____   Date_____
Instructor's signature_____   Date_____

SKILL

PROCEDURE 23-3: Operating an Autoclave

Equipment/Supplies: Sanitized and wrapped instruments or equipment, distilled water, autoclave operating manual

Standards: Given the needed equipment and a place to work, the student will perform this skill with _____% accuracy in a total of _____ minutes. *(Your instructor will tell you what the percentage and time limits will be before you begin practicing.)*

Key: 4 = Satisfactory   0 = Unsatisfactory   NA = This step is not counted

Procedure Steps

	Self	Partner	Instructor
1. Assemble the equipment including the wrapped articles.	☐	☐	☐
2. Check the water level of the autoclave reservoir and add more if needed.	☐	☐	☐
3. Add water to the internal chamber of the autoclave to the fill line.	☐	☐	☐
4. Load the autoclave:	☐	☐	☐

   a. Place trays and packs on their sides, 1 to 3 inches from each other.
   b. Put containers on the sides with the lids off.
   c. In mixed loads, place hard objects on bottom shelf and softer packs on top racks.

	Self	Partner	Instructor
5. Read the instructions, which should be available and close to the machine.	☐	☐	☐

   a. Close the door and secure or lock it.
   b. Turn the machine on.
   c. When the gauge reaches the temperature required for the contents of the load (usually 250°F), set the timer.
   d. When the timer indicates that the cycle is over, vent the chamber.
   e. After pressure has been released to a safe level, crack the door of autoclave to allow additional drying.

	Self	Partner	Instructor
6. When the load has cooled, remove the items.	☐	☐	☐
7. Check the separately wrapped sterilization indicator, if used, for proper sterilization.	☐	☐	☐
8. Store the items in a clean, dry, dust-free area for 30 days.	☐	☐	☐
9. Clean the autoclave following the manufacturer's directions.	☐	☐	☐
10. Rinse the machine thoroughly and allow it to dry.	☐	☐	☐

Calculation

Total Possible Points: _____
Total Points Earned: _____   Multiplied by 100 = _____   Divided by Total Possible Points = _____%

Pass   Fail   Comments:
☐   ☐

Student signature_____   Date_____
Partner signature_____   Date_____
Instructor's signature_____   Date_____

Name_____ Date _____ Time_____

SKILL

PROCEDURE 24-1: Opening Sterile Packs

Equipment/Supplies: Surgical pack, surgical or Mayo stand

Standards: Given the needed equipment and a place to work, the student will perform this skill with _____% accuracy in a total of _____ minutes. *(Your instructor will tell you what the percentage and time limits will be before you begin practicing.)*

Key: 4 = Satisfactory 0 = Unsatisfactory NA = This step is not counted

Procedure Steps

	Self	Partner	Instructor
1. Verify the surgical procedure to be performed and gather supplies.	☐	☐	☐
2. Check the label for contents and the expiration date.	☐	☐	☐
3. Check the package for tears or areas of moisture.	☐	☐	☐
4. Place the package, with the label facing up on Mayo or surgical stand.	☐	☐	☐
5. Wash your hands.	☐	☐	☐
6. Without tearing the wrapper, carefully remove the sealing tape.	☐	☐	☐
7. Open the first flap: pull it up, out, and away; let it fall over the far side of the table.	☐	☐	☐
8. Open the side flaps in a similar manner. Do not touch the sterile inner surface.	☐	☐	☐
9. Pull the remaining flap down and toward you.	☐	☐	☐
10. Repeat steps 4 through 6 for packages with a second or inside wrapper.	☐	☐	☐
11. If you must leave the area after opening the field, cover the tray with a sterile drape.	☐	☐	☐

Calculation

Total Possible Points: _____
Total Points Earned: _____ Multiplied by 100 = _____ Divided by Total Possible Points = _____%

Pass   Fail
☐   ☐

Comments:

Student signature_____ Date_____
Partner signature_____ Date_____
Instructor's signature_____ Date_____

SKILL

PROCEDURE 24-2: Using Sterile Transfer Forceps

Equipment/Supplies: Sterile transfer forceps in a container with sterilization solution, sterile field, sterile items to be transferred

Standards: Given the needed equipment and a place to work, the student will perform this skill with _____% accuracy in a total of _____ minutes. *(Your instructor will tell you what the percentage and time limits will be before you begin practicing.)*

Key: 4 = Satisfactory   0 = Unsatisfactory   NA = This step is not counted

Procedure Steps

	Self	Partner	Instructor
1. Slowly lift the forceps straight up and out of the container without touching the inside above the level of the solution or outside of the container.	☐	☐	☐
2. Hold the forceps with the tips down at all times.	☐	☐	☐
3. Keep the forceps above waist level.	☐	☐	☐
4. With the forceps, pick up the articles to be transferred and drop them onto the sterile field, but do not let the forceps come into contact with the sterile field.	☐	☐	☐
5. Carefully place the forceps back into the sterilization solution.	☐	☐	☐

Calculation

Total Possible Points: _____
Total Points Earned: _____   Multiplied by 100 = _____   Divided by Total Possible Points = _____%

Pass   Fail   Comments:
☐   ☐

Student signature_____ Date_____
Partner signature_____ Date_____
Instructor's signature_____ Date_____

SKILL

PROCEDURE 24-3: Adding Sterile Solution

Equipment/Supplies: Sterile setup, container of sterile solution, sterile bowl or cup

Standards: Given the needed equipment and a place to work, the student will perform this skill with _____% accuracy in a total of _____ minutes. *(Your instructor will tell you what the percentage and time limits will be before you begin practicing.)*

Key: 4 = Satisfactory   0 = Unsatisfactory   NA = This step is not counted

Procedure Steps

	Self	Partner	Instructor
1. Identify the correct solution by carefully reading the label.	☐	☐	☐
2. Check the expiration date on the label.	☐	☐	☐
3. If adding medications into the solution, show medication label to the physician.	☐	☐	☐
4. Remove the cap or stopper; avoid contamination of the inside of the cap.	☐	☐	☐
5. If it is necessary to put the cap down, place on side table with opened end facing up.	☐	☐	☐
6. Retain bottle to track amount added to field.	☐	☐	☐
7. Grasp container with label against the palm of your hand.	☐	☐	☐
8. Pour a small amount of the solution into a separate container or waste receptacle.	☐	☐	☐
9. Slowly pour the desired amount of solution into the sterile container.	☐	☐	☐
10. Recheck the label for the contents and expiration date and replace the cap.	☐	☐	☐
11. Return the solution to its proper storage area or discard the container after rechecking the label again.	☐	☐	☐

Calculation

Total Possible Points: _____
Total Points Earned: _____ Multiplied by 100 = _____ Divided by Total Possible Points = _____%

Pass   Fail   Comments:
☐   ☐

Student signature_____ Date_____
Partner signature_____ Date_____
Instructor's signature_____ Date_____

SKILL

Procedure 24-4: Performing Hair Removal and Skin Preparation

Equipment/Supplies: Nonsterile gloves; shave cream, lotion, or soap; new disposable razor; gauze or cotton balls; warm water; antiseptic; sponge forceps

Standards: Given the needed equipment and a place to work, the student will perform this skill with _____% accuracy in a total of _____ minutes. *(Your instructor will tell you what the percentage and time limits will be before you begin practicing.)*

Key: 4 = Satisfactory   0 = Unsatisfactory   NA = This step is not counted

Procedure Steps

	Self	Partner	Instructor
1. Wash your hands.	☐	☐	☐
2. Assemble the equipment.	☐	☐	☐
3. Greet and identify the patient; explain the procedure and answer any questions.	☐	☐	☐
4. Put on gloves.	☐	☐	☐
5. Prepare the patient's skin.	☐	☐	☐
6. If the patient's skin is to be shaved, apply shaving cream or soapy lather. a. Pull the skin taut and shave in the direction of hair growth. b. Rinse and pat the shaved area thoroughly dry using a gauze square.	☐	☐	☐
7. If the patient's skin is not to be shaved, wash with soap and water; rinse well and pat the area thoroughly dry using a gauze square.	☐	☐	☐
8. Apply antiseptic solution to the operative area using sterile gauze sponges. a. Wipe skin in circular motions starting at the operative site and working outward. b. Discard each sponge after a complete sweep has been made. c. If circles are not appropriate, the sponge may be wiped straight outward from the operative site and discarded. d. Repeat the procedure until the entire area has been thoroughly cleaned.	☐	☐	☐
9. Instruct the patient not to touch or cover the prepared area.	☐	☐	☐
10. Inform the physician that the patient is ready for the surgical procedure.	☐	☐	☐
11. Drape the prepared area with a sterile drape if the physician will be delayed more than 10 or 15 minutes.	☐	☐	☐

Calculation

Total Possible Points: _____

Total Points Earned: _____   Multiplied by 100 = _____   Divided by Total Possible Points = _____%

Pass ☐   Fail ☐

Comments:

Student signature_____ Date_____

Partner signature_____ Date_____

Instructor's signature_____ Date_____

SKILL

PROCEDURE 24-5: Applying Sterile Gloves

Equipment/Supplies: One package of sterile gloves in the appropriate size

Standards: Given the needed equipment and a place to work, the student will perform this skill with _____% accuracy in a total of _____ minutes. *(Your instructor will tell you what the percentage and time limits will be before you begin practicing.)*

Key: 4 = Satisfactory   0 = Unsatisfactory   NA = This step is not counted

Procedure Steps

	Self	Partner	Instructor
1. Remove rings and other jewelry.	☐	☐	☐
2. Wash your hands.	☐	☐	☐

3. Place prepackaged gloves on a clean, dry, flat surface with the cuffed end toward you.
  a. Pull the outer wrapping apart to expose the sterile inner wrap.
  b. With the cuffs toward you, fold back the inner wrap to expose the gloves.
	☐	☐	☐

4. Grasping the edges of the outer paper, open the package out to its fullest.	☐	☐	☐

5. Use your nondominant hand to pick up the dominant hand glove.
  a. Grasp the folded edge of the cuff and lift it up and away from the paper.
  b. Curl your fingers and thumb together and insert them into the glove.
  c. Straighten your fingers and pull the glove on with your nondominant hand still grasping the cuff.
	☐	☐	☐

6. Unfold the cuff by pinching the inside surface and pull it toward your wrist.	☐	☐	☐

7. Place the fingers of your gloved hand under the cuff of the remaining glove.
  a. Lift the glove up and away from the wrapper.
  b. Slide your ungloved hand carefully into the glove with your fingers and thumb curled together.
  c. Straighten your fingers and pull the glove up and over your wrist by carefully unfolding the cuff.
	☐	☐	☐

8. Settle the gloves comfortably onto your fingers by lacing your fingers together	☐	☐	☐
9. Remove contaminated sterile gloves and discard them appropriately.	☐	☐	☐

Calculation

Total Possible Points: _____
Total Points Earned: _____ Multiplied by 100 = _____ Divided by Total Possible Points = _____%

Pass   Fail   Comments:
☐   ☐

Student signature_____ Date_____
Partner signature_____ Date_____
Instructor's signature_____ Date_____

Name_____ Date _____ Time_____

PROCEDURE 24-6: Applying a Sterile Dressing

Equipment/Supplies: Sterile gloves, sterile gauze dressings, scissors, bandage tape, any medication to be applied to the dressing if ordered by the physician

Standards: Given the needed equipment and a place to work, the student will perform this skill with _____% accuracy in a total of _____ minutes. *(Your instructor will tell you what the percentage and time limits will be before you begin practicing.)*

Key: 4 = Satisfactory   0 = Unsatisfactory   NA = This step is not counted

Procedure Steps

	Self	Partner	Instructor
1. Wash your hands.	☐	☐	☐
2. Assemble the equipment and supplies.	☐	☐	☐
3. Greet and identify the patient.	☐	☐	☐
4. Ask about any tape allergies before deciding on what type of tape to use.	☐	☐	☐
5. Cut or tear lengths of tape to secure the dressing.	☐	☐	☐
6. Explain the procedure and instruct the patient to remain still; avoid coughing, sneezing, or talking until the procedure is complete.	☐	☐	☐
7. Open the dressing pack to create a sterile field, maintaining sterile asepsis. a. If sterile gloves are to be used, open and place near dressing pack. b. If using a sterile transfer forceps, place it near the other supplies.	☐	☐	☐
8. Apply topical medication to the sterile dressing that will cover the wound.	☐	☐	☐
9. Apply the number of dressings necessary to properly cover and protect the wound.	☐	☐	☐
10. Apply sufficient cut lengths of tape over the dressing to secure.	☐	☐	☐
11. Remove contaminated gloves and discard in the proper receptacle.	☐	☐	☐
12. Provide patient education and supplies as appropriate.	☐	☐	☐
13. Clean and sanitize the room and equipment.	☐	☐	☐
14. Record the procedure.	☐	☐	☐

Calculation

Total Possible Points: _____
Total Points Earned: _____   Multiplied by 100 = _____   Divided by Total Possible Points = _____%

Pass   Fail
☐   ☐

Comments:

Student signature_____ Date_____

Partner signature_____ Date_____

Instructor's signature_____ Date_____

SKILL

PROCEDURE 24-7: Changing an Existing Dressing

Equipment/Supplies: Sterile gloves, nonsterile gloves, sterile dressing, prepackaged skin antiseptic swabs (or sterile antiseptic solution poured into a sterile basin and sterile cotton balls or gauze), tape, approved biohazard containers

Standards: Given the needed equipment and a place to work, the student will perform this skill with _____% accuracy in a total of _____ minutes. *(Your instructor will tell you what the percentage and time limits will be before you begin practicing.)*

Key: 4 = Satisfactory   0 = Unsatisfactory   NA = This step is not counted

Procedure Steps	Self	Partner	Instructor
1. Wash your hands.	☐	☐	☐
2. Assemble the equipment and supplies.	☐	☐	☐
3. Greet and identify the patient; explain the procedure and answer any questions.	☐	☐	☐
4. Prepare a sterile field including opening sterile dressings.	☐	☐	☐
5. Open a sterile basin and use the inside of the wrapper as the sterile field.	☐	☐	☐
a. Flip the sterile gauze or cotton balls into the basin.			
b. Pour antiseptic solution appropriately into the basin.			
c. If using prepackaged antiseptic swabs, carefully open an adequate number.			
d. Set swabs aside without contaminating them.	☐	☐	☐
6. Instruct the patient not to talk, cough, sneeze, laugh, or move during the procedure.	☐	☐	☐
7. Wear clean gloves and carefully remove tape from the wound dressing by pulling it toward the wound.			
a. Remove the old dressing.			
b. Discard the soiled dressing into a biohazard container.	☐	☐	☐
8. Inspect wound for the degree of healing, amount and type of drainage, and appearance of wound edges.	☐	☐	☐
9. Observing medical asepsis, remove and discard your gloves.	☐	☐	☐
10. Using proper technique, apply sterile gloves.	☐	☐	☐
11. Clean the wound with the antiseptic solution ordered by the physician.	☐	☐	☐
12. Clean in a straight motion with the cotton or gauze or the prepackaged antiseptic swab. Discard the wipe (cotton ball, swab) after each use.			

13. Remove your gloves and wash your hands. ❑ ❑ ❑

14. Change the dressing using the procedure for sterile dressing application and using sterile gloves or sterile transfer forceps (Procedure 6-6). ❑ ❑ ❑

15. Record the procedure. ❑ ❑ ❑

Calculation

Total Possible Points: _____
Total Points Earned: _____ Multiplied by 100 = _____ Divided by Total Possible Points = _____%

Pass ❑   Fail ❑

Comments:

Student signature_____ Date_____
Partner signature_____ Date_____
Instructor's signature_____ Date_____

SKILL

PROCEDURE 24-8: Assisting with Excisional Surgery

Purpose: Prepare for and assist with excisional surgery while maintaining sterile technique

Equipment/Supplies: Sterile gloves, local anesthetic, antiseptic wipes, adhesive tape, specimen container with completed laboratory request. *On the field:* basin for solutions, gauze sponges and cotton balls, antiseptic solution, sterile drape, dissecting scissors, disposable scalpel, blade of physician's choice, mosquito forceps, tissue forceps, needle holder, suture and needle of physician's choice

Standards: Given the needed equipment and a place to work, the student will perform this skill with _____% accuracy in a total of _____ minutes. *(Your instructor will tell you what the percentage and time limits will be before you begin practicing.)*

Key: 4 = Satisfactory   0 = Unsatisfactory   NA = This step is not counted

Procedure Steps	Self	Partner	Instructor
1. Wash your hands.	☐	☐	☐
2. Assemble the equipment.	☐	☐	☐
3. Greet and identify the patient; explain the procedure and answer any questions.	☐	☐	☐
4. Set up a sterile field on a surgical stand with additional equipment close at hand.	☐	☐	☐
5. Cover the field with a sterile drape until the physician arrives.	☐	☐	☐
6. Position the patient appropriately.	☐	☐	☐
7. Put on sterile gloves or use sterile transfer forceps and cleanse the patient's skin (Procedure 6-4).	☐	☐	☐
8. Be ready to assist during the procedure: adding supplies as needed, assisting the physician, comforting the patient.	☐	☐	☐
9. Assist with collecting tissue specimen in an appropriate container.	☐	☐	☐
10. At the end of the procedure, wash your hands and dress the wound using sterile technique (Procedure 6-6).	☐	☐	☐
11. Thank the patient and give appropriate instructions.	☐	☐	☐
12. Sanitize the examining room in preparation for the next patient.	☐	☐	☐
13. Discard all disposables in the appropriate biohazard containers.	☐	☐	☐
14. Record the procedure.	☐	☐	☐

Calculation

Total Possible Points: _____
Total Points Earned: _____ Multiplied by 100 = _____ Divided by Total Possible Points = _____%

Pass   Fail   Comments:
☐   ☐

Student signature_____ Date_____
Partner signature_____ Date_____
Instructor's signature_____ Date_____

PROCEDURE 24-9: Assisting with Incision and Drainage (I & D)

Equipment/Supplies: Sterile gloves, local anesthetic, antiseptic wipes, adhesive tape, sterile dressings, packing gauze, a culture tube if the wound may be cultured. *On the field:* basin for solutions, gauze sponges and cotton balls, antiseptic solution, sterile drape, syringes and needles for local anesthetic, commercial I & D sterile setup OR scalpel, dissecting scissors, hemostats, tissue forceps, 4 × 4 gauze sponges, probe (optional)

Standards: Given the needed equipment and a place to work, the student will perform this skill with _____% accuracy in a total of _____ minutes. *(Your instructor will tell you what the percentage and time limits will be before you begin practicing.)*

Key: 4 = Satisfactory   0 = Unsatisfactory   NA = This step is not counted

Procedure Steps	Self	Partner	Instructor
1. Wash your hands.			
2. Assemble the equipment.	☐	☐	☐
3. Greet and identify the patient. Explain the procedure and answer any questions.	☐ ☐	☐ ☐	☐ ☐
4. Set up a sterile field on a surgical stand with additional equipment close at hand.	☐	☐	☐
5. Cover the field with a sterile drape until the physician arrives.			
6. Position the patient appropriately.	☐	☐	☐
7. Put on sterile gloves or use sterile transfer forceps and cleanse the patient's skin (Procedure 6-4).	☐ ☐	☐ ☐	☐ ☐
8. Be ready to assist during the procedure: adding supplies as needed, assisting the physician, comforting the patient.	☐	☐	☐
9. Assist with collecting culturette specimen for culture and sensitivity.	☐	☐	☐
10. At the end of procedure, wash your hands and dress the wound using sterile technique (Procedure 6-6).	☐	☐	☐
11. Thank the patient and give appropriate instructions.			
12. Sanitize the examining room in preparation for the next patient.	☐	☐	☐
13. Discard all disposables in appropriate biohazard containers.	☐	☐	☐
14. Record the procedure.	☐	☐	☐
	☐	☐	☐

Calculation

Total Possible Points: _____
Total Points Earned: _____   Multiplied by 100 = _____   Divided by Total Possible Points = _____%

Pass   Fail   Comments:
☐   ☐

Student signature_____ Date_____

Partner signature_____ Date_____

Instructor's signature_____ Date_____

SKILL

PROCEDURE 24-10: Removing Sutures

Equipment/Supplies: Skin antiseptic, sterile gloves, prepackaged suture removal kit OR thumb forceps, suture scissors, gauze

Standards: Given the needed equipment and a place to work, the student will perform this skill with _____% accuracy in a total of _____ minutes. *(Your instructor will tell you what the percentage and time limits will be before you begin practicing.)*

Key: 4 = Satisfactory   0 = Unsatisfactory   NA = This step is not counted

Procedure Steps

	Self	Partner	Instructor
1. Wash your hands and apply clean examination gloves.	☐	☐	☐
2. Assemble the equipment.	☐	☐	☐
3. Greet and identify the patient; explain the procedure and answer any questions.	☐	☐	☐
4. If dressings have not been removed previously, remove them from the wound area. a. Properly dispose of the soiled dressings in the biohazard trash container. b. Remove your gloves and wash your hands.	☐	☐	☐
5. Put on another pair of clean examination gloves and cleanse the wound with an antiseptic.	☐	☐	☐
6. Open suture removal packet using sterile asepsis.	☐	☐	☐
7. Put on sterile gloves. a. With the thumb forceps, grasp the end of the knot closest to the skin surface and lift it slightly and gently up from the skin. b. Cut the suture below the knot as close to the skin as possible. c. Use the thumb forceps to pull the suture out of the skin with a smooth motion.	☐	☐	☐
8. Place the suture on the gauze sponge; repeat the procedure for each suture to be removed.	☐	☐	☐
9. Clean the site with an antiseptic solution and cover it with a sterile dressing.	☐	☐	☐
10. Thank the patient.	☐	☐	☐
11. Properly dispose of the equipment and supplies.	☐	☐	☐
12. Clean the work area, remove your gloves, and wash your hands.	☐	☐	☐
13. Record the procedure, including the time, location of sutures, the number removed, and the condition of the wound.	☐	☐	☐

Calculation

Total Possible Points: _____
Total Points Earned: _____ Multiplied by 100 = _____ Divided by Total Possible Points = _____%

Pass Fail Comments:

☐   ☐

Student signature_____ Date_____
Partner signature_____ Date_____
Instructor's signature_____ Date_____

SKILL

PROCEDURE 24-11: Removing Staples

Equipment/Supplies: Antiseptic solution or wipes, gauze squares, sponge forceps, prepackaged sterile staple removal instrument, examination gloves, sterile gloves

Standards: Given the needed equipment and a place to work, the student will perform this skill with _____% accuracy in a total of _____ minutes. *(Your instructor will tell you what the percentage and time limits will be before you begin practicing.)*

Key: 4 = Satisfactory   0 = Unsatisfactory   NA = This step is not counted

Procedure Steps	Self	Partner	Instructor
1. Wash your hands.	☐	☐	☐
2. Assemble the equipment.	☐	☐	☐
3. Greet and identify the patient; explain the procedure and answer any questions.	☐	☐	☐
4. If the dressing has not been removed, put on clean examination gloves and do so.	☐	☐	☐
5. Dispose of the dressing properly in a biohazard container.	☐	☐	☐
6. Clean the incision with antiseptic solution.	☐	☐	☐
7. Pat dry using dry sterile gauze sponges.	☐	☐	☐
8. Put on sterile gloves.	☐	☐	☐
9. Gently slide the end of the staple remover under each staple to be removed; press the handles together to lift the ends of the staple out of the skin and remove the staple.	☐	☐	☐
10. Place each staple on a gauze square as it is removed.	☐	☐	☐
11. When all staples are removed, clean the incision as instructed for all procedures.	☐	☐	☐
12. Pat dry and dress the site if ordered to do so by the physician.	☐	☐	☐
13. Thank the patient and properly care for, or dispose of, all equipment and supplies.	☐	☐	☐
14. Clean the work area, remove your gloves, and wash your hands.	☐	☐	☐
15. Record the procedure.	☐	☐	☐

Calculation

Total Possible Points: _____
Total Points Earned: _____   Multiplied by 100 = _____   Divided by Total Possible Points = _____%

Pass   Fail   Comments:
☐   ☐

Student signature_____ Date_____

Partner signature_____ Date_____

Instructor's signature_____ Date_____

SKILL

PROCEDURE 26-1: Administering Oral Medications

Equipment/Supplies: Physician's order, oral medication, disposable calibrated cup, glass of water, patient's medical record

Standards: Given the needed equipment and a place to work, the student will perform this skill with _____% accuracy in a total of _____ minutes. *(Your instructor will tell you what the percentage and time limits will be before you begin practicing.)*

Key: 4 = Satisfactory   0 = Unsatisfactory   NA = This step is not counted

Procedure Steps	Self	Partner	Instructor
1. Wash your hands.	☐	☐	☐
2. Review the physician's medication order and select the correct oral medication. a. Compare the label with the physician's instructions. b. Note the expiration date. c. Check the label three times: when taking it from the shelf, while pouring, and when returning to the shelf.	☐	☐	☐
3. Calculate the correct dosage to be given if necessary.	☐	☐	☐
4. If using a multidose container, remove cap from container.	☐	☐	☐
5. Remove the correct dose of medication. a. For solid medications: (1) Pour the capsule/tablet into the bottle cap, (2) Transfer the medication to a disposable cup. b. For liquid medications: (1) Open the bottle lid: place it on a flat surface with open end up. (2) Palm the label to prevent liquids from dripping onto the label. (3) With opposite hand, place the thumbnail at the correct calibration. (4) Pour the medication until the proper amount is in the cup.	☐	☐	☐
6. Greet and identify the patient. Explain the procedure.	☐	☐	☐
7. Ask the patient about medication allergies that might not be noted on the chart.	☐	☐	☐
8. Give the patient a glass of water, unless contraindicated. Hand the patient the disposable cup containing the medication or pour the tablets or capsules into the patient's hand.	☐	☐	☐

9. Remain with the patient to be sure that all of the medication is swallowed.
   a. Observe any unusual reactions and report them to the physician
   b. Record in the medical record.

10. Thank the patient and give any appropriate instructions.

11. Wash your hands.

12. Record the procedure in the patient's medical record. Note the date, time, name of medication, dose administered, route of administration, and your name.

Calculation

Total Possible Points: _____
Total Points Earned: _____   Multiplied by 100 = _____   Divided by Total Possible Points = _____%

Pass   Fail   Comments:
☐   ☐

Student signature_____ Date_____

Partner signature_____ Date_____

Instructor's signature_____ Date_____

SKILL

PROCEDURE 26-2: Preparing Injections

Equipment/Supplies: Physician's order, medication for injection in ampule or vial, antiseptic wipes, appropriate-size needle and syringe, small gauze pad, biohazard sharps container, patient's medical record

Standards: Given the needed equipment and a place to work, the student will perform this skill with _____% accuracy in a total of _____ minutes. *(Your instructor will tell you what the percentage and time limits will be before you begin practicing.)*

Key: 4 = Satisfactory   0 = Unsatisfactory   NA = This step is not counted

Procedure Steps

	Self	Partner	Instructor
1. Wash your hands.	☐	☐	☐

2. Review the physician's medication order and select the correct medication.
  a. Compare the label with the physician's instructions. Note the expiration date.
  b. Check the label three times: when taking it from the shelf, while drawing it up into the syringe, and when returning to the shelf.
	☐	☐	☐

3. Calculate the correct dosage to be given, if necessary.	☐	☐	☐
4. Choose the needle and syringe according to the route of administration, type of medication, and size of the patient.	☐	☐	☐
5. Open the needle and syringe package. Assemble if necessary. Secure the needle to the syringe	☐	☐	☐
6. Withdraw the correct amount of medication:	☐	☐	☐

6. Withdraw the correct amount of medication:
  a. From an ampule:
    (1) Tap the stem of the ampule lightly.
    (2) Place a piece of gauze around the ampule neck.
    (3) Grasp the gauze and ampule firmly. Snap the stem off the ampule.
    (4) Dispose of the ampule top in a biohazard sharps container.
    (5) Insert the needle lumen below the level of the medication.
    (6) Withdraw the medication.
    (7) Dispose of the ampule in a biohazard sharps container.
    (8) Remove any air bubbles in the syringe.
    (9) Draw back on the plunger to add a small amount of air; then gently push the plunger forward to eject the air out of the syringe.
  b. From a vial:
    (1) Using the antiseptic wipe, cleanse the rubber stopper of the vial.
    (2) Pull air into the syringe with the amount equivalent to the amount of medication to be removed from the vial.
    (3) Insert the needle into the vial top. Inject the air from the syringe.

(4) With the needle inside the vial, invert the vial.
(5) Hold the syringe at eye level.
(6) Aspirate the desired amount of medication into the syringe.
(7) Displace any air bubbles in the syringe by gently tapping the barrel.
(8) Remove the air by pushing the plunger slowly and forcing the air into the vial.

7. Carefully recap the needle using one-hand technique. ❏ ❏ ❏

Calculation

Total Possible Points: _____
Total Points Earned: _____ Multiplied by 100 = _____ Divided by Total Possible Points = _____%

Pass   Fail   Comments:
❏   ❏

Student signature_____ Date_____
Partner signature_____ Date_____
Instructor's signature_____ Date_____

PROCEDURE 26-3: Administering an Intradermal Injection

Equipment/Supplies: Physician's order, medication for injection in ampule or vial, antiseptic wipes, appropriate-size needle and syringe, small gauze pad, biohazard sharps container, clean examination gloves, patient's medical record

Standards: Given the needed equipment and a place to work, the student will perform this skill with _____% accuracy in a total of _____ minutes. *(Your instructor will tell you what the percentage and time limits will be before you begin practicing.)*

Key: 4 = Satisfactory   0 = Unsatisfactory   NA = This step is not counted

Procedure Steps	Self	Partner	Instructor

1. Wash your hands.
  a. Review the physician's medication order and select the correct medication.
  b. Compare the label with the physician's instructions. Note the expiration date.
  c. Check the label three times: when taking it from the shelf, while drawing it up into the syringe, and when returning it to the shelf.
	❑	❑	❑

2. Prepare the injection according to the steps in Procedure 8-2.	❑	❑	❑
3. Greet and identify the patient. Explain the procedure.	❑	❑	❑
4. Ask patient about medication allergies.	❑	❑	❑
5. Select the appropriate site for the injection.	❑	❑	❑
6. Prepare the site by cleansing with an antiseptic wipe.	❑	❑	❑
7. Put on gloves. Remove the needle guard.	❑	❑	❑
8. Using your nondominant hand, pull the patient's skin taut.	❑	❑	❑

9. With the bevel of the needle facing upward, insert needle at a 10–15° angle into the upper layer of the skin.
  a. When the bevel of the needle is under the skin, stop inserting the needle.
  b. The needle will be slightly visible below the surface of the skin.
  c. It is not necessary to aspirate when performing an intradermal injection.
	❑	❑	❑

10. Inject the medication slowly by depressing the plunger.
  a. A wheal will form as the medication enters the dermal layer of the skin.
  b. Hold the syringe steady for proper administration.
	❑	❑	❑

11. Remove the needle from the skin at the same angle at which it was inserted.
    a. Do not use an antiseptic wipe or gauze pad over the site.
    b. Do not press or massage the site. Do not apply an adhesive bandage.

☐ ☐ ☐

12. Do not recap the needle.

☐ ☐ ☐

13. Dispose of the needle and syringe in an approved biohazard sharps container.

☐ ☐ ☐

14. Remove your gloves, and wash your hands.

☐ ☐ ☐

15. Depending upon the type of skin test administered, the length of time required for the body tissues to react, and the policies of the medical office, perform one of the following:
    a. Read the test results. Inspect and palpate the site for the presence and amount of induration.
    b. Tell the patient when to return (date and time) to the office to have the results read.
    c. Instruct the patient to read the results at home.
    d. Make sure the patient understands the instructions.

☐ ☐ ☐

17. Document the procedure, the site, and the results. If instructions were given to the patient, document these also.

☐ ☐ ☐

Calculation

Total Possible Points: _____
Total Points Earned: _____   Multiplied by 100 = _____   Divided by Total Possible Points = _____%

Pass   Fail
☐   ☐

Comments:

Student signature_____ Date_____

Partner signature_____ Date_____

Instructor's signature_____ Date_____

SKILL

PROCEDURE 26-4: Administering a Subcutaneous Injection

Equipment/Supplies: Physician's order, medication for injection in ampule or vial, antiseptic wipes, appropriate size needle and syringe, small gauze pad, biohazard sharps container, clean examination gloves, adhesive bandage, patient's medical record

Standards: Given the needed equipment and a place to work, the student will perform this skill with _____% accuracy in a total of _____ minutes. *(Your instructor will tell you what the percentage and time limits will be before you begin practicing.)*

Key: 4 = Satisfactory   0 = Unsatisfactory   NA = This step is not counted

Procedure Steps	Self	Partner	Instructor

1. Wash your hands.
  a. Review the physician's medication order and select the correct medication.
  b. Compare the label with the physician's instructions. Note the expiration date.
  c. Check the label three times: when taking it from the shelf, while drawing it up into the syringe, and when returning it to the shelf.
	❑	❑	❑

2. Prepare the injection according to the steps in Procedure 8-2.	❑	❑	❑
3. Greet and identify the patient. Explain the procedure.	❑	❑	❑
4. Ask the patient about medication allergies.	❑	❑	❑
5. Select the appropriate site for the injection.	❑	❑	❑
6. Prepare the site by cleansing with an antiseptic.	❑	❑	❑
7. Put on gloves.	❑	❑	❑
8. Using your nondominant hand, hold the skin surrounding the injection site.	❑	❑	❑
9. With a firm motion, insert the needle into the tissue at a 45° angle to the skin surface.	❑	❑	❑
10. Hold the barrel between the thumb and the index finger of your dominant hand.	❑	❑	❑
11. Insert the needle completely to the hub.	❑	❑	❑
12. Remove your nondominant hand from the skin.	❑	❑	❑
13. Holding the syringe steady, pull back on the syringe gently. If blood appears in the hub or the syringe, do not inject the medication; remove the needle and prepare a new injection.	❑	❑	❑

14. Inject the medication slowly by depressing the plunger.
☐ ☐ ☐

15. Place a gauze pad over the injection site and remove the needle.
☐ ☐ ☐
    a. Gently massage the injection site with the gauze pad.
    b. Do not recap the used needle; place it in the biohazard sharps container.
    c. Apply an adhesive bandage if needed.

16. Remove your gloves and wash your hands.
☐ ☐ ☐

17. An injection given for allergy desensitization requires
☐ ☐ ☐
    a. Keeping the patient in the office for at least 30 minutes for observation.
    b. Notifying the doctor of any reaction. (Be alert, anaphylaxis is possible.)

18. Document the procedure, the site, and the results. If instructions were given to the patient, document these also.
☐ ☐ ☐

Calculation

Total Possible Points: _____
Total Points Earned: _____   Multiplied by 100 = _____   Divided by Total Possible Points = _____%

Pass   Fail
☐   ☐

Comments:

Student signature_____ Date_____
Partner signature_____ Date_____
Instructor's signature_____ Date_____

SKILL

PROCEDURE 26-5: Administering an Intramuscular Injection

Equipment/Supplies: Physician's order, medication for injection in ampule or vial, antiseptic wipes, appropriate-size needle and syringe, small gauze pad, biohazard sharps container, clean examination gloves, adhesive bandage, patient's medical record

Standards: Given the needed equipment and a place to work, the student will perform this skill with _____% accuracy in a total of _____ minutes. (*Your instructor will tell you what the percentage and time limits will be before you begin practicing.*)

Key: 4 = Satisfactory   0 = Unsatisfactory   NA = This step is not counted

Procedure Steps	Self	Partner	Instructor

1. Wash your hands.
    a. Review the physician's order and select the correct medication.
    b. Compare the label with the physician's instructions. Note the expiration date.
    c. Check the label three times: when taking it from the shelf, while drawing it up into the syringe, and when returning to the shelf.
	☐	☐	☐

2. Prepare the injection according to the steps in Procedure 8-2.	☐	☐	☐
3. Greet and identify the patient. Explain the procedure.	☐	☐	☐
4. Ask the patient about medication allergies.	☐	☐	☐
5. Select the appropriate site for the injection.	☐	☐	☐
6. Prepare the site by cleansing with an antiseptic wipe.	☐	☐	☐
7. Put on gloves.	☐	☐	☐
8. Using your nondominant hand, hold the skin surrounding the injection site.	☐	☐	☐
9. While holding the syringe like a dart, use a quick, firm motion to insert the needle at a 90° angle to the skin surface. Hold the barrel between the thumb and the index finger of the dominant hand and insert the needle completely to the hub.	☐	☐	☐
10. Holding the syringe steady, pull back on the syringe gently. If blood appears in the hub or the syringe, do not inject the medication; remove the needle and prepare a new injection.	☐	☐	☐
11. Inject the medication slowly by depressing the plunger.	☐	☐	☐

12. Place a gauze pad over the injection site and remove the needle.
    a. Gently massage the injection site with the gauze pad
    b. Do not recap the used needle. Place in biohazard sharps container.
    c. Apply an adhesive bandage if needed.
	☐	☐	☐

13. Remove your gloves, and wash your hands. ☐ ☐ ☐

14. Notify the doctor of any reaction. (Be alert, anaphylaxis is possible.) ☐ ☐ ☐

15. Document the procedure, the site, and the results. If instructions
were given to the patient, document these also. ☐ ☐ ☐

Calculation

Total Possible Points: _____
Total Points Earned: _____ Multiplied by 100 = _____ Divided by Total Possible Points = _____%

Pass   Fail   Comments:
☐   ☐

Student signature_____ Date_____
Partner signature_____ Date_____
Instructor's signature_____ Date_____

SKILL

ROCEDURE 26-6: Administering an Intramuscular Injection Using the Z-Track Method

Equipment/Supplies: Physician's order, medication for injection in ampule or vial, antiseptic wipes, appropriate size needle and syringe, small gauze pad, biohazard sharps container, clean examination gloves, adhesive bandage, patient's medical record

Standards: Given the needed equipment and a place to work, the student will perform this skill with _____% accuracy in a total of _____ minutes. *(Your instructor will tell you what the percentage and time limits will be before you begin practicing.)*

Key: 4 = Satisfactory   0 = Unsatisfactory   NA = This step is not counted

Procedure Steps

	Self	Partner	Instructor
1. Follow steps 1 through 7 as described in Procedure 8-5.	☐	☐	☐
2. Pull the top layer of skin to the side and hold it with your nondominant hand throughout the injection.	☐	☐	☐
3. While holding the syringe like a dart, use a quick, firm motion to insert the needle at a 90° angle to the skin surface. a. Hold the barrel between the thumb and index finger of the dominant hand. b. Insert the needle completely to the hub.	☐	☐	☐
4. Aspirate by withdrawing the plunger slightly. a. If no blood appears, push the plunger in slowly and steadily. b. Count to 10 before withdrawing the needle.	☐	☐	☐
5. Place a gauze pad over the injection site and remove the needle. a. Gently massage the injection site with the gauze pad. b. Do not recap the used needle. Place in the biohazard sharps container. c. Apply an adhesive bandage if needed.	☐	☐	☐
6. Remove your gloves, and wash your hands.	☐	☐	☐
7. Notify the doctor of any reaction. (Be alert, anaphylaxis is possible.)	☐	☐	☐
8. Document the procedure, the site, and the results. If instructions were given to the patient, document these also.	☐	☐	☐

Calculation

Total Possible Points: _____
Total Points Earned: _____ Multiplied by 100 = _____ Divided by Total Possible Points = _____%

Pass   Fail   Comments:
☐   ☐

Student signature_____ Date_____
Partner signature_____ Date_____
Instructor's signature_____ Date_____

Name _____   Date _____   Time _____

PROCEDURE 26-7: Applying Transdermal Medications

Equipment/Supplies: Physician's order, medication, clean examination gloves, patient's medical record

Standards: Given the needed equipment and a place to work, the student will perform this skill with _____% accuracy in a total of _____ minutes. *(Your instructor will tell you what the percentage and time limits will be before you begin practicing.)*

Key: 4 = Satisfactory   0 = Unsatisfactory   NA = This step is not counted

Procedure Steps	Self	Partner	Instructor
1. Wash your hands.	☐	☐	☐

2. Review the physician's medication order and select the correct medication.
  a. Compare the label with the physician's instructions. Note the expiration date.
  b. Check the label three times: when taking it from the shelf, while drawing it up into the syringe, and when returning to the shelf.
	☐	☐	☐

3. Greet and identify the patient. Explain the procedure.	☐	☐	☐
4. Ask the patient about medication allergies that might not be noted on the medical record.	☐	☐	☐

5. Select the appropriate site and perform any necessary skin preparation. The sites are usually the upper arm, the chest or back surface, or behind the ear.
  a. Ensure that the skin is clean, dry, and free from any irritation.
  b. Do not shave areas with excessive hair; trim the hair closely with scissors.
	☐	☐	☐

6. If there is a transdermal patch already in place, remove it carefully while wearing gloves. Discard the patch in the trash container. Inspect the site for irritation.	☐	☐	☐
7. Open the medication package by pulling the two sides apart. Do not touch the area of medication.	☐	☐	☐

8. Apply the medicated patch to the patient's skin, following the manufacturer's directions.
  a. Press the adhesive edges down firmly all around, starting at the center and pressing outward.
  b. If the edges do not stick, fasten with tape.
	☐	☐	☐

9. Wash your hands.	☐	☐	☐
10. Document the procedure and the site of the new patch in the medical record.	☐	☐	☐

Calculation

Total Possible Points: _____
Total Points Earned: _____   Multiplied by 100 = _____   Divided by Total Possible Points = _____%

Pass   **Fail**   Comments:

☐   ☐

Student signature_____   Date_____
Partner signature_____   Date_____
Instructor's signature_____   Date_____

SKILL

PROCEDURE 26-8: Obtaining and Preparing an Intravenous Site

Equipment/Supplies: Physician's order including the type of fluid to be used and the rate; intravenous solution, infusion administration set, IV pole, blank labels, appropriate size intravenous catheter, antiseptic wipes, tourniquet, small gauze pad, biohazard sharps container, clean examination gloves, bandage tape, adhesive bandage, patient's medical record, intravenous catheter (angiocath)

Standards: Given the needed equipment and a place to work, the student will perform this skill with _____% accuracy in a total of _____ minutes. *(Your instructor will tell you what the percentage and time limits will be before you begin practicing.)*

Key: 4 – Satisfactory   0 – Unsatisfactory   NA = This step is not counted

Procedure Steps	Self	Partner	Instructor
1. Wash your hands.	☐	☐	☐
2. Review the physician's order and select the correct IV catheter, solution, and administration set. a. Compare the label on the infusate solution and administration set with the physician's order. b. Note the expiration dates on the infusion solution and the administration set.	☐	☐	☐
3. Prepare the infusion solution by attaching a label to the solution indicating the date, time and name of the patient who will be receiving the IV. a. Hang the solution on an IV pole. b. Remove the administration set from the package and close the roller clamp.	☐	☐	☐
4. Remove the end of the administration set by removing the cover on the spike (located above the drip chamber). a. Remove the cover from the solution infusion port (located on the bottom of the bag). b. Insert the spike end of the administration set into the IV fluid.	☐	☐	☐
5. Fill the drip chamber on the administration set by squeezing the drip chamber until about half full.	☐	☐	☐
6. Open the roller clamp and allow fluid to flow from the drip chamber through the length of the tubing, displacing any air. Do not remove the cover protecting the end of the tubing. a. Close the roller clamp when the fluid has filled the tubing and no air is noted. b. Drape the filled tubing over the IV pole and proceed to perform a venipuncture.	☐	☐	☐
7. Greet and identify the patient. Explain the procedure.	☐	☐	☐
8. Ask the patient about medication allergies that might not be noted on the medical record.	☐	☐	☐

9. Prepare the IV start equipment by tearing or cutting 2 to 3 strips of tape that will be used to secure the IV catheter after insertion; also, inspect each arm for the best available vein.

❑ ❑ ❑

10. Wearing gloves, apply the tourniquet 1 to 2 inches above the intended venipuncture site.
   a. The tourniquet should be snug, but not too tight.
   b. Ask the patient to open and close the fist of the selected arm to distend the veins.

❑ ❑ ❑

11. Secure the tourniquet by using the half-bow.

❑ ❑ ❑

12. Make sure the ends of the tourniquet extend upward to avoid contaminating the venipuncture site.

❑ ❑ ❑

13. Select a vein by palpating with your gloved index finger to trace the path of the vein and judge its depth.

❑ ❑ ❑

14. Release the tourniquet after palpating the vein if it has been left on for more than 1 minute.

❑ ❑ ❑

15. Prepare the site by cleansing with an antiseptic wipe using a circular motion.

❑ ❑ ❑

16. Place the end of the administration set tubing on the examination table for easy access after the venipuncture.

❑ ❑ ❑

17. Anchor the vein to be punctured by placing the thumb of your non-dominant hand below the intended site and holding the skin taut.

❑ ❑ ❑

18. Remove the needle cover from the IV catheter.
   a. While holding the catheter by the flash chamber, not the hub of the needle, use the dominant hand to insert the needle and catheter unit directly into the top of the vein, with the bevel of the needle up at a 15–20° angle for superficial veins.
   b. Observe for a blood flashback into the flash chamber.

❑ ❑ ❑

19. When the blood flashback is observed, lower the angle of the needle until it is flush with the skin and slowly advance the needle and catheter unit about 1/4 inch.

❑ ❑ ❑

20. Once the needle and catheter unit has been inserted slightly into the lumen of the vein hold the flash chamber of the needle steady with the nondominant hand
   a. Slide the catheter (using the catheter hub) off the needle and into the vein with the dominant hand.
   b. Advance the catheter into the vein up to the hub.

❑ ❑ ❑

21. With the needle partly occluding the catheter, release the tourniquet.

❑ ❑ ❑

22. Remove the needle and discard into a biohazard sharps container.
   a. Connect the end of the administration tubing to the end of the IV catheter that has been inserted into the vein.
   b. Open the roller clamp and adjust the flow according the physician's order.

❑ ❑ ❑

23. Secure the hub of the IV catheter with tape.
   a. Place one small strip, sticky side up, under the catheter.
   b. Cross one end over the hub and adhere onto the skin on the opposite side of the catheter.
   c. Cross the other end of the tape in the same fashion and adhere to the skin on the opposite side of the hub.
   d. A transparent membrane adhesive dressing can then be applied over the entire hub and insertion site.

   ❏   ❏   ❏

24. Make a small loop with the administration set tubing near the IV insertion site and secure with tape.

   ❏   ❏   ❏

25. Remove your gloves, wash your hands, and document the procedure in the medical record indicating the size of the IV catheter inserted, the location, the type of infusion, and the rate.

   ❏   ❏   ❏

Calculation

Total Possible Points: _____
Total Points Earned: _____   Multiplied by 100 = _____   Divided by Total Possible Points = _____%

Pass   Fail   Comments:
❏   ❏

Student signature_____ Date_____
Partner signature_____ Date_____
Instructor's signature_____ Date_____

SKILL

PROCEDURE 29-1: Applying a Warm or Cold Compress

Equipment/Supplies: Warm compresses—appropriate solution (water with possible antiseptic if ordered), warmed to 110°F or recommended temperature; bath thermometer; absorbent material (cloths, gauze); waterproof barriers; hot water bottle (optional); clean or sterile basin; gloves. Cold compresses—appropriate solution; ice bag or cold pack; absorbent material (cloths, gauze); waterproof barriers; gloves

Standards: Given the needed equipment and a place to work, the student will perform this skill with _____% accuracy in a total of _____ minutes. *(Your instructor will tell you what the percentage and time limits will be before you begin practicing.)*

Key: 4 = Satisfactory   0 = Unsatisfactory   NA = This step is not counted

Procedure Steps	Self	Partner	Instructor
1. Wash your hands and put on gloves.	❏	❏	❏
2. Check the physician's order and assemble the equipment and supplies.	❏	❏	❏
3. Pour the appropriate solution into the basin. For hot compresses, check the temperature of the warmed solution.	❏	❏	❏
4. Greet and identify the patient. Explain the procedure.	❏	❏	❏
5. Ask patient to remove appropriate clothing.	❏	❏	❏
6. Gown and drape accordingly.	❏	❏	❏
7. Protect the examination table with a waterproof barrier.	❏	❏	❏
8. Place absorbent material or gauze into the prepared solution. Wring out excess moisture.	❏	❏	❏
9. Place the compress on the patient's skin and ask about comfort of temperature.	❏	❏	❏
10. Observe the skin for changes in color.	❏	❏	❏
11. Arrange the wet compress over the area.	❏	❏	❏
12. Insulate the compress with plastic or another waterproof barrier.	❏	❏	❏
13. Check the compress frequently for moisture and temperature. a. Hot water bottles or ice packs may be used to maintain the temperature. b. Rewet absorbent material as needed.	❏	❏	❏
14. After the prescribed amount of time, usually 20–30 minutes, remove the compress. a. Discard disposable materials. b. Disinfect reusable equipment.	❏	❏	❏

15. Remove your gloves and wash your hands. ❑ ❑ ❑

16. Document the procedure including ❑ ❑ ❑
    a. Length of treatment, type of solution, temperature of solution
    b. Skin color after treatment, assessment of the area, and patient's reactions

Calculation

Total Possible Points: _____
Total Points Earned: _____ Multiplied by 100 = _____ Divided by Total Possible Points = _____%

Pass   **Fail**   Comments:
❑   ❑

Student signature_____ Date_____

Partner signature_____ Date_____

Instructor's signature_____ Date_____

SKILL

PROCEDURE 29-2: Assisting with Therapeutic Soaks

Equipment/Supplies: Clean or sterile basin or container to comfortably contain the body part to be soaked; solution and/or medication; dry towels; bath thermometer; gloves

Standards: Given the needed equipment and a place to work, the student will perform this skill with _____% accuracy in a total of _____ minutes. *(Your instructor will tell you what the percentage and time limits will be before you begin practicing.)*

Key: 4 = Satisfactory   0 = Unsatisfactory   NA = This step is not counted

Procedure Steps	Self	Partner	Instructor
1. Wash your hands and apply your gloves.	☐	☐	☐
2. Assemble the equipment and supplies, including the appropriately sized basin or container. Pad surfaces of container for comfort.	☐	☐	☐
3. Fill the container with solution and check the temperature with a bath thermometer. The temperature should be below 110°F.	☐	☐	☐
4. Greet and identify the patient. Explain the procedure.	☐	☐	☐
5. Slowly lower the patient's extremity or body part into the container.	☐	☐	☐
6. Arrange the part comfortably and in easy alignment.	☐	☐	☐
7. Check for pressure areas and pad the edges as needed for comfort.	☐	☐	☐
8. Check the solution every 5–10 minutes for proper temperature.	☐	☐	☐
9. Soak for the prescribed amount of time, usually 15–20 minutes.	☐	☐	☐
10. Remove the body part from the solution and carefully dry the area with a towel.	☐	☐	☐
11. Properly care for the equipment and appropriately dispose of single-use supplies.	☐	☐	☐

12. Document the procedure including
   a. Length of treatment, type of solution, temperature of solution
   b. Skin color after treatment, assessment of the area, and patient's reactions
	☐	☐	☐

Calculation

Total Possible Points: _____
Total Points Earned: _____   Multiplied by 100 = _____   Divided by Total Possible Points = _____%

Pass   Fail   Comments:
☐   ☐

Student signature_____ Date_____

Partner signature_____ Date_____

Instructor's signature_____ Date_____

SKILL

PROCEDURE 29-3: Applying a Tubular Gauze Bandage

Equipment/Supplies: Tubular gauze; applicator; tape; scissors

Standards: Given the needed equipment and a place to work, the student will perform this skill with _____% accuracy in a total of _____ minutes. *(Your instructor will tell you what the percentage and time limits will be before you begin practicing.)*

Key: 4 = Satisfactory   0 = Unsatisfactory   NA = This step is not counted

Procedure Steps	Self	Partner	Instructor
1. Wash your hands and assemble the equipment.	☐	☐	☐
2. Greet and identify the patient. Explain the procedure.	☐	☐	☐
3. Choose the appropriate-size tubular gauze applicator and gauze width.	☐	☐	☐
4. Select and cut or tear adhesive tape in lengths to secure the gauze ends.	☐	☐	☐
5. Place the gauze bandage on the applicator in the following manner: a. Be sure that the applicator is upright (open end up) and placed on a flat surface. b. Pull a sufficient length of gauze from the stock box; ready to cut. c. Open the end of the length of gauze and slide it over the upper end of the applicator. d. Push estimated amount of gauze needed for this procedure onto the applicator. e. Cut the gauze when the required amount of gauze has been transferred to the applicator.	☐	☐	☐
6. Place applicator over the distal end of the affected part. Hold it in place as you move to step 7.	☐	☐	☐
7. Slide applicator containing the gauze up to the proximal end of the affected part.	☐	☐	☐
8. Pull the applicator 1–2 inches past the end of the affected part if the part is to be completely covered.	☐	☐	☐
9. Turn the applicator one full turn to anchor the bandage.	☐	☐	☐
10. Move the applicator toward the proximal part as before.	☐	☐	☐
11. Move the applicator forward about 1 inch beyond the original starting point.	☐	☐	☐
12. Repeat the procedure until the desired coverage is obtained.	☐	☐	☐

13. The final layer should end at the proximal part of the affected area. Remove the applicator. ❏ ❏ ❏

14. Secure the bandage in place with adhesive tape or cut the gauze into two tails and tie them at the base of the tear. ❏ ❏ ❏

15. Tie the two tails around the closest proximal joint. ❏ ❏ ❏

16. Use the adhesive tape sparingly to secure the end if not using a tie. ❏ ❏ ❏

17. Properly care for or dispose of equipment and supplies. ❏ ❏ ❏

18. Clean the work area. Wash your hands. ❏ ❏ ❏

19. Record the procedure. ❏ ❏ ❏

Calculation

Total Possible Points: _____
Total Points Earned: _____ Multiplied by 100 = _____ Divided by Total Possible Points = _____%

Pass ❏   Fail ❏

Comments:

Student signature_____ Date_____

Partner signature_____ Date_____

Instructor's signature_____ Date_____

SKILL

PROCEDURE 30-1: Applying a Triangular Arm Sling

Equipment/Supplies: A canvas triangular arm sling, 2 safety pins

Standards: Given the needed equipment and a place to work, the student will perform this skill with _____% accuracy in a total of _____ minutes. *(Your instructor will tell you what the percentage and time limits will be before you begin practicing.)*

Key: 4 = Satisfactory   0 = Unsatisfactory   NA = This step is not counted

Procedure Steps	Self	Partner	Instructor
1. Wash your hands.	☐	☐	☐
2. Assemble the equipment and supplies.	☐	☐	☐
3. Greet and identify the patient; explain the procedure.	☐	☐	☐
4. Position the affected limb with the hand at slightly less than a 90° angle.	☐	☐	☐
5. Place the triangle with the uppermost corner at the shoulder on the unaffected side. a. Extend the corner across the nape of the neck. b. The middle angle is at the elbow of the affected side. c. The final lowermost corner is pointing toward the foot of the unaffected side.	☐	☐	☐
6. Bring up the lowermost corner to meet the upper corner at the side of the neck.	☐	☐	☐
7. Tie or pin the sling at the knot.	☐	☐	☐
8. Secure the elbow by fitting any extra fabric neatly around the limb and pinning.	☐	☐	☐
9. Check the patient's level of comfort and distal extremity circulation.	☐	☐	☐
10. Document the appliance in the patient's chart.	☐	☐	☐

Calculation

Total Possible Points: _____
Total Points Earned: _____   Multiplied by 100 = _____   Divided by Total Possible Points = _____%

Pass   Fail | Comments:
☐   ☐

Student signature_____ Date_____
Partner signature_____ Date_____
Instructor's signature_____ Date_____

Name_____ Date _____ Time_____

SKILL

PROCEDURE 30-2: Applying Cold Packs

Equipment/Supplies: Ice bag and ice chips or small cubes, or disposable cold pack; small towel or cover for ice pack; gauze or tape

Standards: Given the needed equipment and a place to work, the student will perform this skill with _____% accuracy in a total of _____ minutes. (*Your instructor will tell you what the percentage and time limits will be before you begin practicing.*)

Key: 4 = Satisfactory   0 = Unsatisfactory   NA = This step is not counted

Procedure Steps	Self	Partner	Instructor
1. Wash your hands.	☐	☐	☐
2. Assemble the equipment and supplies, checking the ice bag, if used, for leaks. If using a commercial cold pack, read the manufacturer's directions.	☐	☐	☐
3. Fill a nondisposable ice bag about two-thirds full. a. Press it flat on a surface to express air from the bag. b. Seal the container.	☐	☐	☐
4. If using a commercial chemical ice pack, activate it now.	☐	☐	☐
5. Cover the bag in a towel or other suitable cover.	☐	☐	☐
6. Greet and identify the patient. Explain the procedure.	☐	☐	☐
7. After assessing skin for color and warmth, place the covered ice pack on the area.	☐	☐	☐
8. Secure the ice pack with gauze or tape.	☐	☐	☐
9. Apply the treatment for the prescribed amount of time, but no longer than 30 minutes.	☐	☐	☐
10. During the treatment, assess the skin under the pack frequently for mottling, pallor, or redness.	☐	☐	☐
11. Properly care for or dispose of equipment and supplies. Wash your hands.	☐	☐	☐
12. Document the procedure, the site of the application, the results including the condition of the skin after the treatment, and the patient's reactions.	☐	☐	☐

Calculation

Total Possible Points: _____
Total Points Earned: _____ Multiplied by 100 = _____ Divided by Total Possible Points = _____%

Pass   Fail   Comments:
☐   ☐

Student signature_____ Date_____
Partner signature_____ Date_____
Instructor's signature_____ Date_____

SKILL

PROCEDURE 30-3: Using a Hot Water Bottle or Commercial Hot Pack

Equipment/Supplies: A hot water bottle or commercial hot pack, towel or other suitable covering for the hot pack

Standards: Given the needed equipment and a place to work, the student will perform this skill with _____% accuracy in a total of _____ minutes. *(Your instructor will tell you what the percentage and time limits will be before you begin practicing.)*

Key: 4 = Satisfactory   0 = Unsatisfactory   NA = This step is not counted

Procedure Steps	Self	Partner	Instructor
1. Wash your hands.	☐	☐	☐
2. Assemble equipment and supplies, checking the hot water bottle for leaks.	☐	☐	☐
3. Fill the hot water bottle about two-thirds full with warm (110°F) water. a. Place the bottle on a flat surface and the opening up; "burp" it by pressing out the air. b. If using a commercial hot pack, follow the manufacturer's directions for activating it.	☐	☐	☐
4. Wrap and secure the pack or bottle before placing it on the patient's skin.	☐	☐	☐
5. Greet and identify the patient. Explain the procedure.	☐	☐	☐
6. After assessing the color of the skin where the treatment is to be applied, place the covered hot pack on the area.	☐	☐	☐
7. Secure the hot pack with gauze or tape.	☐	☐	☐
8. Apply the treatment for the prescribed length of time, but no longer than 30 minutes.	☐	☐	☐
9. During treatment, assess the skin every 10 minutes for pallor (an indication of rebound), excessive redness (indicates temperature may be too high), swelling (indicates possible tissue damage).	☐	☐	☐
10. Properly care for or dispose of equipment and supplies. Wash your hands.	☐	☐	☐
11. Document the procedure, the site of the application, the results including the condition of the skin after the treatment, and the patient's reactions.	☐	☐	☐

Calculation

Total Possible Points: _____
Total Points Earned: _____   Multiplied by 100 = _____   Divided by Total Possible Points = _____%

Pass   Fail   Comments:
☐   ☐

Student signature_____ Date_____
Partner signature_____ Date_____
Instructor's signature_____ Date_____

SKILL

PROCEDURE 30-4: Measuring a Patient for Axillary Crutches

Equipment/Supplies: Axillary crutches with tips, pads for the axillae, and hand rests, as needed; tools to tighten bolts

Standards: Given the needed equipment and a place to work, the student will perform this skill with _____% accuracy in a total of _____ minutes. *(Your instructor will tell you what the percentage and time limits will be before you begin practicing.)*

Key: 4 = Satisfactory   0 = Unsatisfactory   NA = This step is not counted

Procedure Steps	Self	Partner	Instructor
1. Wash your hands.	☐	☐	☐
2. Assemble the equipment including the correct-size crutches.	☐	☐	☐
3. Greet and identify the patient.	☐	☐	☐
4. Ensure that the patient is wearing low-heeled shoes with safety soles.	☐	☐	☐
5. Have the patient stand erect. Support the patient as needed.	☐	☐	☐
6. While standing erect, have the patient hold the crutches in the tripod position.	☐	☐	☐
7. Using the tools as needed, adjust the central support in the base. a. Tighten the bolts for safety when the proper height is reached. b. Adjust the handgrips. Tighten bolts for safety. c. If needed, pad axillary bars and handgrips.	☐	☐	☐
8. Wash your hands and record the procedure.	☐	☐	☐

Calculation

Total Possible Points: _____
Total Points Earned: _____ Multiplied by 100 = _____ Divided by Total Possible Points = _____%

Pass   Fail
☐   ☐

Comments:

Student signature_____ Date_____

Partner signature_____ Date_____

Instructor's signature_____ Date_____

SKILL

PROCEDURE 30-5: Instructing a Patient in Various Crutch Gaits

Equipment/Supplies: Axillary crutches measured appropriately for a patient.

Standards: Given the needed equipment and a place to work, the student will perform this skill with _____% accuracy in a total of _____ minutes. *(Your instructor will tell you what the percentage and time limits will be before you begin practicing.)*

Key: 4 = Satisfactory   0 = Unsatisfactory   NA = This step is not counted

Procedure Steps	Self	Partner	Instructor
1. Wash your hands.	☐	☐	☐
2. Have the patient stand up from a chair: a. The patient holds both crutches on the affected side. b. Then the patient slides to the edge of the chair. c. The patient pushes down on the chair arm on the unaffected side. d. Then the patient pushes to stand.	☐	☐	☐
3. With one crutch in each hand, rest on the crutches until balance is restored.	☐	☐	☐
4. Assist the patient to the tripod position.	☐	☐	☐
5. Depending upon the patient's weight-bearing ability, coordination, and general state of health, instruct the patient in one or more of the following gaits:	☐	☐	☐

a. *Three-point gait:*
   (1) Both crutches are moved forward with the unaffected leg bearing the weight.
   (2) With the weight supported by the crutches on the handgrips, the unaffected leg is brought past the level of the crutches.
   (3) The steps are repeated.
b. *Two-point gait:*
   (1) The right crutch and left foot are moved forward.
   (2) As these points rest, the right foot and left crutch are moved forward.
   (3) The steps are repeated.
c. *Four-point gait:*
   (1) The right crutch moves forward.
   (2) The left foot is moved to a position just ahead of the left crutch.
   (3) The left crutch is moved forward.
   (4) The right foot moves to a position just ahead of the right crutch.
   (5) The steps are repeated.
d. *Swing-through gait:*
   (1) Both crutches are moved forward.
   (2) With the weight on the hands, the body swings through to a position ahead of the crutches with both legs leaving the floor together.

(3) The crutches are moved ahead.

(4) The steps are repeated.

e. *Swing-to gait:*

(1) Both crutches are moved forward.

(2) With the weight on the hands, the body swings to the level of the crutches with both legs leaving the floor.

(3) The crutches are moved ahead.

(4) The steps are repeated.

5. Wash your hands and record the procedure. ❑ ❑ ❑

Calculation

Total Possible Points: _____

Total Points Earned: _____ Multiplied by 100 = _____ Divided by Total Possible Points = _____%

Pass ❑   Fail ❑

Comments:

Student signature_____ Date_____

Partner signature_____ Date_____

Instructor's signature_____ Date_____

Name_____ Date _____ Time_____

PROCEDURE 31-1: Measuring Distance Visual Acuity

Equipment/Supplies: Snellen eye chart, paper cup or eye paddle

Standards: Given the needed equipment and a place to work, the student will perform this skill with _____% accuracy in a total of _____ minutes. *(Your instructor will tell you what the percentage and time limits will be before you begin practicing.)*

Key: 4 = Satisfactory   0 = Unsatisfactory   NA = This step is not counted

Procedure Steps	Self	Partner	Instructor
1. Wash your hands.	☐	☐	☐
2. Prepare the examination area (well lit, distance marker 20 feet from the chart).	☐	☐	☐
3. Make sure the chart is at eye level.	☐	☐	☐
4. Greet and identify the patient. Explain the procedure.	☐	☐	☐
5. Position the patient in a standing or sitting position at the 20-foot marker.	☐	☐	☐
6. If not wearing glasses, ask patient about contact lenses. Mark results accordingly.	☐	☐	☐
7. Have patient cover left eye with eye paddle.	☐	☐	☐
8. Instruct patient not to close the left eye, but to keep both eyes open during the test.	☐	☐	☐
9. Stand beside the chart and point to each row as the patient reads aloud. a. Point to the lines, starting with the 20/200 line. b. Record the smallest line that the patient can read with no errors.	☐	☐	☐
10. Repeat the procedure with the right eye covered and record.	☐	☐	☐
11. Wash your hands and document the procedure.	☐	☐	☐

Calculation

Total Possible Points: _____
Total Points Earned: _____   Multiplied by 100 = _____   Divided by Total Possible Points = _____%

Pass   Fail
☐   ☐

Comments:

Student signature_____ Date_____
Partner signature_____ Date_____
Instructor's signature_____ Date_____

Name_____ Date _____ Time_____

SKILL

PROCEDURE 31-2: Measuring Color Perception

Equipment/Supplies: Ishihara color plates, gloves

Standards: Given the needed equipment and a place to work, the student will perform this skill with _____% accuracy in a total of _____ minutes. *(Your instructor will tell you what the percentage and time limits will be before you begin practicing.)*

Key: 4 = Satisfactory 0 = Unsatisfactory NA = This step is not counted

Procedure Steps	Self	Partner	Instructor
1. Wash your hands, put on gloves, and obtain the Ishihara color plate book.	☐	☐	☐
2. Prepare the examination area (well lit, distance marker 20 feet from the chart).	☐	☐	☐
3. If not wearing glasses, ask patient about contact lenses. Mark results accordingly.	☐	☐	☐
4. Hold the first bookplate about 30 inches from the patient.	☐	☐	☐
5. Ask if the patient can see the "number" within the series of dots. a. Record results of test by noting the number or figure the patient reports. b. If patient cannot distinguish a pattern, record plate number–x (e.g., 4–x).	☐	☐	☐
6. The patient should not take more than 3 seconds when reading the plates. a. The patient should not squint nor guess. These indicate patient is unsure. b. Record as plate number - x.	☐	☐	☐
7. Record the results for plates 1 through 10. a. Plate number 11 requires patient to trace a winding line between x's. b. Patients with a color deficit will not be able to trace the line.	☐	☐	☐
8. Store the book in a closed, protected area to protect the integrity of the colors.	☐	☐	☐
9. Remove your gloves and wash your hands.	☐	☐	☐

Calculation

Total Possible Points: _____
Total Points Earned: _____ Multiplied by 100 = _____ Divided by Total Possible Points = _____%

Pass ☐   Fail ☐   Comments:

Student signature_____ Date_____
Partner signature_____ Date_____
Instructor's signature_____ Date_____

Name_____ Date _____ Time_____

PROCEDURE 31-3: Instilling Eye Medications

Equipment/Supplies: Physician's order and patient record, ophthalmic medications, sterile gauze, tissues, gloves

Standards: Given the needed equipment and a place to work, the student will perform this skill with _____% accuracy in a total of _____ minutes. *(Your instructor will tell you what the percentage and time limits will be before you begin practicing.)*

Key: 4 = Satisfactory   0 = Unsatisfactory   NA = This step is not counted

Procedure Steps	Self	Partner	Instructor
1. Wash your hands.	☐	☐	☐
2. Obtain the physician order, the correct medication, sterile gauze, and tissues.	☐	☐	☐
3. Greet and identify the patient. Explain the procedure.	☐	☐	☐
4. Ask the patient about any allergies not recorded in the chart.	☐	☐	☐
5. Position the patient comfortably.	☐	☐	☐
6. Put on gloves. Ask the patient to look upward.	☐	☐	☐

7. Use sterile gauze to gently pull lower lid down. Instill the medication.
  a. *Ointment:* Discard first bead of ointment without touching the end of the tube.
    (1) Place a thin line of ointment across inside of lower eyelid.
    (2) Move from the inner canthus outward.
    (3) Release ointment by twisting the tube slightly.
    (4) Do not touch the tube to the eye.
  b. *Drops:* Hold dropper close to conjunctival sac, but do not touch the patient.
    (1) Release the proper number of drops into the sac.
    (2) Discard any medication left in the dropper.
	☐	☐	☐

8. Release the lower lid. Have patient gently close the eyelid and roll the eye.	☐	☐	☐
9. Wipe off any excess medication with tissue.	☐	☐	☐
10. Instruct patient to apply light pressure on puncta lacrimale for several minutes.	☐	☐	☐
11. Properly care for or dispose of equipment and supplies. Clean the work area.	☐	☐	☐
12. Wash your hands.	☐	☐	☐
13. Record the procedure.	☐	☐	☐

Calculation

Total Possible Points: _____
Total Points Earned: _____   Multiplied by 100 = _____   Divided by Total Possible Points = _____%

Pass   Fail
☐   ☐

Comments:

Student signature_____ Date_____

Partner signature_____ Date_____

Instructor's signature_____ Date_____

PROCEDURE 31-4: Irrigating the Eye

Equipment/Supplies: Physician's order and patient record, small sterile basin, irrigating solution and medication if ordered, protective barrier or towels, emesis basin, sterile bulb syringe, tissues, gloves

Standards: Given the needed equipment and a place to work, the student will perform this skill with _____% accuracy in a total of _____ minutes. (*Your instructor will tell you what the percentage and time limits will be before you begin practicing.*)

Key: 4 = Satisfactory   0 = Unsatisfactory   NA = This step is not counted

Procedure Steps

	Self	Partner	Instructor
1. Wash your hands and put on your gloves.	☐	☐	☐
2. Assemble the equipment, supplies, and medication if ordered by the physician. a. Check solution label three times. b. Make sure that the label indicates for ophthalmic use.	☐	☐	☐
3. Greet and identify the patient. Explain the procedure.	☐	☐	☐
4. Position the patient comfortably. a. Sitting with head tilted with the affected eye lower. b. Lying with the affected eye downward.	☐	☐	☐
5. Drape patient with the protective barrier or towel to avoid wetting the clothing.	☐	☐	☐
6. Place emesis basin against upper cheek near eye with the towel under the basin. a. Wipe the eye from the inner canthus outward with gauze to remove debris. b. Separate the eyelids with your thumb and forefinger. c. Lightly support your hand, holding the syringe, on bridge of patient's nose.	☐	☐	☐
7. Holding syringe 1 inch above the eye, gently irrigate from inner to outer canthus. a. Use gentle pressure and do not touch the eye. b. Physician will order the period of time or amount of solution required.	☐	☐	☐
8. Use tissues to wipe any excess solution from the patient's face.	☐	☐	☐
9. Properly dispose of equipment or sanitize as recommended.	☐	☐	☐
10. Remove your gloves. Wash your hands.	☐	☐	☐
11. Record procedure, including amount, type, and strength of solution; which eye was irrigated; and any observations.	☐	☐	☐

Calculation

Total Possible Points: _____
Total Points Earned: _____   Multiplied by 100 = _____   Divided by Total Possible Points = _____%

Pass   Fail   Comments:
☐   ☐

Student signature_____ Date_____
Partner signature_____ Date_____
Instructor's signature_____ Date_____

SKILL

PROCEDURE 31-5: Audiometry Testing

Equipment/Supplies: Audiometer, otoscope

Standards: Given the needed equipment and a place to work, the student will perform this skill with _____% accuracy in a total of _____ minutes. *(Your instructor will tell you what the percentage and time limits will be before you begin practicing.)*

Key: 4 = Satisfactory   0 = Unsatisfactory   NA = This step is not counted

Procedure Steps	Self	Partner	Instructor
1. Wash your hands.	☐	☐	☐
2. Greet and identify patient. Explain the procedure.	☐	☐	☐
3. Take patient to a quiet area or room for testing.	☐	☐	☐
4. Visually inspect the ear canal and tympanic membrane before the examination.	☐	☐	☐
5. Choose the correct-size tip for the end of the audiometer.	☐	☐	☐
6. Attach a speculum to fit the patient's external auditory meatus.	☐	☐	☐

7. With the specula in the ear canal, retract the pinna:
  a. *Adults:* Gently pull up and back to straighten the auditory canal.
  b. *Children:* Gently pull slightly down and back to straighten the auditory canal.
	☐	☐	☐

8. Follow audiometer instrument directions for use:
  a. Screen right ear
  b. Screen left ear
	☐	☐	☐

9. If the patient fails to respond at any frequency, rescreening is required.	☐	☐	☐
10. If the patient fails rescreening, notify the physician.	☐	☐	☐
11. Record the results in the medical record.	☐	☐	☐

Calculation

Total Possible Points: _____
Total Points Earned: _____   Multiplied by 100 = _____   Divided by Total Possible Points = _____%

Pass   Fail   Comments:
☐   ☐

Student signature_____   Date_____
Partner signature_____   Date_____
Instructor's signature_____   Date_____

PROCEDURE 31-6: Irrigating the Ear

Equipment/Supplies: Physician's order and patient record, emesis basin or ear basin, waterproof barrier or towels, otoscope, irrigation solution, bowl for solution, gauze

Standards: Given the needed equipment and a place to work, the student will perform this skill with _____% accuracy in a total of _____ minutes. *(Your instructor will tell you what the percentage and time limits will be before you begin practicing.)*

Key: 4 = Satisfactory   0 = Unsatisfactory   NA = This step is not counted

Procedure Steps	Self	Partner	Instructor
1. Wash your hands.	☐	☐	☐
2. Assemble the equipment and supplies.	☐	☐	☐
3. Greet and identify the patient. Explain the procedure.	☐	☐	☐
4. Position the patient comfortably in an erect position.	☐	☐	☐

5. View the affected ear with an otoscope to locate the foreign matter or cerumen.
  a. *Adults:* Gently pull up and back to straighten the auditory canal.
  b. *Children:* Gently pull slightly down and back to straighten the auditory canal.
	☐	☐	☐

6. Drape the patient with a waterproof barrier or towel.	☐	☐	☐
7. Tilt the patient's head toward the affected side.	☐	☐	☐
8. Place the drainage basin under the affected ear.	☐	☐	☐
9. Fill the irrigating syringe or turn on the irrigating device.	☐	☐	☐
10. Gently position the auricle as described above using your nondominant hand.	☐	☐	☐
11. With dominant hand, place the tip of the syringe into the auditory meatus.	☐	☐	☐
12. Direct the flow of the solution gently upward toward the roof of the canal.	☐	☐	☐
13. Irrigate for the prescribed period of time or until the desired results are obtained.	☐	☐	☐
14. Dry the patient's external ear with gauze.	☐	☐	☐
15. Have patient sit for a while with the affected ear downward to drain the solution.	☐	☐	☐
16. Inspect the ear with the otoscope to determine the results.	☐	☐	☐
17. Properly care for or dispose of equipment and supplies. Clean the work area.	☐	☐	☐
18. Wash your hands.	☐	☐	☐
19. Record the procedure in the patient's chart.			

Calculation

Total Possible Points: _____
Total Points Earned: _____   Multiplied by 100 = _____   Divided by Total Possible Points = _____%

Pass   Fail   Comments:

☐   ☐

Student signature_____ Date_____

Partner signature_____ Date_____

Instructor's signature_____ Date_____

SKILL

PROCEDURE 31-7: Instilling Ear Medication

Equipment/Supplies: Physician's order and patient record, otic medication with dropper, cotton balls

Standards: Given the needed equipment and a place to work, the student will perform this skill with _____% accuracy in a total of _____ minutes. *(Your instructor will tell you what the percentage and time limits will be before you begin practicing.)*

Key: 4 = Satisfactory   0 = Unsatisfactory   NA = This step is not counted

Procedure Steps	Self	Partner	Instructor
1. Wash your hands.	☐	☐	☐
2. Assemble the equipment, supplies, and medication if ordered by the physician. a. Check solution label three times. b. Make sure that the label indicates for otic use.	☐	☐	☐
3. Greet and identify the patient. Explain the procedure.	☐	☐	☐
4. Ask patient about any allergies not documented.	☐	☐	☐
5. Have the patient seated with the affected ear tilted upward.	☐	☐	☐
6. Draw up the ordered amount of medication. a. *Adults:* Pull the auricle slightly up and back to straighten S-shaped canal. b. *Children:* Pull the auricle slightly down and back to straighten S-shaped canal.	☐	☐	☐
7. Insert the tip of dropper without touching the patient's skin. a. Let the medication flow along the side of the canal. b. Have patient sit or lie with affected ear upward for about 5 minutes.	☐	☐	☐
8. To keep medication in the canal, gently insert a moist cotton ball into the external auditory meatus.	☐	☐	☐
9. Properly care for or dispose of equipment and supplies. Clean the work area.	☐	☐	☐
10. Wash your hands.	☐	☐	☐
11. Record the procedure in the patient record.	☐	☐	☐

Calculation

Total Possible Points: _____
Total Points Earned: _____   Multiplied by 100 = _____   Divided by Total Possible Points = _____%

Pass ☐   Fail ☐

Comments:

Student signature_____ Date_____

Partner signature_____ Date_____

Instructor's signature_____ Date_____

Name_____ Date _____ Time_____

SKILL

PROCEDURE 31-8: Instilling Nasal Medication

Equipment/Supplies: Physician's order and patient record; nasal medication, drops, or spray; tissues; gloves

Standards: Given the needed equipment and a place to work, the student will perform this skill with _____% accuracy in a total of _____ minutes. *(Your instructor will tell you what the percentage and time limits will be before you begin practicing.)*

Key: 4 = Satisfactory   0 = Unsatisfactory   NA = This step is not counted

Procedure Steps

	Self	Partner	Instructor
1. Wash your hands and put on gloves.	☐	☐	☐
2. Assemble the equipment and supplies. Check the medication label three times.	☐	☐	☐
3. Greet and identify the patient. Explain the procedure.	☐	☐	☐
4. Ask patient about any allergies not documented.	☐	☐	☐
5. Position the patient in a comfortable recumbent position.	☐	☐	☐

   a. Extend patient's head beyond edge of examination table
   b. Or place a pillow under the patient's shoulders.
   c. Support the patient's neck to avoid strain as the head is tilted back.

	Self	Partner	Instructor
6. Administering nasal medication:	☐	☐	☐

   a. Nasal drops
     (1) Hold the dropper upright just above each nostril.
     (2) Drop the medication one drop at a time without touching the nares.
     (3) Keep the patient in a recumbent position for 5 minutes.
   b. Nasal spray
     (1) Place tip of the bottle at the naris opening without touching the patient.
     (2) Spray as the patient takes a deep breath.

	Self	Partner	Instructor
7. Wipe any excess medication from the patient's skin with tissues.	☐	☐	☐
8. Properly care for or dispose of equipment and supplies. Clean the work area.	☐	☐	☐
9. Remove your gloves and wash your hands.	☐	☐	☐
10. Record the procedure in the patient's chart.	☐	☐	☐

Calculation

Total Possible Points: _____
Total Points Earned: _____   Multiplied by 100 = _____   Divided by Total Possible Points = _____%

Pass   Fail   Comments:
☐   ☐

Student signature_____ Date_____
Partner signature_____ Date_____
Instructor's signature_____ Date_____

Name_____ Date _____ Time_____

PROCEDURE 31-9: Collecting a Specimen for Throat Culture

Equipment/Supplies: Physician's order and patient record, tongue blade, sterile specimen container and swab, gloves, commercial throat culture kit (if being done in the office) or completed laboratory request form and bio-hazard bag for transport (if being sent to the laboratory for analysis)

Standards: Given the needed equipment and a place to work, the student will perform this skill with _____% accuracy in a total of _____ minutes. (*Your instructor will tell you what the percentage and time limits will be before you begin practicing.*)

Key: 4 = Satisfactory   0 = Unsatisfactory   NA = This step is not counted

Procedure Steps	Self	Partner	Instructor
1. Wash your hands.	❏	❏	❏
2. Assemble the equipment and supplies. Put on gloves.	❏	❏	❏
3. Greet and identify the patient. Explain the procedure.	❏	❏	❏
4. Have the patient sit with a light source directed at the throat.	❏	❏	❏
5. Carefully remove the sterile swab from the container.	❏	❏	❏
6. Have the patient say "AHHHHH" with the mouth wide open.	❏	❏	❏
7. Press down on the midpoint of the tongue with the tongue depressor.	❏	❏	❏
8. Swab areas of concern: a. Mucous membranes, especially the tonsillar area. b. Crypts and the posterior pharynx.	❏	❏	❏
9. Turn the swab to expose all of its surfaces to the membranes. Avoid touching areas other than those suspected of infection.	❏	❏	❏
10. Maintain tongue depressor position and withdraw swab from the patient's mouth.	❏	❏	❏
11. Follow the instructions on the specimen container for transferring the swab.	❏	❏	❏
12. Properly dispose of the equipment and supplies in a biohazard waste container.	❏	❏	❏
13. Remove your gloves and wash your hands.	❏	❏	❏
14. Route the specimen or store it appropriately until routing can be completed.	❏	❏	❏
15. Document the procedure.	❏	❏	❏

Calculation

Total Possible Points: _____
Total Points Earned: _____   Multiplied by 100 = _____   Divided by Total Possible Points = _____%

Pass   Fail   Comments:
❏   ❏

Student signature_____ Date_____
Partner signature_____ Date_____
Instructor's signature_____ Date_____

PROCEDURE 32-1: Collecting a Sputum Specimen

Equipment/Supplies: Labeled sterile specimen container, gloves, laboratory request, biohazard bag for transporting the specimen

Standards: Given the needed equipment and a place to work, the student will perform this skill with _____% accuracy in a total of _____ minutes. *(Your instructor will tell you what the percentage and time limits will be before you begin practicing.)*

Key: 4 = Satisfactory   0 = Unsatisfactory   NA = This step is not counted

Procedure Steps	Self	Partner	Instructor
1. Wash your hands and put on clean examination gloves.	☐	☐	☐
2. Assemble the equipment, greet and identify the patient, and explain the procedure. Also, write the name of the patient on a label and affix to the outside of the container.	☐	☐	☐
3. Ask the patient to cough deeply, using the abdominal muscles as well as the accessory muscles to bring secretions from the lungs and not just the upper airways.	☐ ☐	☐ ☐	☐ ☐
4. Ask the patient to expectorate directly into the specimen container without touching the inside and without getting sputum on the outsides of the container. About 5–10 mL is sufficient for most sputum studies.	☐	☐	☐
5. Handle the specimen container, observing standard precautions. Cap the container immediately and put it into the biohazardous bag for transport to the laboratory. Complete a laboratory requisition slip to accompany the specimen to the laboratory.	☐	☐	☐
6. Properly care for or dispose of equipment and supplies, clean the work area, remove your gloves, and wash your gloves.	☐	☐	☐
7. Send the specimen to the laboratory immediately to avoid compromising the test results.	☐	☐	☐
8. Document the procedure.	☐	☐	☐

Calculation

Total Possible Points: _____
Total Points Earned: _____   Multiplied by 100 = _____   Divided by Total Possible Points = _____%

Pass   Fail   Comments:
☐   ☐

Student signature_____ Date_____

Partner signature_____ Date_____

Instructor's signature_____ Date_____

SKILL

PROCEDURE 32-2: Instructing a Patient on Using the Peak Flowmeter

Equipment/Supplies: Peak flowmeter, recording documentation form

Standards: Given the needed equipment and a place to work, the student will perform this skill with _____% accuracy in a total of _____ minutes. *(Your instructor will tell you what the percentage and time limits will be before you begin practicing.)*

Key: 4 = Satisfactory   0 = Unsatisfactory   NA = This step is not counted

Procedure Steps	Self	Partner	Instructor
1. Wash your hands.	☐	☐	☐
2. Assemble the peak flowmeter, disposable mouthpiece, and patient documentation form.	☐	☐	☐
3. Greet and identify the patient, explain the procedure.	☐	☐	☐
4. Holding the peak flowmeter upright, explain how to read and reset the gauge after each reading.	☐	☐	☐
5. Instruct the patient to place the peak flowmeter mouthpiece into the mouth, forming a tight seal with the lips. After taking a deep breath, the patient should blow hard into the mouthpiece without blocking the back of the flowmeter.	☐	☐	☐
6. Note the number on the flowmeter denoting the level at which the sliding gauge stopped after the hard blowing into the mouthpiece. Reset the gauge to zero.	☐	☐	☐
7. Instruct the patient to perform this procedure a total of three times consecutively, in both the morning and at night, and to record the highest reading on the form.	☐	☐	☐
8. Explain to the patient the procedure for cleaning the mouthpiece of the flowmeter by washing with soapy water and rinsing without immersing the flowmeter in water.	☐	☐	☐
9. Document the procedure.	☐	☐	☐

Calculation

Total Possible Points: _____
Total Points Earned: _____   Multiplied by 100 = _____   Divided by Total Possible Points = _____%

Pass   Fail   Comments:

☐   ☐

Student signature_____ Date_____
Partner signature_____ Date_____
Instructor's signature_____ Date_____

Name_____ Date _____ Time_____

PROCEDURE 32-3: Performing a Nebulized Breathing Treatment

Equipment/Supplies: Physician's order and patient's medical record, inhalation medication, saline for inhalation, nebulizer disposable setup, nebulizer machine

Standards: Given the needed equipment and a place to work, the student will perform this skill with _____% accuracy in a total of _____ minutes. *(Your instructor will tell you what the percentage and time limits will be before you begin practicing.)*

Key: 4 = Satisfactory   0 = Unsatisfactory   NA = This step is not counted

Procedure Steps	Self	Partner	Instructor
1. Wash your hands.	☐	☐	☐
2. Assemble the equipment and medication, checking the medication label three times as indicated when administering any medications.	☐	☐	☐
3. Greet and identify the patient and explain the procedure.	☐	☐	☐
4. Remove the nebulizer treatment cup from the setup and add the exact amount of medication ordered by the physician.	☐	☐	☐
5. Add 2–3 mL of saline for inhalation therapy to the cup that contains the medication.	☐	☐	☐
6. Place the top on the cup securely, attach the "T" piece to the top of the cup, and position the mouthpiece firmly on one end of the "T" piece.	☐	☐	☐
7. Attach one end of the tubing securely to the connector on the cup and the other end to the connector on the nebulizer machine.	☐	☐	☐
8. Ask the patient to place the mouthpiece into the mouth and make a seal with the lips, without biting the mouthpiece. Instruct the patient to breathe normally during the treatment, occasionally taking a deep breath.	☐	☐	☐
9. Turn the machine on using the on/off switch. The medication in the reservoir cup will become a fine mist that is inhaled by the patient breathing through the mouthpiece.	☐	☐	☐
10. Before, during, and after the breathing treatment, take and record the patient's pulse.	☐	☐	☐
11. When the treatment is over and the medication/saline is gone from the cup, turn the machine off and have the patient remove the mouthpiece.	☐	☐	☐
12. Disconnect the disposable treatment setup and dispose of all parts into a biohazard container. Properly put away the machine.	☐	☐	☐
13. Wash your hands and document the procedure, including the patient's pulse before, during, and after the treatment.	☐	☐	☐

Calculation

Total Possible Points: _____
Total Points Earned: _____ Multiplied by 100 = _____ Divided by Total Possible Points = _____%

Pass   Fail   Comments:
☐   ☐

Student signature_____ Date_____
Partner signature_____ Date_____
Instructor's signature_____ Date_____

Name_____ Date _____ Time_____

PROCEDURE 32-4: Perform a Pulmonary Function Test (PFT)

Equipment/Supplies: Physician's order and patient's medical record, spirometer and appropriate cables, calibration syringe and log book, disposable mouthpiece, printer, nose clip

Standards: Given the needed equipment and a place to work, the student will perform this skill with _____% accuracy in a total of _____ minutes. *(Your instructor will tell you what the percentage and time limits will be before you begin practicing.)*

Key: 4 = Satisfactory   0 = Unsatisfactory   NA = This step is not counted

Procedure Steps	Self	Partner	Instructor
1. Wash your hands.	☐	☐	☐
2. Assemble the equipment, greet and identify the patient, and explain the procedure.	☐	☐	☐
3. Turn the PFT machine on and if the spirometer has not been calibrated according to the office policy, calibrate the machine using the calibration syringe according to the manufacturer's instructions, and record the calibration in the appropriate log book.	☐	☐	☐
4. With the machine on and calibrated, attach the appropriate cable, tubing, and mouthpiece for the type of machine being used.	☐	☐	☐
5. Using the keyboard on the machine, input patient data into the machine including the patient's name or identification number, age, weight, height, sex, race, and smoking history.	☐	☐	☐
6. Ask the patient to remove any restrictive clothing such as a necktie and instruct the patient in applying the nose clip.	☐	☐	☐
7. Ask the patient to stand, breathe in deeply, and blow into the mouthpiece as hard as possible. He or she should continue to blow into the mouthpiece until the machine indicates that it is appropriate to stop blowing. A chair should be available in case the patient becomes dizzy or lightheaded.	☐	☐	☐
8. During the procedure, coach the patient as needed to obtain an adequate reading.	☐	☐	☐
9. Continue the procedure until three adequate readings or maneuvers are performed.	☐	☐	☐
10. After printing the results, properly care for the equipment and dispose of the mouthpiece into the biohazard container. Wash your hands.	☐	☐	☐
11. Document the procedure and place the printed results in the patient's medical record.	☐	☐	☐

Calculation

Total Possible Points: _____
Total Points Earned: _____   Multiplied by 100 = _____   Divided by Total Possible Points = _____%

Pass   Fail
☐   ☐

Comments:
_____

Student signature_____ Date_____
Partner signature_____ Date_____
Instructor's signature_____ Date_____

SKILL

PROCEDURE 33-1: Performing a 12-Lead Electrocardiogram (ECG)

Equipment/Supplies: Physician order, ECG machine with cable and lead wires, ECG paper, disposable electrodes that contain coupling gel, patient gown and drape, skin preparation materials including a razor and antiseptic wipes

Standards: Given the needed equipment and a place to work, the student will perform this skill with _____% accuracy in a total of _____ minutes. (*Your instructor will tell you what the percentage and time limits will be before you begin practicing.*)

Key: 4 = Satisfactory   0 = Unsatisfactory   NA = This step is not counted

Procedure Steps	Self	Partner	Instructor
1. Wash your hands.	☐	☐	☐
2. Assemble the equipment.	☐	☐	☐
3. Greet and identify the patient. Explain the procedure.	☐	☐	☐
4. Turn the ECG machine on and enter appropriate data into it. Include the patient's name and/or identification number, age, sex, height, weight, blood pressure, and medications.	☐	☐	☐
5. Instruct the patient to disrobe above the waist. a. Provide a gown for privacy. b. Female patients should also be instructed to remove any nylons or tights.	☐	☐	☐
6. Position patient comfortably in a supine position. a. Provide pillows as needed for comfort. b. Drape the patient for warmth and privacy.	☐	☐	☐
7. Prepare the skin as needed. a. Wipe away skin oil and lotions with the antiseptic wipes. b. Shave hair that will interfere with good contact between skin and electrodes.	☐	☐	☐
8. Apply the electrodes snugly against the fleshy, muscular parts of upper arms and lower legs according to the manufacturer's directions. Apply the chest electrodes, V_1 through V_6.	☐	☐	☐
9. Connect the lead wires securely according to the color codes. a. Untangle the wires before applying them to prevent electrical artifacts. b. Each lead must lie unencumbered along the contours of the patient's body to decrease the incidence of artifacts. c. Double-check the placement.	☐	☐	☐
10. Determine the sensitivity and paper speed settings on the ECG machine.	☐	☐	☐
11. Depress the automatic button on the ECG machine to obtain the 12-lead ECG.	☐	☐	☐
12. When tracing is printed, check the ECG for artifacts and standardization mark.	☐	☐	☐

13. If the tracing is adequate, turn off the machine. ☐ ☐ ☐
   a. Remove the electrodes from the patient's skin.
   b. Assist the patient to a sitting position and help with dressing if needed.

14. For a single-channel machine, roll the ECG strip. ☐ ☐ ☐
   a. Do not secure the roll with clips.
   b. This ECG will need to be mounted on an 8 × 11-inch paper or form.

15. Record the procedure in the patient's medical record. ☐ ☐ ☐

16. Place the ECG tracing and the patient's medical record on the ☐ ☐ ☐
   physician's desk or give it directly to the physician as instructed.

Calculation

Total Possible Points: _____
Total Points Earned: _____ Multiplied by 100 = _____ Divided by Total Possible Points = _____%

Pass   Fail   Comments:
☐   ☐

Student signature_____ Date_____
Partner signature_____ Date_____
Instructor's signature_____ Date_____

PROCEDURE 33-2: Applying a Holter Monitor

Equipment/Supplies: Physician's order, Holter monitor with appropriate lead wires, fresh batteries, carrying case with strap, disposable electrodes that contain coupling gel, adhesive tape, patient gown and drape, skin preparation materials including a razor and antiseptic wipes, patient diary

Standards: Given the needed equipment and a place to work, the student will perform this skill with _____% accuracy in a total of _____ minutes. *(Your instructor will tell you what the percentage and time limits will be before you begin practicing.)*

Key: 4 = Satisfactory   0 = Unsatisfactory   NA = This step is not counted

Procedure Steps	Self	Partner	Instructor
1. Wash your hands.	❑	❑	❑
2. Assemble the equipment.	❑	❑	❑
3. Greet and identify the patient.	❑	❑	❑
4. Explain the procedure and importance of carrying out all normal activities.	❑	❑	❑
5. Explain the reason for the incident diary, emphasizing the need for the patient to carry it at all times during the test.	❑	❑	❑
6. Ask the patient to remove all clothing from the waist up; gown and drape appropriately for privacy.	❑	❑	❑
7. Prepare the patient's skin for electrode attachment. a. Provide privacy and have the patient in a sitting position. b. Shave the skin if necessary and cleanse with antiseptic wipes.	❑	❑	❑
8. Apply the Holter electrodes at the specified sites: a. The right manubrium border b. The left manubrium border c. The right sternal border at the fifth rib level d. The fifth rib at the anterior axillary line e. The right lower rib cage over the cartilage as a ground lead.	❑	❑	❑
9. To do this, expose the adhesive backing of the electrodes and follow the manufacturer's instructions to attach each firmly. Check the security of the attachments.	❑	❑	❑
10. Position electrode connectors downward toward the patient's feet.	❑	❑	❑
11. Attach the lead wires and secure with adhesive tape.	❑	❑	❑
12. Connect the cable and run a baseline ECG by hooking the Holter monitor to the ECG machine with the cable hookup.	❑	❑	❑
13. Assist the patient to carefully redress with the cable extending through the garment opening. Clothing that buttons down the front is more convenient.	❑	❑	❑
14. Plug the cable into the recorder and mark the diary. a. If needed, explain the purpose of the diary to the patient again. b. Give instructions for a return appointment to evaluate the recording and the diary.	❑	❑	❑
15. Record the procedure in the patient's medical record.	❑	❑	❑

Calculation

Total Possible Points: _____
Total Points Earned: _____   Multiplied by 100 = _____   Divided by Total Possible Points = _____%

Pass   Fail   Comments:

☐   ☐

Student signature_____ Date_____

Partner signature_____ Date_____

Instructor's signature_____ Date_____

SKILL

PROCEDURE 34-1: Assisting with Colon Procedures

Equipment/Supplies: Appropriate instrument (flexible or rigid sigmoidoscope, anoscope, or proctoscope); water-soluble lubricant; patient gown and drape; cotton swabs; suction (if not part of the scope), biopsy forceps, specimen container with preservative; completed laboratory requisition form; personal wipes or tissues; equipment for assessing vital signs; examination gloves

Standards: Given the needed equipment and a place to work, the student will perform this skill with _____% accuracy in a total of _____ minutes. *(Your instructor will tell you what the percentage and time limits will be before you begin practicing.)*

Key: 4 = Satisfactory   0 = Unsatisfactory   NA = This step is not counted

Procedure Steps	Self	Partner	Instructor
1. Wash your hands.	☐	☐	☐
2. Assemble the equipment and supplies.	☐	☐	☐
a. Place the name of the patient on label on outside of specimen container.			
b. Complete the laboratory requisition.			
3. Check the illumination of the light source if a flexible sigmoidoscope. Turn off the power after checking for working order.	☐	☐	☐
4. Greet and identify the patient and explain the procedure.	☐	☐	☐
a. Inform patient that a sensation of pressure may be felt.			
b. Tell the patient that the pressure is from the instrument.			
c. Gas pressure may be felt when air is insufflated during the sigmoidoscopy.			
5. Instruct the patient to empty the urinary bladder.	☐	☐	☐
6. Assess the vital signs and record in the medical record.	☐	☐	☐
7. Have the patient undress from the waist down and gown and drape appropriately.	☐	☐	☐
8. Assist the patient onto the examination table.	☐	☐	☐
a. If the instrument is an anoscope or a fiberoptic device, Sims' position or a side-lying position is most comfortable.			
b. If a rigid instrument is used, position patient when doctor is ready: knee-chest position or on a proctological table. Drape the patient.			
9. Assist the physician with lubricant, instruments, power, swabs, suction, etc.	☐	☐	☐
10. Monitor the patient's response and offer reassurance.	☐	☐	☐
a. Instruct the patient to breathe slowly through pursed lips			
b. Encourage relaxing as much as possible.			
11. When the physician is finished:	☐	☐	☐
a. Assist the patient into a comfortable position and allow a rest period.			
b. Offer personal cleaning wipes or tissues.			
c. Take the vital signs before allowing the patient to stand.			
d. Assist the patient from the table and with dressing as needed.			
e. Give the patient any instructions regarding postprocedure care.			

12. Clean the room and route the specimen to the laboratory with the requisition. ☐ ☐ ☐

13. Disinfect or dispose of the supplies and equipment as appropriate. ☐ ☐ ☐

14. Wash your hands. ☐ ☐ ☐

15. Document the procedure. ☐ ☐ ☐

Calculation

Total Possible Points: _____
Total Points Earned: _____   Multiplied by 100 = _____   Divided by Total Possible Points = _____%

Pass   Fail   Comments:
☐   ☐

Student signature_____ Date_____

Partner signature_____ Date_____

Instructor's signature_____ Date_____

SKILL

PROCEDURE 34-2: Collecting a Stool Specimen

Equipment/Supplies: Stool specimen container (ova and parasite testing), occult blood test kit (occult blood testing), wooden spatulas or tongue blades

Standards: Given the needed equipment and a place to work, the student will perform this skill with _____% accuracy in a total of _____ minutes. *(Your instructor will tell you what the percentage and time limits will be before you begin practicing.)*

Key: 4 = Satisfactory   0 = Unsatisfactory   NA = This step is not counted

Procedure Steps	Self	Partner	Instructor
1. Wash your hands.	☐	☐	☐
2. Assemble the equipment and supplies.	☐	☐	☐
3. Place patient's name on the label on the outside of each container or test slide kit.	☐	☐	☐
4. Greet and identify the patient and explain the procedure.	☐	☐	☐
5. Instruct patient to collect a sample for ova and parasite testing. a. Collect a small amount of the first and last portion of the stool after the bowel movement. b. Use a wooden spatula and place it in specimen container. c. Do not contaminate the spatula on the outside of the container.	☐	☐	☐
6. Instruct patient to collect a stool specimen for the occult blood test with a test kit. a. Label slide with name, doctor, and date of collection. b. Place only a small smear on slide windows after opening. c. Close window after the smear is applied.	☐	☐	☐
7. Explain dietary, medication, and other restrictions to follow during the collection process.	☐	☐	☐
8. After obtaining the stool sample, store the specimen as directed. a. Some samples require refrigeration; others are kept at room temperature. b. Some must be placed in an incubator at a laboratory as soon as possible.	☐	☐	☐
9. Document that instructions were given including the routing procedure.	☐	☐	☐

Calculation

Total Possible Points: _____
Total Points Earned: _____   Multiplied by 100 = _____   Divided by Total Possible Points = _____%

Pass   Fail   Comments:
☐   ☐

Student signature_____ Date_____
Partner signature_____ Date_____
Instructor's signature_____ Date_____

PROCEDURE 34-3: Testing a Stool Specimen for Occult Blood

Equipment/Supplies: Gloves, patient's labeled specimen pack, developer or reagent drops

Standards: Given the needed equipment and a place to work, the student will perform this skill with _____% accuracy in a total of _____ minutes. *(Your instructor will tell you what the percentage and time limits will be before you begin practicing.)*

Key: 4 = Satisfactory   0 = Unsatisfactory   NA = This step is not counted

Procedure Steps

	Self	Partner	Instructor
1. Wash your hands and put on clean examination gloves.	☐	☐	☐
2. Assemble the supplies including patient's prepared test pack and the developer. Check the expiration date on the developing solution.	☐	☐	☐
3. Open the test window on the back of the pack: a. Apply one drop of the developer or testing reagent to each window. b. Read the color change within the specified time, usually 60 seconds. c. Apply one drop of developer as directed onto the control monitor section. d. Note whether quality control results are positive or negative.	☐	☐	☐
5. Properly dispose of the test pack and gloves. Wash your hands.	☐	☐	☐
6. Record the procedure.	☐	☐	☐

Calculation

Total Possible Points: _____
Total Points Earned: _____   Multiplied by 100 = _____   Divided by Total Possible Points = _____%

Pass   Fail   Comments:
☐   ☐

Student signature_____ Date_____
Partner signature_____ Date_____
Instructor's signature_____ Date_____

PROCEDURE 35-1: Assisting with a Lumbar Puncture

Equipment/Supplies: Sterile gloves, examination gloves, 3- to 5-inch lumbar needle with a stylet (physician will specify gauge and length), sterile gauze sponges, specimen containers, local anesthetic and syringe, needle, adhesive bandages, fenestrated drape, sterile drape, antiseptic, skin preparation supplies (razor), biohazard sharps container, biohazard waste container

Standards: Given the needed equipment and a place to work, the student will perform this skill with _____% accuracy in a total of _____ minutes. *(Your instructor will tell you what the percentage and time limits will be before you begin practicing.)*

Key: 4 = Satisfactory   0 = Unsatisfactory   NA = This step is not counted

Procedure Steps	Self	Partner	Instructor
1. Wash your hands.	☐	☐	☐
2. Assemble the equipment, identify the patient, and explain the procedure.	☐	☐	☐
3. Check that the consent form is signed and available in the chart.	☐	☐	☐
4. Explain the importance of not moving during the procedure and explain that the area will be numbed but pressure may still be felt.	☐	☐	☐
5. Have the patient void.	☐	☐	☐
6. Direct the patient to disrobe and put on a gown with the opening in the back.	☐	☐	☐
7. Prepare the skin unless this is to be done as part of the sterile preparation. a. Use a sterile forceps after gloving. b. You may be required to add sterile solutions to the field.	☐	☐	☐
8. Assist as needed with administration of the anesthetic.	☐	☐	☐

9. Assist the patient into the appropriate position.
a. For the side-lying position:
  (1) Stand in front of the patient and help by holding the patient's knees and top shoulder.
  (2) Ask the patient to move, so the back is close to the edge of the table.
b. For the forward-leaning, supported position:
  (1) Stand in front of the patient and rest your hands on the patient's shoulders.
  (2) Ask the patient to breathe slowly and deeply.
	☐	☐	☐

10. Throughout the procedure, observe the patient closely for signs such as dyspnea or cyanosis. a. Monitor the pulse at intervals and record the vital signs after the procedure. b. Note the patient's mental alertness. c. Watch for any signs of leakage at the site, nausea, or vomiting. d. Assess lower limb mobility.	☐	☐	☐

11. When the physician has the needle securely in place, if specimens are to be taken
   a. Put on gloves to receive the potentially hazardous body fluid.
   b. Label the tubes in sequence as you receive them.
   c. Label with the patient's identification and place them in biohazard bags.

□ □ □

12. If the Queckenstedt test is to be performed, you may be required to press against the patient's jugular veins in the neck, either, right, left, or both, while the physician monitors the CSF pressure.

□ □ □

13. At the completion of the procedure:
   a. Cover the site with an adhesive bandage and assist the patient to a flat position.
   b. The physician will determine when the patient is ready to leave.

□ □ □

14. Route the specimens as required.

□ □ □

15. Clean the examination room and care for or dispose of the equipment as needed.

□ □ □

16. Wash your hands.

□ □ □

17. Chart all observations and record the procedure.

□ □ □

Calculation

Total Possible Points: _____
Total Points Earned: _____ Multiplied by 100 = _____ Divided by Total Possible Points = _____%

Pass   Fail   Comments:
□   □

Student signature_____ Date_____
Partner signature_____ Date_____
Instructor's signature_____ Date_____

SKILL

PROCEDURE 37-1: Female Urinary Catheterization

Equipment/Supplies: Straight catheterization tray that includes a #14 or #16 French catheter, a sterile tray, sterile gloves, antiseptic, a specimen cup with a lid, lubricant, and a sterile drape; an examination light, an anatomically correct female torso model for performing the catheterization, a biohazard container

Standards: Given the needed equipment and a place to work, the student will perform this skill with _____% accuracy in a total of _____ minutes. *(Your instructor will tell you what the percentage and time limits will be before you begin practicing.)*

Key: 4 = Satisfactory   0 = Unsatisfactory   NA = This step is not counted

Procedure Steps	Self	Partner	Instructor
1. Wash your hands.	❑	❑	❑
2. Identify the patient. a. Explain the procedure and have the patient disrobe from the waist down. b. Provide adequate gowning and draping materials.	❑	❑	❑
3. Place the patient in the dorsal recumbent or lithotomy position. a. Drape carefully to prevent unnecessary exposure. b. Open the tray and place it between the legs of the patient. c. Adjust examination light to allow adequate visualization of the perineum.	❑	❑	❑
4. Remove the sterile glove package and put on the sterile gloves.	❑	❑	❑
5. Remove sterile drape and place it under buttocks of the patient.	❑	❑	❑
6. Open the antiseptic swabs and place them upright inside the catheter tray.	❑	❑	❑
7. Open lubricant and squeeze a generous amount onto tip of the catheter.	❑	❑	❑
8. Remove sterile urine specimen cup and lid and place them to the side of the tray.	❑	❑	❑
9. Using your nondominant hand, carefully expose the urinary meatus.	❑	❑	❑
10. Using your sterile dominant hand, pick up the catheter. a. Carefully insert the lubricated tip into the urinary meatus approximately 3 inches. b. The other end of the catheter should be left in the tray.	❑	❑	❑
11. Once the urine begins to flow into the catheter tray, hold the catheter in position with your nondominant hand.	❑	❑	❑
12. Use your dominant hand to direct the flow of urine into the specimen cup.	❑	❑	❑
13. Remove catheter when urine flow slows or stops or 1000 mL has been obtained.	❑	❑	❑
14. Wipe the perineum carefully with the drape that was placed under the buttocks.	❑	❑	❑

15. Dispose of urine appropriately and discard supplies in a biohazard container.

    a. Label the specimen container and complete the necessary laboratory requisition.

    b. Process the specimen according to the guidelines of the laboratory.

16. Remove your gloves and wash your hands.

17. Instruct patient to dress and give any follow-up information.

18. Document the procedure in the patient's medical record.

Calculation

Total Possible Points: _____
Total Points Earned: _____ Multiplied by 100 = _____ Divided by Total Possible Points = _____%

Pass   Fail   Comments:

Student signature_____ Date_____

Partner signature_____ Date_____

Instructor's signature_____ Date_____

PROCEDURE 37-2: Male Urinary Catheterization

Equipment/Supplies: Straight catheterization tray that includes a #14 or #16 French catheter, a sterile tray, sterile gloves, antiseptic, a specimen cup with a lid, lubricant, a sterile drape, an examination light, an anatomically correct male torso model for performing the catheterization, a biohazard container

Standards: Given the needed equipment and a place to work, the student will perform this skill with _____% accuracy in a total of _____ minutes. *(Your instructor will tell you what the percentage and time limits will be before you begin practicing.)*

Key: 4 = Satisfactory   0 = Unsatisfactory   NA = This step is not counted

Procedure Steps	Self	Partner	Instructor
1. Wash your hands.	❑	❑	❑
2. Identify the patient.	❑	❑	❑
a. Explain the procedure and have the patient disrobe from the waist down.			
b. Provide adequate gowning and draping materials.			
4. Place the patient in the supine position.	❑	❑	❑
a. Drape carefully to prevent unnecessary exposure.			
b. Open the tray and place it to the side or on the patient's thighs.			
c. Adjust examination light to allow adequate visualization of the perineum.			
5. Remove the sterile glove package and put on the sterile gloves.	❑	❑	❑
6. Carefully remove the sterile drape and place it under the glans penis.	❑	❑	❑
7. Open the antiseptic swabs and place them upright inside the catheter tray.	❑	❑	❑
8. Open lubricant and squeeze a generous amount onto the tip of the catheter.	❑	❑	❑
9. Remove sterile urine specimen cup and lid and place them to the side of the tray.	❑	❑	❑
10. Using your nondominant hand, pick up the penis, to expose the urinary meatus.	❑	❑	❑
11. Using your sterile dominant hand, pick up the catheter.	❑	❑	❑
a. Carefully insert the lubricated tip into the meatus approximately 4 to 6 inches.			
b. The other end of the catheter should be left in the tray.			
12. Once the urine begins to flow into the catheter tray, hold the catheter in position.	❑	❑	❑
13. Use your dominant hand to direct the flow of urine into the specimen cup.	❑	❑	❑
14. Remove the catheter when urine flow slows or stops or 1000 mL has been obtained.	❑	❑	❑

15. Wipe the glans penis carefully with the drape that was placed under the buttocks.

16. Dispose of urine appropriately and discard supplies in a biohazard container.

17. Label the specimen container and complete the necessary laboratory requisition.

18. Process specimen according to the guidelines of the laboratory.

19. Remove your gloves and wash your hands.

20. Instruct patient to dress and give any follow-up information.

21. Document the procedure in the patient's medical record.

Calculation

Total Possible Points: _____
Total Points Earned: _____ Multiplied by 100 = _____ Divided by Total Possible Points = _____ %

Pass   Fail   Comments:
☐   ☐

Student signature_____ Date_____
Partner signature_____ Date_____
Instructor's signature_____ Date_____

SKILL

PROCEDURE 37-3: Instructing a Male Patient on Testicular Self-Examination

Equipment/Supplies: A patient instruction sheet if available; a testicular examination model or pictures

Standards: Given the needed equipment and a place to work, the student will perform this skill with _____% accuracy in a total of _____ minutes. *(Your instructor will tell you what the percentage and time limits will be before you begin practicing.)*

Key: 4 = Satisfactory   0 = Unsatisfactory   NA = This step is not counted

Procedure Steps

	Self	Partner	Instructor
1. Wash your hands.	☐	☐	☐
2. Identify the patient and explain the procedure.	☐	☐	☐
3. Using the testicular model or pictures, explain the procedure. 　a. Tell the patient to examine each testicle by gently rolling between the fingers and the thumb with both hands. 　b. Check for lumps or thickenings.	☐	☐	☐
4. Explain that the epididymis is located on top of each testicle. 　a. Palpate to avoid incorrectly identifying it as an abnormal growth or lump. 　b. Instruct patient to report abnormal lumps or thickenings to the physician.	☐	☐	☐
5. Allow the patient to ask questions related to the testicular self-examination.	☐	☐	☐
6. Document the procedure in the patient's medical record.	☐	☐	☐

Calculation

Total Possible Points: _____
Total Points Earned: _____   Multiplied by 100 = _____   Divided by Total Possible Points = _____%

Pass   Fail
☐   ☐

Comments:

Student signature_____   Date_____
Partner signature_____   Date_____
Instructor's signature_____   Date_____

SKILL

PROCEDURE 38-1: Instructing the Patient on Breast Self-Examination.

Equipment/Supplies: Patient education instruction sheet, if available; breast examination model, if available

Standards: Given the needed equipment and a place to work, the student will perform this skill with _____% accuracy in a total of _____ minutes. *(Your instructor will tell you what the percentage and time limits will be before you begin practicing.)*

Key: 4 = Satisfactory   0 = Unsatisfactory   NA = This step is not counted

Procedure Steps	Self	Partner	Instructor
1. Wash your hands.	☐	☐	☐
2. Explain the purpose and frequency of examining the breasts.	☐	☐	☐
3. Describe three positions necessary for the patient to examine the breasts: in front of a mirror, in the shower, and while lying down.	☐	☐	☐
4. In front of a mirror: a. Disrobe and inspect the breasts with her arms at sides and with arms raised above her head. b. Look for any changes in contour, swelling, dimpling of the skin, or changes in the nipple.	☐	☐	☐
5. In the shower: a. Feel each breast with hands over wet skin using the flat part of the first three fingers. b. Check for any lumps, hard knots, or thickenings. c. Use right hand to lightly press over all areas of left breast. d. Use left hand to examine right breast.	☐	☐	☐
6. Lying down: a. Place a pillow or folded towel under the right shoulder and place right hand behind head to examine the right breast. b. With left hand, use flat part of the fingers to palpate the breast tissue. c. Begin at the outermost top of the right breast. d. Work in a small circular motion around the breast in a clockwise rotation.	☐	☐	☐
7. Encourage patient to palpate the breast carefully moving her fingers inward toward the nipple and palpating every part of the breast including the nipple.	☐	☐	☐
8. Repeat the procedure for the left breast. Place a pillow or folded towel under the left shoulder with the left hand behind the head.	☐	☐	☐
9. Gently squeeze each nipple between the thumb and index finger. a. Report any clear or bloody discharge to the physician. b. Promptly report any abnormalities found in the self-breast examination to the physician.	☐	☐	☐
10. Document the patient education.	☐	☐	☐

Calculation

Total Possible Points: _____
Total Points Earned: _____   Multiplied by 100 = _____   Divided by Total Possible Points = _____%

Pass   Fail   Comments:

☐   ☐

Student signature_____   Date_____
Partner signature_____   Date_____
Instructor's signature_____   Date_____

SKILL

PROCEDURE 38-2: Assisting with the Pelvic Examination and Pap Smear

Equipment/Supplies: Patient gown and drape, appropriate size vaginal speculum, cotton-tipped applicators, water-soluble lubricant, exam gloves, examination light, tissues. *Materials for Pap smear*: Cervical spatula and/or brush, glass slides, fixative solution, laboratory request form, identification labels OR the materials required according to the laboratory, biohazard container

Standards: Given the needed equipment and a place to work, the student will perform this skill with _____% accuracy in a total of _____ minutes. *(Your instructor will tell you what the percentage and time limits will be before you begin practicing.)*

Key: 4 = Satisfactory   0 = Unsatisfactory   NA = This step is not counted

Procedure Steps	Self	Partner	Instructor
1. Wash your hands.	❑	❑	❑
2. Assemble the equipment and supplies. 　a. Warm vaginal speculum by running under warm water. 　b. Do not use lubricant on the vaginal speculum before insertion.	❑	❑	❑
3. Label each slide with date and type of specimen on the frosted end with a pencil.	❑	❑	❑
4. Greet and identify the patient. Explain the procedure.	❑	❑	❑
5. Ask the patient to empty her bladder and if necessary, collect a urine specimen.	❑	❑	❑
6. Provide a gown and drape and ask patient to disrobe from the waist down.	❑	❑	❑
7. Position patient in the dorsal lithotomy position—buttocks at bottom edge of table.	❑	❑	❑
8. Adjust drape to cover patient's abdomen and knees—expose the genitalia	❑	❑	❑
9. Adjust light over the genitalia for maximum visibility.	❑	❑	❑
10. Assist physician with the examination as needed.	❑	❑	❑
11. Put on examination gloves 　a. Hold microscope slides while the physician obtains and makes the smears. 　b. Spray or cover each slide with fixative solution.	❑	❑	❑
12. Have a basin or other container ready to receive the now contaminated speculum.	❑	❑	❑
13. Apply lubricant across the physician's two fingers.	❑	❑	❑
14. Encourage the patient to relax during the bimanual examination as needed.	❑	❑	❑
15. After the examination, assist the patient in sliding up to the top of the examination table and remove both feet at the same time from the stirrups.	❑	❑	❑

16. Offer the patient tissues to remove excess lubricant. ☐ ☐ ☐
    a. Assist her to a sitting position if necessary.
    b. Watch for signs of vertigo.
    c. Ask the patient to get dressed and assist as needed.
    d. Provide for privacy as the patient dresses.

17. Reinforce any physician instructions regarding follow-up appoint- ☐ ☐ ☐
    ments needed.
    a. Advise patient on the procedure for obtaining results from the
       Pap smear.

18. Properly care for or dispose of equipment and clean the examina- ☐ ☐ ☐
    tion room.

19. Wash your hands. ☐ ☐ ☐

20. Document your responsibilities during the procedure. ☐ ☐ ☐

Calculation

Total Possible Points: _____
Total Points Earned: _____   Multiplied by 100 = _____   Divided by Total Possible Points = _____%

Pass   Fail   Comments:
☐   ☐

Student signature_____ Date_____

Partner signature_____ Date_____

Instructor's signature_____ Date_____

SKILL

PROCEDURE 38-3: Assisting with the Colposcopy and Cervical Biopsy

Equipment/Supplies: Patient gown and drape, vaginal speculum, colposcope, specimen container with preservative (10% formalin), sterile gloves, appropriate size, sterile cotton-tipped applicators, sterile normal saline solution, sterile 3% acetic acid, sterile povidone-iodine (Betadine), silver nitrate sticks or ferric subsulfate (Monsel's solution), sterile biopsy forceps or punch biopsy instrument, sterile uterine curet, sterile uterine dressing forceps, sterile 4 × 4 gauze pad, sterile towel, sterile endocervical curet, sterile uterine tenaculum, sanitary napkin, examination gloves, examination light, tissues, biohazard container

Standards: Given the needed equipment and a place to work, the student will perform this skill with _____% accuracy in a total of _____ minutes. *(Your instructor will tell you what the percentage and time limits will be before you begin practicing.)*

Key: 4 = Satisfactory   0 = Unsatisfactory   NA = This step is not counted

Procedure Steps	Self	Partner	Instructor
1. Wash your hands.	☐	☐	☐
2. Verify that the patient has signed the consent form.	☐	☐	☐
3. Assemble the equipment and supplies.	☐	☐	☐
4. Check the light on the colposcope.	☐	☐	☐
5. Set up the sterile field without contaminating it.	☐	☐	☐
6. Pour sterile normal saline and acetic acid into their respective sterile containers.	☐	☐	☐
7. Cover the field with a sterile drape.	☐	☐	☐
8. Greet and identify the patient. Explain the procedure.	☐	☐	☐
9. When the physician is ready to proceed with the procedure: a. Assist the patient into the dorsal lithotomy position. b. Put on sterile gloves after positioning the patient if necessary.	☐	☐	☐
10. Hand the physician a. The applicator immersed in normal saline. b. Followed by the applicator immersed in acetic acid. c. Hand the physician the applicator with the antiseptic solution (Betadine).	☐	☐	☐
11. If you did not apply sterile gloves to assist the physician: a. Apply clean examination gloves. b. Accept the biopsy specimen into a container of 10% formalin preservative.	☐	☐	☐
12. Provide the physician with Monsel's solution or silver nitrate sticks.	☐	☐	☐
13. When the physician is finished with the procedure: a. Assist the patient from the stirrups and into a sitting position. b. Explain to the patient that a small amount of bleeding may occur. c. Have a sanitary napkin available for the patient. d. Ask the patient to get dressed and assist as needed. e. Provide for privacy as the patient dresses.	☐	☐	☐

f. Reinforce any physician instructions regarding follow-up appointments.

g. Advise the patient on how to obtain the biopsy results.

14. Label the specimen container with the patient's name and date.
    a. Prepare the laboratory request.
    b. Transport the specimen and form to the laboratory.

15. Properly care for, or dispose of, equipment and clean the examination room.

16. Wash your hands.

17. Document your responsibilities during the procedure.

Calculation

Total Possible Points: _____
Total Points Earned: _____ Multiplied by 100 = _____ Divided by Total Possible Points = _____%

Pass ☐   **Fail** ☐   Comments:

Student signature_____ Date_____

Partner signature_____ Date_____

Instructor's signature_____ Date_____

SKILL

PROCEDURE 39-1: Obtaining an Infant's Length and Weight

Equipment/Supplies: Examining table with clean paper, tape measure, infant scale, protective paper for the scale, appropriate growth chart

Standards: Given the needed equipment and a place to work, the student will perform this skill with _____% accuracy in a total of _____ minutes. *(Your instructor will tell you what the percentage and time limits will be before you begin practicing.)*

Key: 4 = Satisfactory   0 = Unsatisfactory   NA = This step is not counted

Procedure Steps	Self	Partner	Instructor
1. Wash your hands.	☐	☐	☐
2. Explain the procedure to the parent. Ask parent to remove the infant's clothing except for the diaper.	☐	☐	☐
3. Place the child on a firm examination table covered with clean table paper.	☐	☐	☐
4. Fully extend the child's body by holding the head in the midline.	☐	☐	☐
5. Grasp the knees and press flat onto the table gently but firmly.	☐	☐	☐
6. Make a mark on table paper with pen at the top of the head and heel of the feet.	☐	☐	☐
7. Measure between marks in either inches or centimeters.	☐	☐	☐
8. Record the child's length on the growth chart and in the patient's chart.	☐	☐	☐
9. Either carry the infant or have the parent carry the infant to the scale.	☐	☐	☐
10. Place a protective paper on the scale and balance the scale.	☐	☐	☐
11. Remove the diaper just before laying the infant on the scale.	☐	☐	☐
12. Place the child gently on the scale. Keep one of your hands over or near the child on the scale at all times.	☐	☐	☐
13. Balance the scale quickly but carefully.	☐	☐	☐
14. Pick infant up and instruct the parent to replace the diaper if removed.	☐	☐	☐
15. Record the infant's weight on the growth chart and in the patient chart.	☐	☐	☐
16. Wash your hands.	☐	☐	☐

Calculation

Total Possible Points: _____
Total Points Earned: _____ Multiplied by 100 = _____ Divided by Total Possible Points = _____%

Pass ☐   Fail ☐

Comments:

Student signature_____ Date_____
Partner signature_____ Date_____
Instructor's signature_____ Date_____

SKILL

PROCEDURE 39-2: Obtaining the Head and Chest Circumference

Equipment/Supplies: Paper or cloth measuring tape, growth chart

Standards: Given the needed equipment and a place to work, the student will perform this skill with _____% accuracy in a total of _____ minutes. *(Your instructor will tell you what the percentage and time limits will be before you begin practicing.)*

Key: 4 = Satisfactory   0 = Unsatisfactory   NA = This step is not counted

Procedure Steps	Self	Partner	Instructor
1. Wash your hands.	☐	☐	☐
2. Place the infant in the supine position on the examination table or ask the parent to hold.	☐	☐	☐
3. Measure around the head above the eyebrow and posteriorly at the largest part of the occiput.	☐	☐	☐
4. Record the child's head circumference on the growth chart.	☐	☐	☐
5. With clothing removed from chest, measure around the chest at the nipple line, keeping the measuring tape at the same level anteriorly and posteriorly.	☐	☐	☐
6. Record the child's chest circumference on the growth chart.	☐	☐	☐
7. Wash your hands.	☐	☐	☐

Calculation

Total Possible Points: _____
Total Points Earned: _____   Multiplied by 100 = _____   Divided by Total Possible Points = _____%

Pass   Fail
☐   ☐

Comments:

Student signature_____ Date_____

Partner signature_____ Date_____

Instructor's signature_____ Date_____

SKILL

PROCEDURE 39-3: Applying a Urinary Collection Device

Equipment/Supplies: Gloves, personal antiseptic wipes, pediatric urine collection bag, completed laboratory request slip, biohazard transport container

Standards: Given the needed equipment and a place to work, the student will perform this skill with _____% accuracy in a total of _____ minutes. *(Your instructor will tell you what the percentage and time limits will be before you begin practicing.)*

Key: 4 = Satisfactory   0 = Unsatisfactory   NA = This step is not counted

Procedure Steps	Self	Partner	Instructor
1. Wash your hands and assemble the equipment and supplies.	☐	☐	☐
2. Explain the procedure to the child's parents.	☐	☐	☐
3. Place the child in a supine position. Ask for help from the parents as needed.	☐	☐	☐

4. After putting on gloves, clean the genitalia with the antiseptic wipes:
a. For females:
  (1) Cleanse front to back with separate wipes for each downward stroke on the outer labia.
  (2) The last clean wipe should be used between the inner labia.
b. For males:
  (1) Retract the foreskin if the baby has not been circumcised.
  (2) Cleanse the meatus in an ever-widening circle.
  (3) Discard the wipe and repeat the procedure.
  (4) Return the foreskin to its proper position.
	☐	☐	☐

5. Holding the collection device: a. Remove the upper portion of the paper backing and press it around the mons pubis. b. Remove the second section and press it against the perineum. c. Loosely attach the diaper.	☐	☐	☐
6. Give the baby fluids unless contraindicated and check the diaper frequently.	☐	☐	☐
7. When the child has voided, remove the device, clean the skin of residual adhesive, and rediaper.	☐	☐	☐
8. Prepare the specimen for transport to the laboratory.	☐	☐	☐
9. Remove your gloves and wash your hands.	☐	☐	☐
10. Record the procedure.	☐	☐	☐

Calculation

Total Possible Points: _____
Total Points Earned: _____ Multiplied by 100 = _____ Divided by Total Possible Points = _____%

Pass ☐   **Fail** ☐

Comments:

Student signature_____ Date_____

Partner signature_____ Date_____

Instructor's signature_____ Date_____

Name_____ Date _____ Time_____

PROCEDURE 41-1: Caring for a Microscope

Equipment/Supplies: Lens paper, lens cleaner, gauze, mild soap solution, microscope

Standards: Given the needed equipment and a place to work, the student will perform this skill with _____% accuracy in a total of _____ minutes. *(Your instructor will tell you what the percentage and time limits will be before you begin practicing.)*

Key: 4 = Satisfactory   0 = Unsatisfactory   NA = This step is not counted

Procedure Steps	Self	Partner	Instructor
1. Wash your hands.	❑	❑	❑
2. Assemble the equipment.	❑	❑	❑
3. If necessary to move the microscope, carry it in both hands, one holding the base and the other holding the arm.	❑	❑	❑

4. Clean the ocular areas, following these steps:
 a. Place a drop or two of lens cleaner on a piece of lens paper.
   (1) Never use tissue or gauze because these may scratch the ocular areas.
   (2) Wipe each eyepiece thoroughly with the lens paper.
   (3) Avoid touching the ocular areas with your fingers.
 	
 b. Wipe each objective lens.
   (1) Start with the lowest power and continue to the highest power.
   (2) If the lens paper has dirt or oil on it, use a clean section of the lens paper.
 	
 c. Remove cleaner: using a new piece of dry lens paper, wipe each eyepiece and objective lens.
	❑	❑	❑

5. Clean the nonocular areas, following these steps: a. Moisten gauze with mild soap solution and wipe all nonocular areas, including the stage, base, and adjustment knobs. b. Moisten another gauze pad with water and rinse the washed areas.	❑	❑	❑
6. To store the cleaned microscope, make sure that the light source is turned off. a. Rotate the nosepiece, so the low power objective is pointed down toward the stage. b. Cover the microscope with the plastic that came with it or a small trash bag.	❑	❑	❑

Calculation

Total Possible Points: _____
Total Points Earned: _____   Multiplied by 100 = _____   Divided by Total Possible Points = _____%

Pass   Fail   Comments:
❑   ❑

Student signature_____ Date_____
Partner signature_____ Date_____
Instructor's signature_____ Date_____

SKILL

PROCEDURE 42-1: Preparing a Specimen for Transport

Equipment/Supplies: Appropriate laboratory requisition, specimen container/mailing container

Standards: Given the needed equipment and a place to work, the student will perform this skill with _____% accuracy in a total of _____ minutes. *(Your instructor will tell you what the percentage and time limits will be before you begin practicing.)*

Key: 4 = Satisfactory   0 = Unsatisfactory   NA = This step is not counted

Procedure Steps

	Self	Partner	Instructor
1. Assemble the equipment.	☐	☐	☐
2. Complete the laboratory request form.	☐	☐	☐
3. Wash your hands and put on gloves.	☐	☐	☐
4. Check expiration date and the condition of the transport medium.	☐	☐	☐
5. Peel envelope away from the transport tube about one-third of the way and remove tube.	☐	☐	☐
6. Label the tube with date, patient's name, source of the specimen, and initials of the person processing the specimen.	☐	☐	☐
7. Obtain specimen as directed or obtained by the physician.	☐	☐	☐
8. Return the swab to the tube and follow the manufacturer's recommendation for immersion in the medium.	☐	☐	☐
9. Remove and dispose of gloves and wash hands.	☐	☐	☐
10. Package for transport as directed by the manufacturer's recommendations.	☐	☐	☐
11. Route the specimen.	☐	☐	☐

Calculation

Total Possible Points: _____
Total Points Earned: _____   Multiplied by 100 = _____   Divided by Total Possible Points = _____%

Pass   **Fail**   Comments:
☐   ☐

Student signature_____   Date_____
Partner signature_____   Date_____
Instructor's signature_____   Date_____

SKILL

PROCEDURE 42-2: Preparing a Dry Smear

Equipment/Supplies: Specimen, Bunsen burner, slide forceps, slide, sterile swab or inoculating loop, pencil or diamond-tipped pen

Standards: Given the needed equipment and a place to work, the student will perform this skill with _____% accuracy in a total of _____ minutes. *(Your instructor will tell you what the percentage and time limits will be before you begin practicing.)*

Key: 4 = Satisfactory   0 = Unsatisfactory   NA = This step is not counted

Procedure Steps	Self	Partner	Instructor
1. Wash your hands.	☐	☐	☐
2. Assemble the equipment.	☐	☐	☐
3. Label slide with the patient's name and date on the frosted edge with a pencil.	☐	☐	☐

4. Put on gloves and face shield.
  a. Hold the edges of the slide between the thumb and index finger.
  b. Gently and evenly spread the material from the specimen over the slide, starting at the right side of slide.
  c. Use a rolling motion of the swab or a sweeping motion of the inoculating loop.
  d. The material should thinly fill the center of the slide within 1/2 inch of each end.
	☐	☐	☐

5. Do not rub the material vigorously over the slide.	☐	☐	☐
6. Dispose of contaminated swab or inoculating loop in a biohazard container.	☐	☐	☐

7. If you are not using a disposable loop, sterilize it as follows:
  a. Hold loop in the colorless part of the Bunsen burner flame for 10 seconds.
  b. Raise the loop slowly to the blue part of the flame until loop and connecting wire glow red.
  c. If reusing the loop, cool so the heat will not kill bacteria that must be allowed to grow.
  d. Do not wave loop in the air; doing so may expose it to contamination.
  e. Do not stab the medium with a hot loop to cool; this creates an aerosol.
	☐	☐	☐

8. Allow the smear to air dry in a flat position for at least 1/2 hour.
  a. Do not blow on the slide or wave it about in the air.
  b. Heat should not be applied until the specimen has been allowed to dry.
  c. Some specimens require a fixative spray (eg, Pap smears).
	☐	☐	☐

9. Hold the dried smear slide with the slide forceps. a. Pass the slide quickly through the flame of a Bunsen burner three or four times.	☐	☐	☐

b. The slide has been fixed properly when the back of the slide feels slightly uncomfortably warm to the back of the gloved hand. It should not feel hot.

9. Examine the smear under the microscope or stain it according to office policy.   ❑   ❑   ❑

10. Dispose of equipment and supplies in appropriate containers.   ❑   ❑   ❑

11. Remove and dispose of gloves and wash your hands.   ❑   ❑   ❑

Calculation

Total Possible Points: _____
Total Points Earned: _____ Multiplied by 100 = _____ Divided by Total Possible Points = _____%

Pass   Fail   Comments:

❑   ❑

Student signature_____ Date_____

Partner signature_____ Date_____

Instructor's signature_____ Date_____

SKILL

PROCEDURE 42-3: Gram Staining a Smear Slide

Equipment/Supplies: Crystal violet stain, staining rack, Gram's iodine solution, wash bottle with distilled water alcohol-acetone solution, counterstain (e.g., safranin), absorbent (bibulous) paper pad, specimen on a glass slide labeled with a diamond-tipped pen, immersion oil, microscope, Bunsen burner, slide forceps, stop watch or timer

Standards: Given the needed equipment and a place to work, the student will perform this skill with _____% accuracy in a total of _____ minutes. *(Your instructor will tell you what the percentage and time limits will be before you begin practicing.)*

Key: 4 = Satisfactory   0 = Unsatisfactory   NA = This step is not counted

Procedure Steps	Self	Partner	Instructor
1. Wash your hands.	❑	❑	❑
2. Assemble the equipment.	❑	❑	❑
3. Make sure the specimen is heat fixed to the labeled slide and the slide is at room temperature.	❑	❑	❑
4. Put on gloves.	❑	❑	❑
5. Place the slide on the staining rack with the smear side upward.	❑	❑	❑
6. Flood the smear with crystal violet. Time with the stopwatch or timer for 30 to 60 seconds.	❑	❑	❑
7. Hold the slide with slide forceps. a. Tilt the slide to an angle of about 45° to drain the excess dye. b. Rinse slide with distilled water for about 5 seconds and drain off the excess water.	❑	❑	❑
8. Replace the slide on the slide rack. Flood the slide with Gram's iodine solution and time for 30 to 60 seconds.	❑	❑	❑
9. Using the forceps, tilt the slide at a 45° angle to drain the iodine solution. a. With the slide tilted, rinse the slide with distilled water for about 5 to 10 seconds. b. Gently wash with the alcohol–acetone solution until no more purple stain runs off.	❑	❑	❑
10. Immediately rinse the slide with distilled water for 5 seconds and return the slide to the rack.	❑	❑	❑
11. Flood with the safranin or a suitable counterstain. Time the process for 30 to 60 seconds.	❑	❑	❑
12. Drain the excess counterstain from the slide by tilting it at a 45° angle. a. Rinse the slide with distilled water for 5 seconds to remove counterstain. b. Gently blot the smear dry using absorbent bibulous paper. c. Take care not to disturb the smeared specimen. d. Wipe the back of the slide clear of any solution. e. It may be placed between the pages of a bibulous paper pad and gently pressed.	❑	❑	❑

13. Inspect the slide using the oil immersion objective lens for greatest magnification. ☐ ☐ ☐

14. Properly care for, or dispose of, equipment and supplies. Clean the work area. ☐ ☐ ☐

15. Remove gloves and wash your hands. ☐ ☐ ☐

Calculation

Total Possible Points: _____
Total Points Earned: _____ Multiplied by 100 = _____ Divided by Total Possible Points = _____%

Pass   Fail   Comments:
☐   ☐

Student signature_____ Date_____
Partner signature_____ Date_____
Instructor's signature_____ Date_____

SKILL

PROCEDURE 42-4: Inoculating a Culture

Equipment/Supplies: Specimen on a swab or loop, china marker or permanent laboratory markers, sterile or disposable loops, Bunsen burner, labeled Petri dish (The patient's name should be on the side of the plate containing the medium because it is always placed upward to prevent condensation from dripping onto the culture.)

Standards: Given the needed equipment and a place to work, the student will perform this skill with _____% accuracy in a total of _____ minutes. *(Your instructor will tell you what the percentage and time limits will be before you begin practicing.)*

Key: 4 – Satisfactory   0 = Unsatisfactory   NA = This step is not counted

Procedure Steps	Self	Partner	Instructor
1. Assemble the equipment.	☐	☐	☐
2. Put on gloves and face shield.	☐	☐	☐
3. Label the medium side of the plate with a. Patient's name, identification number. b. Source of specimen, time collected, time inoculated. c. Your initials and date.	☐	☐	☐
4. Remove the Petri plate from the cover. a. Place the cover with the opening upward on the work surface. b. Do not open the cover unnecessarily.	☐	☐	☐
5. Streak the specimen swab completely across 1/2 of the plate a. Start at the top and work to a midpoint or the diameter of the plate. b. Use a rolling and sliding motion. c. Dispose of the swab in a biohazard container. d. If the inoculating loop is used to lift a secondary culture, streak in the same manner.	☐	☐	☐
6. Dispose of this loop. If your office does not use disposable inoculating loops, sterilize the loop as described in step 6 of Procedure 24-2.	☐	☐	☐
7. Turn the plate 1/4 turn from its previous position. a. Pass the loop a few times in the original inoculum, then downward into the medium approximately 1/4 of the surface of the plate. b. Do not enter the originally streaked area after the first few sweeps.	☐	☐	☐
8. Dispose of this loop. If you are not using a disposable loop, flame the loop and allow it to cool again.	☐	☐	☐
9. Turn the plate another 1/4 turn so that now it is 180° to the original smear. a. Working in the previous manner, draw the loop at right angles through the most recently streaked area. b. Do not enter the originally streaked area after the first few sweeps.	☐	☐	☐

10. If the plate is to be used for sensitivity, follow these steps:
    a. Use a sterile forceps or an automatic dispenser.
    b. Place specified disks on areas of the plate equidistant from each other.
    c. Press them gently with a sterilized loop or forceps until good contact is made with the surface.

11. Properly care for, or dispose of, equipment and supplies.

12. Remove gloves and wash your hands.

Calculation

Total Possible Points: _____
Total Points Earned: _____ Multiplied by 100 = _____ Divided by Total Possible Points = _____%

Pass   Fail   Comments:
☐   ☐

Student signature_____ Date_____

Partner signature_____ Date_____

Instructor's signature_____ Date_____

SKILL

PROCEDURE 43-1: Obtaining a Clean-Catch Midstream Urine Specimen

Equipment/Supplies: Sterile urine container labeled with patient's name, bedpan or urinal (if necessary), gloves if you are to assist patient

Standards: Given the needed equipment and a place to work, the student will perform this skill with _____% accuracy in a total of _____ minutes. *(Your instructor will tell you what the percentage and time limits will be before you begin practicing.)*

Key: 4 = Satisfactory   0 = Unsatisfactory   NA = This step is not counted

Procedure Steps	Self	Partner	Instructor
1. Wash your hands. If you are to assist the patient, put on gloves.	☐	☐	☐
2. Assemble the equipment.	☐	☐	☐
3. Identify the patient and explain the procedure. Ask for and answer any questions.	☐	☐	☐
4. If the patient is to perform the procedure, provide the necessary supplies.	☐	☐	☐
5. Have the patient perform the procedure.	☐	☐	☐

5. Have the patient perform the procedure.
   a. Instruct the male patient to
      (1) If uncircumcised, expose the glans penis by retracting the foreskin.
          (a) Clean the meatus with an antiseptic wipe, using a circular motion away from the meatus.
          (b) A new wipe should be used for each cleaning sweep.
      (2) Keeping the foreskin retracted, initially void for a few seconds into the toilet or urinal.
      (3) Bring the sterile container into the urine stream.
          (a) Avoid touching the inside of the container with the penis.
          (b) Collect a sufficient amount (about 30–100 mL).
      (4) Finish voiding into the toilet or urinal.
   b. Instruct the female patient to
      (1) Using either toilet bowl or bedpan, spread legs wide apart.
          (a) Spread the labia minora widely to expose the meatus.
          (b) Using a new wipe for each side, cleanse on either side of the meatus.
          (c) Using a new wipe, cleanse the meatus.
      (2) Keeping the labia separated, initially void for a few seconds into the toilet.
      (3) Bring the sterile container into the urine stream.
      (4) Collect a sufficient amount (about 30–100 mL).
      (5) Finish voiding into the toilet or bedpan.

6. Cap the filled container and place it in a designated area.	☐	☐	☐
7. Properly care for or dispose of equipment and supplies.	☐	☐	☐
8. Clean the work area. Remove gloves and wash your hands.	☐	☐	☐

Calculation

Total Possible Points: _____
Total Points Earned: _____   Multiplied by 100 = _____   Divided by Total Possible Points = _____%

Pass   Fail

☐   ☐   Comments:

Student signature_____   Date_____
Partner signature_____   Date_____
Instructor's signature_____   Date_____

SKILL

PROCEDURE 43-2: Obtaining a 24-Hour Urine Specimen

Equipment/Supplies: Chemical hazard labels, clean random urine container, volumetric cylinder (that holds at least 1 L), serological or volumetric pipettes, gloves, fresh 10% bleach solution, patient log form

Standards: Given the needed equipment and a place to work, the student will perform this skill with _____% accuracy in a total of _____ minutes. *(Your instructor will tell you what the percentage and time limits will be before you begin practicing.)*

Key: 4 = Satisfactory   0 = Unsatisfactory   NA = This step is not counted

Procedure Steps	Self	Partner	Instructor
1. Wash your hands.	☐	☐	☐
2. Assemble the equipment.	☐	☐	☐

3. Identify the type of 24-hour urine collection requested.
   a. Check for any special requirements (i.e., acid or preservative to be added).
   b. Label the container appropriately.
	☐	☐	☐

4. Add the correct amount of acid or preservative required; use a serological or volumetric pipette to the 24-hour urine container.	☐	☐	☐

5. Use a label provided or write on the 24-hour urine container.
   a. "Beginning Time _____ and Date _____."
   b. "Ending Time _____ and Date _____."
   c. The patient can fill in the appropriate information.
	☐	☐	☐

6. Instruct the patient to collect a 24-hour urine sample as follows:
   a. Void into the toilet and note this time and date as "beginning."
   b. After the first voiding, collect each voiding and add it to the urine container.
   c. Precisely 24 hours after beginning collection, empty the bladder (even if there is no urge to void).
   d. Note on the label the "ending" time and date.
	☐	☐	☐

7. Explain the following to the patient:
   a. The 24-hour urine sample may need to be refrigerated the entire time.
   b. Return the specimen to you as soon as possible after collection is complete.
	☐	☐	☐

8. Record in the patient's chart:
   a. Supplies and instructions were given to collect a 24-hour urine specimen.
   b. Test request was sent to the laboratory.
	☐	☐	☐

9. After receiving the 24-hour urine specimen from the patient:
   a. Verify beginning and ending times and dates before the patient leaves.
   b. Check for required acids or preservatives that need to be added before transporting specimen.
	☐	☐	☐

10. Put on gloves.	☐	☐	☐

11. Pour the urine into a cylinder to record the total volume collected during the 24-hour period. ❑ ❑ ❑

   a. Pour an aliquot of the urine into a clean container to be sent to the laboratory.

   b. Label the specimen with the patient's identification.

   c. On the sample container and on the laboratory requisition, record:

     (1) Volume of urine collected (and amount of added acid or preservative)

     (2) If permissible, you may dispose of the remainder of the urine.

12. Record the volume on the patient log form. ❑ ❑ ❑

13. Clean the cylinder with fresh 10% bleach solution, rinse with water, and let it air dry. ❑ ❑ ❑

14. If you are using a disposable container be sure to dispose of it in the proper biohazard container. ❑ ❑ ❑

15. Clean the work area and dispose of waste properly. Remove PPE and wash your hands. ❑ ❑ ❑

Calculation

Total Possible Points: _____

Total Points Earned: _____ Multiplied by 100 = _____ Divided by Total Possible Points = _____%

Pass ❑   Fail ❑

Comments:

Student signature_____ Date_____

Partner signature_____ Date_____

Instructor's signature_____ Date_____

Name_____ Date _____ Time_____

PROCEDURE 43-3: Determining Color and Clarity of Urine

Equipment/Supplies: Patient's labeled urine specimen, clear tube, usually a centrifuge, white paper scored with black lines, gloves, impervious gown, face shield, 10% bleach solution

Standards: Given the needed equipment and a place to work, the student will perform this skill with _____% accuracy in a total of _____ minutes. *(Your instructor will tell you what the percentage and time limits will be before you begin practicing.)*

Key: 4 = Satisfactory   0 = Unsatisfactory   NA = This step is not counted

Procedure Steps

	Self	Partner	Instructor
1. Wash your hands.	☐	☐	☐
2. Assemble the equipment.	☐	☐	☐
3. Put on gloves, impervious gown, and face shield.	☐	☐	☐
4. Verify that the names on the specimen container and the report form are the same.	☐	☐	☐
5. Pour 10–15 mL of urine into the tube.	☐	☐	☐
6. In bright light against a white background, examine the urine for color.	☐	☐	☐
7. Determine urine clarity. Hold the urine tube in front of the white paper scored with black lines.	☐	☐	☐
a. If you see the lines clearly (not obscured), record as *clear*.			
b. If you see the lines but they are not well delineated, record as *hazy*.			
c. If you cannot see the lines at all, record as *cloudy*.			
8. Properly care for or dispose of equipment and supplies.	☐	☐	☐
9. Clean the work area using a 10% bleach solution.	☐	☐	☐
10. Remove gloves, gown, and face shield. Wash your hands.	☐	☐	☐

Calculation

Total Possible Points: _____
Total Points Earned: _____   Multiplied by 100 = _____   Divided by Total Possible Points = _____%

Pass ☐   Fail ☐

Comments:

Student signature_____ Date_____

Partner signature_____ Date_____

Instructor's signature_____ Date_____

Name_____   Date _____   Time_____

PROCEDURE 43-4: Chemical Reagent Strip Analysis

Equipment/Supplies: Patient's labeled urine specimen, chemical strip (such as Multistix or Chemstrip), manufacturer's color comparison chart, stopwatch or timer, gloves, impervious gown, face shield, 10% bleach solution

Standards: Given the needed equipment and a place to work, the student will perform this skill with _____% accuracy in a total of _____ minutes. *(Your instructor will tell you what the percentage and time limits will be before you begin practicing.)*

Key: 4 = Satisfactory   0 = Unsatisfactory   NA = This step is not counted

Procedure Steps

	Self	Partner	Instructor
1. Wash your hands.	☐	☐	☐
2. Assemble the equipment.	☐	☐	☐
3. Put on gloves, impervious gown, and face shield.	☐	☐	☐
4. Verify that the names on the specimen container and the report form are the same.	☐	☐	☐
5. Mix the patient's urine by gently swirling the covered container.	☐	☐	☐
6. Remove the reagent strip from its container and replace the lid.	☐	☐	☐
7. Immerse the reagent strip in the urine completely, then immediately remove. Slide the side edge of strip along the lip of the urine container to remove excess urine.	☐	☐	☐
8. Start your stopwatch or timer immediately.	☐	☐	☐
9. Compare reagent pads to the color chart and determine results at correct time intervals.	☐	☐	☐
10. Read all reactions at the times indicated and record the results.	☐	☐	☐
11. Discard the reagent strips in the proper receptacle. Discard urine unless more testing is required.	☐	☐	☐
12. Clean the work area with 10% bleach solution.	☐	☐	☐
13. Remove gown, gloves, and face shield. Wash your hands.	☐	☐	☐

Calculation

Total Possible Points: _____
Total Points Earned: _____   Multiplied by 100 = _____   Divided by Total Possible Points = _____%

Pass   Fail   Comments:
☐   ☐

Student signature_____   Date_____
Partner signature_____   Date_____
Instructor's signature_____   Date_____

SKILL

PROCEDURE 43-5: Clinitest for Reducing Sugars

Equipment/Supplies: Patient's labeled urine specimen, positive and negative controls, Clinitest tablets (tightly sealed or new bottle), 16 × 125 mm glass test tubes, test tube rack, transfer pipettes, distilled water, stopwatch or timer, five-drop Clinitest color comparison chart, daily sample log, patient report form or data form, impervious gown, gloves, face shield, 10% bleach solution

Standards: Given the needed equipment and a place to work, the student will perform this skill with _____% accuracy in a total of _____ minutes. *(Your instructor will tell you what the percentage and time limits will be before you begin practicing.)*

Key: 4 = Satisfactory   0 – Unsatisfactory   NA = This step is not counted

Procedure Steps	Self	Partner	Instructor
1. Wash your hands.	☐	☐	☐
2. Assemble the equipment.	☐	☐	☐
3. Put on impervious gown, gloves, and face shield.	☐	☐	☐
4. Identify the patient's specimen to be tested and record patient and sample information on the daily log.	☐	☐	☐
5. Record the patient's identification information. a. Catalog and lot numbers for all test and control materials b. Expiration dates on report or data form.	☐	☐	☐
6. Label test tubes with patient and control identification, and place them in the test tube rack.	☐	☐	☐
7. Using a different transfer pipette for each: a. Add 10 drops of distilled water to each labeled test tube in the rack. b. Add drops by holding the dropper vertically to ensure proper delivery. c. Add 5 drops of the patient's urine or control sample to the appropriately labeled tube.	☐	☐	☐
9. Open the Clinitest bottle, and shake a Clinitest tablet into the lid without touching it.	☐	☐	☐
10. Drop the tablet from the lid into the sample in the test tube rack.	☐	☐	☐
11. Observe reactions in the test tubes as the mixture boils.	☐	☐	☐
12. After the reaction stops, wait 15 seconds, then gently swirl the test tubes.	☐	☐	☐
13. Compare results for patient specimen and controls with the color chart immediately after shaking.	☐	☐	☐
14. Clean the work area with 10% bleach and dispose of all waste properly.	☐	☐	☐
15. Remove gown, gloves, and face shield. Wash your hands.	☐	☐	☐

Calculation

Total Possible Points: _____
Total Points Earned: _____   Multiplied by 100 = _____   Divided by Total Possible Points = _____%

Pass   **Fail**   Comments:

☐   ☐

Student signature_____   Date_____
Partner signature_____   Date_____
Instructor's signature_____   Date_____

SKILL

PROCEDURE 43-6: Nitroprusside Reaction (Acetest) for Ketones

Equipment/Supplies: Patient's labeled urine specimen, white filter paper, plastic transfer pipette, Acetest tablet, manufacturer's color comparison chart, gloves, impervious gown, face shield, 10% bleach solution

Standards: Given the needed equipment and a place to work, the student will perform this skill with _____% accuracy in a total of _____ minutes. *(Your instructor will tell you what the percentage and time limits will be before you begin practicing.)*

Key: 4 = Satisfactory   0 = Unsatisfactory   NA = This step is not counted

Procedure Steps	Self	Partner	Instructor
1. Wash your hands.	☐	☐	☐
2. Assemble the equipment.	☐	☐	☐
3. Put on gloves, impervious gown, and face shield.	☐	☐	☐
4. Identify the patient's specimen to be tested and record patient and sample information in the daily log.	☐	☐	☐
5. Record the patient's identification information. a. Catalog and lot numbers for all test and control materials. b. Expiration dates on report or data form.	☐	☐	☐
6. Place an Acetest tablet on the filter paper by shaking one into the cap and dispensing onto the paper. Replace the cap.	☐	☐	☐
7. Swirl urine specimen to mix. a. Using a transfer pipette, place 1 drop of well-mixed urine on top of the tablet. b. Wait 30 seconds for the complete reaction.	☐	☐	☐
8. Compare the color of the tablet with the color chart, and record the results.	☐	☐	☐
9. Properly care for or dispose of equipment and supplies.	☐	☐	☐
10. Clean the work area with 10% bleach solution.	☐	☐	☐
11. Remove gloves, gown, and face shield, and wash hands.	☐	☐	☐

Calculation

Total Possible Points: _____
Total Points Earned: _____   Multiplied by 100 = _____   Divided by Total Possible Points = _____%

Pass   Fail
☐   ☐

Comments:

Student signature_____ Date_____
Partner signature_____ Date_____
Instructor's signature_____ Date_____

Name_____   Date _____   Time_____

PROCEDURE 43-7: Acid Precipitation Test for Protein

Equipment/Supplies: Patient's labeled urine specimen, positive and negative controls, 3% sulfosalicylic acid (SSA) solution, clear test tubes, test tube rack, transfer pipettes, stopwatch or timer, daily sample log, patient report form or data form, impervious gown, gloves, face shield, 10% bleach solution

Standards: Given the needed equipment and a place to work, the student will perform this skill with _____% accuracy in a total of _____ minutes. *(Your instructor will tell you what the percentage and time limits will be before you begin practicing.)*

Key: 4 = Satisfactory   0 = Unsatisfactory   NA = This step is not counted

Procedure Steps	Self	Partner	Instructor
1. Wash your hands.	☐	☐	☐
2. Assemble the equipment.	☐	☐	☐
3. Put on impervious gown, gloves, and face shield.	☐	☐	☐
4. Identify the patient's specimen to be tested.	☐	☐	☐
5. Record patient and sample information in the daily log.	☐	☐	☐
6. Record the patient's name or identification information. a. Catalog and lot numbers for all test and control materials. b. Expiration dates on report or data form.	☐	☐	☐
7. Label the test tube with patient and control identification, and place in test tube rack.	☐	☐	☐
8. Centrifuge the patient sample at 1,500 rotations per minute for 5 minutes.	☐	☐	☐
9. Add 1 to 3 mL of supernatant urine or control sample to appropriately labeled tube in rack.	☐	☐	☐
10. Add an equal amount of 3% SSA solution to sample amount in each tube.	☐	☐	☐
11. Mix contents of the tube and let stand for a minimum of 2 minutes—no longer than 10 minutes.	☐	☐	☐
12. Mix contents of tube again and observe degree of turbidity seen and assign a score as follows: NEG: No turbidity or cloudiness; urine remains clear TRACE: Slight turbidity 1+: Turbidity with no precipitation 2+: Heavy turbidity with fine granulation 3+: Heavy turbidity with granulation and flakes 4+: Clumps of precipitated protein The specimen may be matched against a McFarland standard to decrease the degree of subjective interpretation.	☐	☐	☐
13. Clean the work area with 10% bleach solution and dispose of all waste properly.	☐	☐	☐
14. Remove gown, gloves, and face shield. Wash your hands.			

Calculation

Total Possible Points: _____
Total Points Earned: _____   Multiplied by 100 = _____   Divided by Total Possible Points = _____%

Pass   **Fail**

☐   ☐

Comments:

Student signature_____ Date_____

Partner signature_____ Date_____

Instructor's signature_____ Date_____

PROCEDURE 43-8: The Diazo Tablet Test (Ictotest) for Bilirubin

Equipment/Supplies: Patient's labeled urine specimen, Ictotest (diazo) tablets, Ictotest white mats, clean paper towel, transfer pipette, stopwatch or timer, impervious gown, gloves, face shield, 10% bleach solution

Standards: Given the needed equipment and a place to work, the student will perform this skill with _____% accuracy in a total of _____ minutes. *(Your instructor will tell you what the percentage and time limits will be before you begin practicing.)*

Key: 4 = Satisfactory   0 = Unsatisfactory   NA = This step is not counted

Procedure Steps

	Self	Partner	Instructor
1. Wash your hands.	☐	☐	☐
2. Assemble the equipment.	☐	☐	☐
3. Put on impervious gown, gloves, and face shield.	☐	☐	☐
4. Verify that the names on the specimen container and the report form are the same.	☐	☐	☐
5. Place an Ictotest white mat on a clean, dry paper towel.	☐	☐	☐
6. Using a clean transfer pipette, add 10 drops of the patient's urine to the center of the mat.	☐	☐	☐
7. Shake a tablet into the bottle cap, and dispense onto the center of the mat.	☐	☐	☐
8. Recap the bottle immediately.	☐	☐	☐
9. Using a clean transfer pipette, place 1 drop of water on the tablet and wait 5 seconds.	☐	☐	☐
10. Add another drop of water to the tablet, so that the solution formed by the first drop runs onto the mat.	☐	☐	☐
11. Within 60 seconds, observe for either a blue or purple color on the mat around the tablet.	☐	☐	☐
12. Clean the work area with 10% bleach solution and dispose of waste properly.	☐	☐	☐
13. Remove gown, gloves, and face shield. Wash your hands.	☐	☐	☐

Calculation

Total Possible Points: _____
Total Points Earned: _____   Multiplied by 100 = _____   Divided by Total Possible Points = _____%

Pass   Fail   Comments:
☐   ☐

Student signature_____   Date_____

Partner signature_____   Date_____

Instructor's signature_____   Date_____

SKILL

PROCEDURE 43-9: Preparing Urine Sediment

Equipment/Supplies: Patient's labeled urine specimen; urine centrifuge tubes; transfer pipette; centrifuge (1,500–2,000 rotations per minute [RPM]); impervious gown; gloves; face shield; 10% bleach solution

Standards: Given the needed equipment and a place to work, the student will perform this skill with _____% accuracy in a total of _____ minutes. *(Your instructor will tell you what the percentage and time limits will be before you begin practicing.)*

Key: 4 = Satisfactory   0 = Unsatisfactory   NA = This step is not counted

Procedure Steps	Self	Partner	Instructor
1. Wash your hands.	☐	☐	☐
2. Assemble the equipment.	☐	☐	☐
3. Put on an impervious gown, gloves, and face shield.	☐	☐	☐
4. Verify that the names on the specimen container and the report form are the same.	☐	☐	☐
5. Swirl patient's specimen to mix. a. Pour 10–15 mL of the patient's well-mixed urine into a labeled centrifuge tube. b. Cap the tube with a plastic cap or Parafilm.	☐	☐	☐
6. Centrifuge the patient's sample at 1,500 RPM for 5 minutes.	☐	☐	☐
7. When the centrifuge has stopped, remove the tubes. a. Make sure no tests are to be performed first on the supernatant. b. Remove the caps and pour off the supernatant, leaving a small portion of it (0.5–1.0 mL). c. Resuspend the sediment by aspirating up and down with a transfer pipette.	☐	☐	☐
9. Properly care for and dispose of equipment and supplies.	☐	☐	☐
10. Clean the work area with 10% bleach solution. Remove gown, gloves, and shield.	☐	☐	☐
11. Wash your hands.	☐	☐	☐

Calculation

Total Possible Points: _____
Total Points Earned: _____   Multiplied by 100 = _____   Divided by Total Possible Points = _____%

Pass   Fail   Comments:
☐   ☐

Student signature_____ Date_____
Partner signature_____ Date_____
Instructor's signature_____ Date_____

SKILL

PROCEDURE 44-1: Obtaining a Blood Specimen by Venipuncture

Equipment/Supplies: Needle, syringe, and tube(s) or evacuated tubes; tourniquet; sterile gauze pads; bandages; needle and adaptor; sharps container; 70% alcohol pad or alternate antiseptic; permanent marker or pen; appropriate biohazard barriers (e.g., gloves, impervious gown, face shield)

Standards: Given the needed equipment and a place to work, the student will perform this skill with _____% accuracy in a total of _____ minutes. *(Your instructor will tell you what the percentage and time limits will be before you begin practicing.)*

Key: 4 = Satisfactory   0 = Unsatisfactory   NA = This step is not counted

Procedure Steps	Self	Partner	Instructor
1. Check the requisition slip to determine the tests ordered and specimen requirements.	☐	☐	☐
2. Wash your hands.	☐	☐	☐
3. Assemble the equipment. Check the expiration date on the tubes.	☐	☐	☐
4. Greet and identify the patient. a. Explain the procedure. b. Ask for and answer any questions.	☐	☐	☐
5. If a fasting specimen is required, ask the patient when the last food was eaten.	☐	☐	☐
6. Put on nonsterile latex or vinyl gloves.	☐	☐	☐
7. Break the seal of the needle cover. a. Thread sleeved needle into the adaptor. Use the needle cover as a wrench. b. Tap tubes that contain additives to dislodge from stopper and wall of the tube. c. Insert tube into adaptor until the needle slightly enters the stopper. d. Do not push the top of the tube stopper beyond the indentation mark. e. If the tube retracts slightly, leave it in the retracted position. f. If using a syringe, tighten the needle on the hub, and breathe the syringe.	☐	☐	☐
8. Tell the patient to sit with a well-supported arm. a. Apply the tourniquet around the patient's arm 3–4 inches above the elbow. b. Apply the tourniquet snugly, but not too tightly. c. Secure the tourniquet by using the half-bow. d. Tails of tourniquet extend upward (avoid contaminating venipuncture site). e. Ask patient to close the hand into a fist and hold it (not pump the fist).	☐	☐	☐
9. Select a vein by palpating. Use your gloved index finger to trace the path of the vein and judge its depth.	☐	☐	☐

10. Release the tourniquet after palpating the vein (if left on for more than 1 minute).   ❑ ❑ ❑

11. Cleanse the venipuncture site with an alcohol pad.   ❑ ❑ ❑
    a. Start in center of puncture site and work outward in a circular motion.
    b. Allow site to dry or dry the site with sterile gauze.
    c. Do not touch the area after cleansing.

12. A sterile specimen is required for blood to be cultured to diagnose septic conditions.   ❑ ❑ ❑
    a. To do this, apply alcohol to the area for 2 full minutes.
    b. Then apply a 2% iodine solution in ever-widening circles.
    c. Use a new wipe for each sweep across the area.

13. Reapply the tourniquet if it was removed after palpation and ask the patient to make a fist.   ❑ ❑ ❑

14. Remove the needle cover.   ❑ ❑ ❑
    a. Hold the syringe or evacuated assembly in your dominant hand.
    b. With nondominant hand, grasp patient's arm to draw the skin taut over the site.
    c. This anchors the vein about 1–2 inches below the puncture site.

15. Bevel up, line up the needle with the vein approximately 1/4–1/2 inch below the site where the vein is to be entered.   ❑ ❑ ❑
    a. At a 15–30° angle, rapidly and smoothly insert the needle through the skin.
    b. Remove your nondominant hand, slowly pull back the plunger of the syringe or place two fingers on the flanges of the adapter and, with the thumb, push the tube onto the needle inside the adapter.
    c. When blood flow begins in the tube or syringe, release the tourniquet.
    d. Allow patient to release the fist. Allow the syringe or tube(s) to fill to capacity.
    e. When blood flow ceases, remove the tube from the adapter by gripping the tube with the nondominant hand, placing the thumb against the flange during removal.
       (1) Twist and gently pull out the tube. Steady the needle in the vein.
       (2) Try not to pull up or press down on the needle while it is in the vein.
    f. Insert any other necessary tubes into adapter and allow each to fill to capacity.

16. Release the tourniquet. Remove the tube from the adapter.   ❑ ❑ ❑
    a. Place a sterile gauze pad over the puncture site during needle withdrawal.
    b. Do not apply any pressure to the site until the needle is completely removed.
    c. After needle is removed, apply pressure or have patient apply direct pressure for 3–5 minutes.
    d. Do not bend the arm at the elbow.

17. Transfer the blood from a syringe into tubes via the transfer device.   ❑ ❑ ❑
    a. In the proper order of draw, allow the vacuum to fill the tubes.
    b. Place the tubes in tube rack and carefully insert the device through the stopper.

c. If the vacuum tubes contain an anticoagulant,
 (1) Mix immediately by gently inverting the tube 8–10 times.
 (2) Do not shake the tube.
 d. Label the tubes with the proper information.

18. Check the puncture site for bleeding.
 a. Apply a bandage, a clean 2 × 2 gauze pad folded in quarters.
 b. Hold in place by a Band-Aid or 3-inch strip of tape.

19. Thank the patient.

20. Tell the patient to leave the bandage in place at least 15 minutes and not to carry a heavy object (such as a purse) or lift heavy objects with that arm for 1 hour.

21. Properly care for, or dispose of, all equipment and supplies.

22. Clean the work area.

23. Remove gloves and wash your hands.

24. Test, transfer, or store the blood specimen according to the medical office policy.

25. Record the procedure.

Charting Example

Calculation

Total Possible Points: _____
Total Points Earned: _____ Multiplied by 100 = _____ Divided by Total Possible Points = _____%

Pass   Fail   Comments:
☐   ☐

Student signature_____ Date_____

Partner signature_____ Date_____

Instructor's signature_____ Date_____

SKILL

PROCEDURE 44-2: Obtaining a Blood Specimen by Skin Puncture

Equipment/Supplies: Sterile disposable lancet or automated skin puncture device; 70% alcohol or alternate antiseptic; sterile gauze pads; microcollection tubes or containers; heel-warming device, if needed; appropriate bio-hazard barriers (e.g., gloves, impervious gown, face shield)

Standards: Given the needed equipment and a place to work, the student will perform this skill with _____% accuracy in a total of _____ minutes. *(Your instructor will tell you what the percentage and time limits will be before you begin practicing.)*

Key: 4 = Satisfactory   0 = Unsatisfactory   NA = This step is not counted

Procedure Steps	Self	Partner	Instructor
1. Check the requisition slip to determine the tests ordered and specimen requirements.	☐	☐	☐
2. Wash your hands.	☐	☐	☐
3. Assemble the equipment.	☐	☐	☐

4. Greet and identify the patient.
  a. Explain the procedure.
  b. Ask for and answer any questions.
	☐	☐	☐

5. Put on gloves.	☐	☐	☐

6. Select the puncture site.
  a. Middle or ring finger of the nondominant hand.
  b. Lateral curved surface of the heel, or the great toe of an infant.
  c. Make sure that the site chosen is warm and not cyanotic or edematous.
  d. Gently massage the finger from the base to the tip.
  e. Identify the exact location to make the puncture.
	☐	☐	☐

7. Grasp the finger firmly or grasp the infant's heel firmly.	☐	☐	☐
8. Cleanse the ball of the selected finger or heel with 70% isopropyl alcohol.	☐	☐	☐
9. Wipe it dry with a sterile gauze pad or allow it to air dry.	☐	☐	☐

10. Hold the patient's finger or heel firmly and make a swift, firm puncture.
  a. Perform the puncture perpendicular to the whorls of the fingerprint or footprint.
  b. Dispose of the used puncture device in a sharps container.
  c. Wipe away the first drop of blood with sterile dry gauze.
  d. Apply pressure toward the site but do not "milk" the site.
	☐	☐	☐

11. Collect the required specimen in the chosen containers or slides.
  a. Touch only the tip of the collection device to the drop of blood.
  b. Blood flow is encouraged if the puncture site is held in a downward, or dependent, angle and gentle pressure is applied near the site.
	☐	☐	☐

12. Cap microcollection tubes with caps provided and mix the additives by gently tilting or inverting the tubes 8–10 times. ☐ ☐ ☐

13. When collection is complete, apply clean gauze to the site with pressure. ☐ ☐ ☐
    a. Hold pressure or have the patient hold pressure until the bleeding stops.
    b. Label the containers with the proper information.
    c. Do not apply bandages to skin punctures of infants less than 2 years of age.
    d. Never release a patient until the bleeding has stopped.

14. Thank the patient. ☐ ☐ ☐

15. Tell the patient to leave the bandage in place at least 15 minutes. ☐ ☐ ☐

16. Properly care for or dispose of equipment and supplies. ☐ ☐ ☐

17. Clean the work area. Remove gloves and wash your hands. ☐ ☐ ☐

18. Test, transfer, or store the blood specimen according to the medical office policy. ☐ ☐ ☐

19. Record the procedure.

Calculation

Total Possible Points: _____
Total Points Earned: _____ Multiplied by 100 = _____ Divided by Total Possible Points = _____%

Pass ☐   Fail ☐

Comments:

Student signature_____ Date_____

Partner signature_____ Date_____

Instructor's signature_____ Date_____

PROCEDURE 45-1: Preparing a Whole Blood Dilution Using the Unopette System

Equipment/Supplies: Unopette system, gauze

Standards: Given the needed equipment and a place to work, the student will perform this skill with _____% accuracy in a total of _____ minutes. *(Your instructor will tell you what the percentage and time limits will be before you begin practicing.)*

Key: 4 = Satisfactory   0 = Unsatisfactory   NA = This step is not counted

Procedure Steps	Self	Partner	Instructor
1. Wash your hands.	☐	☐	☐
2. Assemble the equipment.	☐	☐	☐
3. Using the shield on the capillary pipette pierce the diaphragm in the neck of the reservoir. a. Push tip of the shield firmly through the diaphragm before removing it. b. Remove the shield from the capillary pipette using a twisting motion. c. Fill the pipette with free-flowing whole blood obtained through skin puncture or from a properly obtained, well-mixed EDTA (lavender top) tube specimen.	☐	☐	☐
4. If filling from a tube, place the tip of Unopette just below the surface of the blood and allow capillary action to fill the Unopette system completely.	☐	☐	☐
5. Wipe off the pipette with gauze, being careful not to draw it across the tip.	☐	☐	☐
6. Squeeze the reservoir gently to press out air. a. Don't expel any of the specimen. b. Place your finger over the opening of the overflow chamber of the pipette.	☐	☐	☐
7. Maintain pressure on the reservoir and your finger position on the pipette. a. Insert the pipette into the reservoir. b. Release the reservoir pressure. c. Then remove your finger from the pipette. d. Gently press and release the reservoir several times, forcing diluent into, but not out of, the overflow chamber.	☐	☐	☐
8. Place your index finger over the opening of the overflow chamber. a. Gently invert or swirl the container several times. b. Remove your finger, and cover the opening with the pipette shield.	☐	☐	☐
9. Label with the required patient information.	☐	☐	☐

Calculation

Total Possible Points: _____
Total Points Earned: _____   Multiplied by 100 = _____   Divided by Total Possible Points = _____%

Pass   Fail   Comments:
☐   ☐

Student signature_____ Date_____
Partner signature_____ Date_____
Instructor's signature_____ Date_____

SKILL

PROCEDURE 45-2: Performing a Manual White Blood Cell Count

Equipment/Supplies: Unopette system for white blood cell (WBC) count, moist filter paper or moist cotton ball, Neubauer hemacytometer, Petri dish, cover glass, hand tally counter, gauze

Standards: Given the needed equipment and a place to work, the student will perform this skill with _____% accuracy in a total of _____ minutes. *(Your instructor will tell you what the percentage and time limits will be before you begin practicing.)*

Key: 4 = Satisfactory   0 = Unsatisfactory   NA = This step is not counted

Procedure Steps	Self	Partner	Instructor
1. Wash your hands.	☐	☐	☐
2. Assemble the equipment.	☐	☐	☐
3. Prepare a whole blood dilution using Procedure 27-1.	☐	☐	☐
4. At proper interval, mix the contents again by gently swirling the assembly.	☐	☐	☐
5. Remove pipette from the Unopette reservoir, and replace it as a dropper assembly.	☐	☐	☐
6. Invert the reservoir and gently squeeze the sides, discarding the first 3–4 drops.	☐	☐	☐

7. Charge the hemacytometer:
  a. Touch tip of assembly to the V-shaped loading area of the covered chamber.
  b. Control the flow gently and do not overfill.
  c. Do not allow the specimen to flow into the H-shaped moats surrounding the platform loading area.
	☐	☐	☐

8. Place the hemacytometer and moistened filter paper or cotton ball in the Petri dish and cover the entire assembly for 5–10 minutes.	☐	☐	☐
9. Place the prepared hemacytometer on the microscope stage and turn to 1002 magnification.	☐	☐	☐

10. Use a zigzag counting pattern, and start at the top far left.
  a. Count the top row left to right.
  b. At the end of the top row, drop to the second row and count from right to left.
	☐	☐	☐

11. Using the tally counter,
  a. Count all of the WBCs within the boundaries and those that touch the top and left borders.
  b. Do not count those that touch the bottom or right borders.
	☐	☐	☐

12. Record the number.
  a. Return the tally counter to 0.
  b. Move to the next square until all nine squares have been counted.
	☐	☐	☐

Note: If the numbers do not match within 10%, the hemacytometer was improperly charged, and the test must be repeated. Count the opposite side of the hemacytometer.

13. Add the total from both sides of the hemacytometer and divide by 2.
    a. Add 10% to the averaged total.
    b. Multiply this figure by 100.

☐ ☐ ☐

14. Clean the hemacytometer cover glass with 10% bleach solution. Wipe dry with lens paper.

☐ ☐ ☐

15. Clean the work area.

☐ ☐ ☐

16. Remove your PPE, and wash your hands.

☐ ☐ ☐

Calculation

Total Possible Points: _____
Total Points Earned: _____ Multiplied by 100 = _____ Divided by Total Possible Points = _____%

Pass   Fail   Comments:
☐   ☐

Student signature_____ Date_____

Partner signature_____ Date_____

Instructor's signature_____ Date_____

SKILL

PROCEDURE 45-3: Making a Peripheral Blood Smear

Equipment/Supplies: Clean glass slides with frosted ends, pencil, transfer pipette, well-mixed patient specimen, whole blood

Standards: Given the needed equipment and a place to work, the student will perform this skill with _____% accuracy in a total of _____ minutes. *(Your instructor will tell you what the percentage and time limits will be before you begin practicing.)*

Key: 4 = Satisfactory   0 = Unsatisfactory   NA = This step is not counted

Procedure Steps

	Self	Partner	Instructor
1. Wash your hands.	☐	☐	☐
2. Assemble the equipment.	☐	☐	☐
3. Greet and identify the patient. a. Explain the procedure. b. Ask for and answer any questions.	☐	☐	☐
4. Put on the gloves, impervious gown, and face shield.	☐	☐	☐
5. Obtain an EDTA blood specimen following the steps for venipuncture (Chapter 26).	☐	☐	☐
6. Label the slide on the frosted area.	☐	☐	☐
7. Place a drop of blood 1 cm from the frosted end of the slide.	☐	☐	☐
8. Place the slide on a flat surface. a. With thumb and forefinger of the dominant hand, hold second (spreader) slide against the surface of the first at a 30° angle. b. Draw the spreader slide back against the drop of blood until contact is established. c. Allow the blood to spread out under the edge. d. Then push the spreader slide at moderate speed toward other end of the slide. e. Keep contact between the two slides at all times.	☐	☐	☐
9. Allow the slide to air dry.	☐	☐	☐
10. Properly care for or dispose of equipment and supplies.	☐	☐	☐
11. Clean the work area.	☐	☐	☐
12. Remove gloves, gown, and face shield, and wash your hands.	☐	☐	☐

Calculation

Total Possible Points: _____

Total Points Earned: _____   Multiplied by 100 = _____   Divided by Total Possible Points = _____%

Pass	Fail	Comments:
☐	☐	

Student signature_____ Date_____

Partner signature_____ Date_____

Instructor's signature_____ Date_____

SKILL

PROCEDURE 45-4: Staining a Peripheral Blood Smear

Equipment/Supplies: Staining rack, Wright's stain, Giemsa stain, prepared slide, tweezers

Standards: Given the needed equipment and a place to work, the student will perform this skill with _____% accuracy in a total of _____ minutes. *(Your instructor will tell you what the percentage and time limits will be before you begin practicing.)*

Key: 4 = Satisfactory   0 = Unsatisfactory   NA = This step is not counted

Procedure Steps	Self	Partner	Instructor
1. Wash your hands.	☐	☐	☐
2. Assemble the equipment.	☐	☐	☐
3. Put on the gloves, impervious gown, and face shield.	☐	☐	☐
4. Obtain a recently made dried blood smear.	☐	☐	☐
5. Place the slide on a stain rack, blood side up.	☐	☐	☐
6. Flood the slide with Wright's stain and allow the stain to remain on the slide for 3–5 minutes.	☐	☐	☐

7. Using tweezers, tilt the slide so that the stain drains off.
    a. Apply equal amounts of Giemsa stain and water.
    b. A green sheen will appear on the surface.
    c. Allow the stain to remain on the slide for 5 minutes.
	☐	☐	☐

8. Holding the slide with tweezers, gently rinse the slide with water.
    a. Wipe off the back of the slide with gauze.
    b. Stand the slide upright and allow it to dry.
	☐	☐	☐

9. Properly care for or dispose of equipment and supplies.	☐	☐	☐
10. Clean the work area.	☐	☐	☐
11. Remove gloves, gown, and face shield, and wash your hands.	☐	☐	☐

Calculation

Total Possible Points: _____
Total Points Earned: _____   Multiplied by 100 = _____   Divided by Total Possible Points = _____%

Pass   **Fail**
☐   ☐

Comments:

Student signature_____   Date_____
Partner signature_____   Date_____
Instructor's signature_____   Date_____

Name_____ Date _____ Time_____

SKILL

PROCEDURE 45-5: Performing a White Blood Cell Differential

Equipment/Supplies: Stained peripheral blood smear, microscope, immersion oil, paper, recording tabulator

Standards: Given the needed equipment and a place to work, the student will perform this skill with _____% accuracy in a total of _____ minutes. *(Your instructor will tell you what the percentage and time limits will be before you begin practicing.)*

Key: 4 = Satisfactory   0 = Unsatisfactory   NA = This step is not counted

Procedure Steps	Self	Partner	Instructor
1. Wash your hands.	❏	❏	❏
2. Assemble the equipment.	❏	❏	❏
3. Put on gloves.	❏	❏	❏
4. Place the stained slide on the microscope. a. Focus on the feathered edge of the smear. b. Scan to ensure an even distribution of cells and proper staining. c. Use the low-power objective.	❏	❏	❏
5. Carefully turn the nosepiece to the high-power objective. a. Bring the slide into focus using the fine adjustment. b. Place a drop of oil on the slide. c. Rotate the oil immersion lens into place. d. Focus and begin to identify any leukocytes present.	❏	❏	❏
6. Record on a tally sheet or tabulator the types of white cells found.	❏	❏	❏
7. Move the stage, so that the next field is in view. a. Identify any white cells in this field. b. Continue to next field to identify all that are present until 100 are counted.	❏	❏	❏
8. Calculate the number of each type of leukocyte as a percentage.	❏	❏	❏
9. Properly care for or dispose of equipment and supplies.	❏	❏	❏
10. Clean the work area.	❏	❏	❏
11. Remove gloves and wash your hands.	❏	❏	❏

Calculation

Total Possible Points: _____
Total Points Earned: _____ Multiplied by 100 = _____ Divided by Total Possible Points = _____%

Pass   Fail   Comments:
❏   ❏

Student signature_____ Date_____
Partner signature_____ Date_____
Instructor's signature_____ Date_____

PROCEDURE 45-6: Performing a Manual Red Blood Cell Count

Equipment/Supplies: Unopette system for red blood cell (RBC) count; clean, lint-free hemacytometer; cover glass; gauze; moist filter paper or moist cotton ball; Petri dish; microscope; hand tally counter

Standards: Given the needed equipment and a place to work, the student will perform this skill with _____% accuracy in a total of _____ minutes. *(Your instructor will tell you what the percentage and time limits will be before you begin practicing.)*

Key: 4 = Satisfactory   0 = Unsatisfactory   NA = This step is not counted

Procedure Steps	Self	Partner	Instructor
1. Wash your hands.	☐	☐	☐
2. Assemble the equipment.	☐	☐	☐
3. Prepare a whole blood dilution using Procedure 27-1.	☐	☐	☐
4. At proper interval, mix the contents again by gently swirling the assembly.	☐	☐	☐
5. Remove pipette from the Unopette reservoir, and replace it as a dropper assembly.	☐	☐	☐
6. Invert the reservoir and gently squeeze the sides, discarding the first 3–4 drops.	☐	☐	☐
7. Charge the hemacytometer: a. Touch the tip of assembly to V-shaped loading area of the covered chamber. b. Control the flow gently, and do not overfill. c. Do not allow the specimen to flow into the H-shaped moats surrounding the platform loading area.	☐	☐	☐
8. Place the hemacytometer and moistened filter paper or cotton ball in the Petri dish.	☐	☐	☐
9. Cover the entire assembly for 5–10 minutes.	☐	☐	☐
10. Place the hemacytometer on the microscope stage, so the ruled area can be surveyed with the low-power objective. a. Focus the microscope. b. Progress to 400× magnification to count the RBCs.	☐	☐	☐
11. Count RBCs in the four corner squares and center square following a zigzag pattern. a. Starting at the top far left, count the top row left to right. b. At the end of top row, drop to second row, and count from right to left. c. Continue this pattern until all of the rows are counted. d. Count cells touching the upper and left sides. e. Do not count those on the lower and right sides.	☐	☐	☐
12. Tally the count and record the number. a. Return the counter to 0 and count the next grid. b. Count the opposite side of the hemacytometer.	☐	☐	☐

Note: The count within the squares should not vary by more than 20 cells. If the variance is greater, the test must be repeated.

13. Average the counts on the two sides and multiply the result by 10,000. ❑ ❑ ❑

14. Clean the hemacytometer and cover glass with 10% bleach; wipe dry with lens paper. ❑ ❑ ❑

15. Dispose of, or care for, any other equipment and supplies appropriately. ❑ ❑ ❑

16. Clean the work area. ❑ ❑ ❑

17. Remove gloves and gown, and wash your hands. ❑ ❑ ❑

Calculation

Total Possible Points: _____
Total Points Earned: _____ Multiplied by 100 = _____ Divided by Total Possible Points = _____%

Pass ❑   Fail ❑

Comments:

Student signature_____ Date_____

Partner signature_____ Date_____

Instructor's signature_____ Date_____

SKILL

PROCEDURE 45-7: Performing a Hemoglobin Determination

Equipment/Supplies: Hemoglobinometer, applicator sticks, whole blood

Standards: Given the needed equipment and a place to work, the student will perform this skill with _____% accuracy in a total of _____ minutes. *(Your instructor will tell you what the percentage and time limits will be before you begin practicing.)*

Key: 4 = Satisfactory   0 = Unsatisfactory   NA = This step is not counted

Procedure Steps	Self	Partner	Instructor
1. Wash your hands.	☐	☐	☐
2. Assemble the necessary equipment.	☐	☐	☐
3. Put on the gloves, gown, and face shield.	☐	☐	☐
4. Obtain an EDTA blood specimen from the patient. Follow steps for capillary puncture described in Chapter 26.	☐	☐	☐
5. Place a drop of well-mixed whole blood (skin puncture) on the glass chamber of hemoglobinometer. a. Place the coverslip into the holding clip over the chamber. b. Slide it into the holding clip.	☐	☐	☐
6. At one of the open edges, push the applicator stick into the chamber and gently move the stick around until the specimen no longer appears cloudy.	☐	☐	☐
7. Slide the chamber into the hemoglobinometer and remove the face shield.	☐	☐	☐
8. With your nondominant hand, hold the meter and press the light button. a. View the field through the eyepiece. b. With your dominant hand, move the dial until the right and left sides match in color intensity. c. Note the hemoglobin level indicated on the dial.	☐	☐	☐
9. Clean the chamber and work area with 10% bleach solution.	☐	☐	☐
10. Dispose of equipment and supplies appropriately.	☐	☐	☐
11. Remove gloves and gown, and wash your hands.	☐	☐	☐

Calculation

Total Possible Points: _____
Total Points Earned: _____   Multiplied by 100 = _____   Divided by Total Possible Points = _____%

Pass   Fail   Comments:

Student signature_____   Date_____

Partner signature_____   Date_____

Instructor's signature_____   Date_____

SKILL

PROCEDURE 45-8: Performing a Manual Microhematocrit Determination

Equipment/Supplies: Microcollection tubes, sealing clay, microhematocrit centrifuge, microhematocrit reading device

Standards: Given the needed equipment and a place to work, the student will perform this skill with _____ % accuracy in a total of _____ minutes. *(Your instructor will tell you what the percentage and time limits will be before you begin practicing.)*

Key: 4 = Satisfactory   0 = Unsatisfactory   NA = This step is not counted

Procedure Steps

	Self	Partner	Instructor
1. Wash your hands.	☐	☐	☐
2. Assemble the equipment.	☐	☐	☐
3. Put on the gloves, gown, and face shield.	☐	☐	☐
4. Draw blood into the capillary tube by one of two methods: a. Directly from a capillary puncture where tip of the capillary tube is touched to the blood at the wound and allowed to fill three-fourths of the tube or to the indicated mark (see Chapter 26). b. OR, from a well mixed anticoagulated (EDTA) tube of whole blood where, again, the tip is touched to the blood and allowed to fill three-fourths of the tube. c. Place the forefinger over the top of the tube. d. Wipe excess blood off the sides and push the bottom into the sealing clay. e. Draw a second specimen in the same manner.	☐	☐	☐
5. Place tubes (clay-sealed end out) in radial grooves of the microhematocrit centrifuge opposite each other. a. Place the cover on top of the grooved area. b. Tighten by turning the knob clockwise. c. Close the lid. Spin for 5 minutes or as directed by the manufacturer.	☐	☐	☐
6. Remove tubes from the centrifuge and read results from the available reading device. a. Results should match within 5% of each other. b. Take the average and report as a percentage.	☐	☐	☐
7. Dispose of the microhematocrit tubes in a biohazard container.	☐	☐	☐
8. Properly care for or dispose of other equipment and supplies.	☐	☐	☐
9. Clean the work area.	☐	☐	☐
10. Remove gloves, gown, and face shield, and wash your hands.	☐	☐	☐

Calculation

Total Possible Points: _____
Total Points Earned: _____ Multiplied by 100 = _____ Divided by Total Possible Points = _____%

Pass Fail Comments:

☐ ☐

Student signature_____ Date_____
Partner signature_____ Date_____
Instructor's signature_____ Date_____

PROCEDURE 45-9: Wintrobe Erythrocyte Sedimentation Rate

Equipment/Supplies: Anticoagulation tube, Wintrobe tube, transfer pipette, timer

Standards: Given the needed equipment and a place to work, the student will perform this skill with _____% accuracy in a total of _____ minutes. *(Your instructor will tell you what the percentage and time limits will be before you begin practicing.)*

Key: 4 = Satisfactory   0 = Unsatisfactory   NA = This step is not counted

Procedure Steps

	Self	Partner	Instructor
1. Wash your hands.	☐	☐	☐
2. Assemble the necessary equipment.	☐	☐	☐
3. Put on the gloves, impervious gown, and face shield.	☐	☐	☐
4. Draw blood (see Chapter 26) into an EDTA anticoagulation tube.	☐	☐	☐
5. Fill a graduated Wintrobe tube to the 0 mark with the well-mixed whole (EDTA) blood. using the provided transfer pipette. Be sure to eliminate any trapped bubbles and fill exactly to the 0 line.	☐	☐	☐
6. Place the tube in a holder that will allow the tube to remain in a vertical position.	☐	☐	☐
7. Wait exactly 1 hour. a. Use a timer for accuracy. b. Keep the tube straight upright and undisturbed during the hour.	☐	☐	☐
8. Record the level of the top of the red blood cells after 1 hour. Normal results for men are 0–10 mL/h; for women, 0–15 mL/h.	☐	☐	☐
9. Properly care for or dispose of equipment and supplies.	☐	☐	☐
10. Clean the work area.	☐	☐	☐
11. Remove gloves, gown, and face shield. Wash your hands.	☐	☐	☐

Calculation

Total Possible Points: _____
Total Points Earned: _____   Multiplied by 100 = _____   Divided by Total Possible Points = _____%

Pass   Fail   Comments:
☐   ☐

Student signature_____ Date_____
Partner signature_____ Date_____
Instructor's signature_____ Date_____

PROCEDURE 45-10: Determining Bleeding Time

Equipment/Supplies: Blood pressure cuff, filter paper, Simplate device, butterfly bandage, alcohol or antiseptic wipe, stopwatch

Standards: Given the needed equipment and a place to work, the student will perform this skill with _____% accuracy in a total of _____ minutes. *(Your instructor will tell you what the percentage and time limits will be before you begin practicing.)*

Key: 4 = Satisfactory   0 = Unsatisfactory   NA = This step is not counted

Procedure Steps	Self	Partner	Instructor
1. Wash your hands.	☐	☐	☐
2. Assemble the equipment.	☐	☐	☐
3. Greet and identify the patient. a. Explain the procedure. b. Ask for and answer any questions.	☐	☐	☐
4. Put on the gloves, impervious gown, and face shield.	☐	☐	☐
5. Position patient so the arm is extended in a manner that is comfortable and stable.	☐	☐	☐
6. Have the patient turn the palm upward so the inner aspect of the arm is exposed. a. Select a site several inches below the antecubital area. b. The area should be free of lesions and have no visible veins. c. Clean the site with alcohol or an antiseptic wipe.	☐	☐	☐
7. Apply the pressure cuff and set it at 40 mm Hg for the length of the test.	☐	☐	☐
8. Twist the tear-away tab on the Simplate. a. Make an incision 1 mm deep on the cleaned skin surface by placing the Simplate bleeding time device on the site and pressing the trigger button on the side. b. This will spring the blade to make the incision. c. At the same time, start the stopwatch.	☐	☐	☐
9. At 30-second intervals, a. Bring filter paper near edge of wound to draw off some accumulating blood. b. Avoid touching the wound with the filter paper.	☐	☐	☐
10. The test is complete when the blood flow stops completely. a. Stop the watch when the blood no longer stains the filter paper. b. Note the time to the nearest 30 seconds.	☐	☐	☐
11. Apply a butterfly bandage across the wound to keep it sealed. a. Cover the site with a waterproof bandage. b. Tell the patient to keep the site dry and to keep the bandage on for 24 hours.	☐	☐	☐
12. Properly care for or dispose of all equipment and supplies.	☐	☐	☐
13. Clean the work area.	☐	☐	☐
14. Remove gloves, gown, and face shield, and wash your hands.	☐	☐	☐

Calculation

Total Possible Points: _____
Total Points Earned: _____ Multiplied by 100 = _____ Divided by Total Possible Points = _____%

Pass   Fail   Comments:

☐   ☐

Student signature_____ Date_____

Partner signature_____ Date_____

Instructor's signature_____ Date_____

SKILL

PROCEDURE 46-1: Performing a Mononucleosis Test

Equipment/Supplies: Patient's labeled specimen (whole blood, plasma, or serum depending on the kit); stopwatch or timer; saline, test tubes, pipettes (if titration is required); mononucleosis kit (slide or card, controls, reagents, capillary tubes, bulb, stirrers)

Standards: Given the needed equipment and a place to work, the student will perform this skill with _____% accuracy in a total of _____ minutes. *(Your instructor will tell you what the percentage and time limits will be before you begin practicing.)*

Key: 4 = Satisfactory   0 = Unsatisfactory   NA = This step is not counted

Procedure Steps	Self	Partner	Instructor
1. Wash your hands.	❑	❑	❑
2. Verify that the name on the specimen container and the laboratory form is the same.	❑	❑	❑
3. Assemble equipment and ensure that the materials in the kit are at room temperature before beginning the procedure.	❑	❑	❑
4. Label the slide or card with the patient's name, positive control, and negative control. One circle or space is provided per patient and control.	❑	❑	❑
5. Place the rubber bulb on the capillary tube. a. Aspirate the patient's specimen up to the marked line. b. Dispense the sample in the middle of the circle labeled with the patient's name. c. Avoid air bubbles to ensure accurate results.	❑	❑	❑
6. Gently mix the positive control. a. Using a capillary tube, aspirate the positive control up to the marked line. b. Dispense the control in the middle of the circle labeled "negative control." c. Avoid air bubbles.	❑	❑	❑
7. Mix the latex reagent. a. Add 1 drop to each circle or space. b. Avoid splashing the reagents.	❑	❑	❑
8. Using a clean stirrer for each test, mix reagent with the patient sample and controls. a. Mix only one circle at a time, keeping within each circle. b. Going outside a circle may lead to cross-contamination and incorrect results.	❑	❑	❑
9. Gently rock the slide for 2 minutes. a. Observe for agglutination (clumping). b. Testing time may vary if you are using a disposable card.	❑	❑	❑
10. Verify results of controls before documenting the patient's results, then log controls and patient information on the worksheet.	❑	❑	❑

11. Read the kit's instructions if titration is required.

12. Clean the work area and dispose of waste properly.
    a. Wash the slide thoroughly with bleach and rinse with water before using again.
    b. Remove gown, gloves and shield. Wash your hands.

Calculation

Total Possible Points: _____
Total Points Earned: _____ Multiplied by 100 = _____ Divided by Total Possible Points = _____%

Pass Fail Comments:

Student signature_____ Date_____
Partner signature_____ Date_____
Instructor's signature_____ Date_____

PROCEDURE 46-2: Performing an HCG Pregnancy Test

Equipment/Supplies: Liquid soap, disposable paper towels, an orangewood manicure stick, a waste can

Standards: Given the needed equipment and a place to work, the student will perform this skill with _____% accuracy in a total of _____ minutes. *(Your instructor will tell you what the percentage and time limits will be before you begin practicing.)*

Key: 4 = Satisfactory   0 = Unsatisfactory   NA = This step is not counted

Procedure Steps	Self	Partner	Instructor
1. Wash your hands.	☐	☐	☐
2. Assemble the equipment.	☐	☐	☐
3. Verify that the names on the specimen container and the laboratory form are the same.	☐	☐	☐
4. Label the test pack with the patient's name. a. Label positive control and negative control. b. Use one test pack per patient and control.	☐	☐	☐
5. Note in patient's information and in control log whether you are testing urine, plasma, or serum.	☐	☐	☐
6. Be sure that the kit and controls are at room temperature for accurate testing.	☐	☐	☐
7. Aspirate the patient's specimen using a transfer pipette and place three drops (180 mL) on the sample well of the test pack labeled with the patient's name.	☐	☐	☐
8. Aspirate the positive control using a transfer pipette and place three drops (180 mL) on the sample well. Avoid splashing to eliminate cross-contamination.	☐	☐	☐
9. Aspirate the negative control using a transfer pipette, and place three drops (180 mL) on the sample well. Avoid splashing to eliminate cross-contamination.	☐	☐	☐
10. Report the results when the "End of Assay Window" is red. a. This will take approximately 7 minutes for serum samples and 4 minutes for urine samples. b. Check to verify controls before reporting the results. c. Repeat test if the "End of Assay Window" does not appear and if the controls do not work.	☐	☐	☐
11. Record control and patient information on the worksheet and log form.	☐	☐	☐
12. Clean the work area and dispose of waste properly.	☐	☐	☐
13. Remove gown, gloves, and shield. Wash your hands.	☐	☐	☐

Calculation

Total Possible Points: _____
Total Points Earned: _____ Multiplied by 100 = _____ Divided by Total Possible Points = _____%

Pass   Fail   Comments:

☐   ☐

Student signature_____   Date_____

Partner signature_____   Date_____

Instructor's signature_____   Date_____

SKILL

PROCEDURE 46-3: Performing a Group A Rapid Strep Test

Equipment/Supplies: Patient's labeled throat specimen, beta-strep agar culture (use a Culturette with two swabs provided), bacitracin disks, group A strep kit (controls may be included, depending on the kit), timer

Standards: Given the needed equipment and a place to work, the student will perform this skill with _____% accuracy in a total of _____ minutes. *(Your instructor will tell you what the percentage and time limits will be before you begin practicing.)*

Key: 4 = Satisfactory   0 = Unsatisfactory   NA = This step is not counted

Procedure Steps	Self	Partner	Instructor
1. Wash your hands.	❏	❏	❏
2. Verify that the names on the specimen container and the laboratory form are the same.	❏	❏	❏
3. Label one extraction tube with the patient's name, one with the positive control, and one with the negative control.	❏	❏	❏
4. Follow the directions for the kit. Add the appropriate reagents and drops to each of the extraction tubes. Avoid splashing, and use the correct number of drops.	❏	❏	❏
5. Insert the patient's swab (one of the two swabs) into the labeled extraction tube. If only one culture swab was submitted, first swab a beta strep agar plate, then use the swab for the rapid strep test.	❏	❏	❏
6. Add the appropriate controls to each of the labeled extraction tubes.	❏	❏	❏
7. Set the timer for the appropriate time to ensure accuracy.	❏	❏	❏
8. Add the appropriate reagent and drops to each of the extraction tubes.	❏	❏	❏
9. Use the swab to mix the reagents. Then press out any excess fluid on the swab against the inside of the tube.	❏	❏	❏
10. Add three drops from the well-mixed extraction tube to the sample window of the strep A test unit labeled with the patient's name. Do the same for each control.	❏	❏	❏
11. Set the timer for the appropriate time.	❏	❏	❏
12. A positive result appears as a line in the result window within 5 minutes. The strep A test unit has an internal control; if a line appears in the control window, the test is valid.	❏	❏	❏
13. Read a negative result at exactly 5 minutes to avoid a false negative.	❏	❏	❏
14. Verify results of the controls before recording test results. Log the controls and the patient's information on the worksheet.	❏	❏	❏
15. Depending on laboratory protocol, you may have to culture all negative rapid strep screens on beta-strep agar. A bacitracin disk may	❏	❏	❏

be added to the first quadrant when you set up or after 24 hours if a beta-hemolytic colony appears. A culture is more sensitive than a rapid immunoasssay test.

16. Clean the work area and dispose of waste properly. Remove gown, gloves, and shield. Wash your hands.

❑   ❑   ❑

Calculation

Total Possible Points: _____
Total Points Earned: _____   Multiplied by 100 = _____   Divided by Total Possible Points = _____%

Pass   Fail   Comments:

❑   ❑

Student signature_____ Date_____
Partner signature_____ Date_____
Instructor's signature_____ Date_____

SKILL

PROCEDURE 47-1: Determining Blood Glucose

Equipment/Supplies: Glucose reagent strips, gloves, sterile gauze, glucose meter, paper towel, Band-Aid, lancet, alcohol pad (*Note:* These are generic instructions for using a glucose meter. Refer to the manufacturer's instructions shipped with the meter for instructions specific for the instrument in use.)

Standards: Given the needed equipment and a place to work, the student will perform this skill with _____% accuracy in a total of _____ minutes. *(Your instructor will tell you what the percentage and time limits will be before you begin practicing.)*

Key: 4 = Satisfactory   0 = Unsatisfactory   NA = This step is not counted

Procedure Steps	Self	Partner	Instructor
1. Wash your hands.	☐	☐	☐
2. Assemble the equipment and supplies.	☐	☐	☐
3. Put on gloves before removing reagent strip.	☐	☐	☐
4. Turn on the instrument, and ensure that it is calibrated.	☐	☐	☐
5. Remove one reagent strip, lay it on the paper towel, and recap the container.	☐	☐	☐
6. Greet and identify the patient. Explain the procedure. Ask for and answer any questions.	☐	☐	☐
7. Have the patient wash his or her hands in warm water.	☐	☐	☐
8. Cleanse the selected puncture site (finger) with alcohol.	☐	☐	☐
9. Perform a capillary puncture, following the steps described in Chapter 26, Phlebotomy.	☐	☐	☐
10. Wipe away the first drop of blood.	☐	☐	☐
11. Turn the patient's hand palm down, and gently squeeze the finger to form a large drop of blood.	☐	☐	☐
12. Bring the reagent strip up to the finger and touch the pad to the blood. a. Do not touch the finger. b. Completely cover the pad with blood.	☐	☐	☐
13. Insert the reagent strip into the analyzer. a. Meanwhile, apply pressure to the puncture wound with gauze. b. The meter will continue to incubate the strip and measure the reaction.	☐	☐	☐
14. The instrument reads the reaction strip and displays the result on the screen in mg/dL.	☐	☐	☐
15. If the glucose level is higher or lower than expected, refer to the troubleshooting guide provided by the manufacturer.	☐	☐	☐

16. Apply a small Band-Aid to the patient's fingertip.

17. Properly care for or dispose of equipment and supplies.

18. Clean the work area. Remove gloves and wash your hands.

☐ ☐ ☐
☐ ☐ ☐
☐ ☐ ☐

Calculation

Total Possible Points: _____
Total Points Earned: _____ Multiplied by 100 = _____ Divided by Total Possible Points = _____%

Pass Fail
☐   ☐

Comments:

Student signature_____ Date_____

Partner signature_____ Date_____

Instructor's signature_____ Date_____

SKILL

PROCEDURE 47-2: Glucose Tolerance Test (GTT)

Equipment/Supplies: Calibrated amount of glucose solution per physician's order, glucose meter equipment, phlebotomy equipment, glucose test strips, alcohol wipes, stopwatch, gloves

Standards: Given the needed equipment and a place to work, the student will perform this skill with _____% accuracy in a total of _____ minutes. *(Your instructor will tell you what the percentage and time limits will be before you begin practicing.)*

Key: 4 = Satisfactory   0 = Unsatisfactory   NA = This step is not counted

Procedure Steps	Self	Partner	Instructor
1. Wash your hands.	☐	☐	☐
2. Assemble the equipment and supplies.	☐	☐	☐
3. Greet and identify the patient. a. Explain the procedure. b. Ask for and answer any questions.	☐	☐	☐
4. Put on gloves.	☐	☐	☐
5. Obtain a fasting glucose (FBS) specimen from the patient. a. Use the venipuncture or capillary puncture procedure (see Chapter 26). b. Test the blood sample before administering the glucose drink.	☐	☐	☐
6. Give the glucose drink to the patient to consume within a 5-minute period. a. Note time the patient finishes the drink; this is the "START" of the test. b. Ensure that the patient remains fairly sedentary throughout this procedure. c. The patient should avoid smoking. d. Encourage the patient to drink water to increase blood volume.	☐	☐	☐
7. If patient experiences any severe symptoms, a. Obtain a blood specimen at this time. b. End the test and notify the physician.	☐	☐	☐
8. Exactly 30 minutes after patient finished the glucose drink a. Obtain another blood specimen. b. Label the specimen with the patient's name and time of collection.	☐	☐	☐
9. Follow precaution guidelines in steps 5, 6, and 7.	☐	☐	☐
10. Exactly 1 hour after the glucose drink, repeat step 8.	☐	☐	☐
11. Exactly 2 hours after the glucose drink, repeat step 8.	☐	☐	☐
12. Exactly 3 hours after the glucose drink, repeat step 8. a. Testing is complete at this time. b. For a longer GTT, continue specimen collection in the same manner.	☐	☐	☐

13. If specimens are to be tested by an outside laboratory, package as required.

☐ ☐ ☐

14. Properly care for or dispose of equipment and supplies.
   a. Clean the work area.
   b. Remove gloves and gown, and wash your hands.

☐ ☐ ☐

Calculation

Total Possible Points: _____
Total Points Earned: _____ Multiplied by 100 = _____ Divided by Total Possible Points = _____%

Pass   Fail

☐   ☐

Comments:

Student signature_____ Date_____

Partner signature_____ Date_____

Instructor's signature_____ Date_____